In Vitro Propagation and Secondary Metabolite Production from Medicinal Plants: Current Trends

(Part 1)

Edited by

Mohammad Anis
Plant Biotechnology Laboratory
Department of Botany
Aligarh Muslim University
Aligarh-202-002, India

&

Mehrun Nisha Khanam
Plant Biotechnology Laboratory
Department of Botany
Aligarh Muslim University
Aligarh-202-002, India

University Centre for Research & Development
Chandigarh University
Mohali-140-413
Punjab, India

In Vitro Propagation and Secondary Metabolite Production from Medicinal Plants: Current Trends (Part 1)

Editors: Mohammad Anis and Mehrun Nisha Khanam

ISBN (Online): 978-981-5165-22-7

ISBN (Print): 978-981-5165-23-4

ISBN (Paperback): 978-981-5165-24-1

need for a court order if at any point you breach any terms of this License Agreement. In no event will any delay or failure by Bentham Science Publishers in enforcing your compliance with this License Agreement constitute a waiver of any of its rights.

3. You acknowledge that you have read this License Agreement, and agree to be bound by its terms and conditions. To the extent that any other terms and conditions presented on any website of Bentham Science Publishers conflict with, or are inconsistent with, the terms and conditions set out in this License Agreement, you acknowledge that the terms and conditions set out in this License Agreement shall prevail.

Bentham Science Publishers Pte. Ltd.
80 Robinson Road #02-00
Singapore 068898
Singapore
Email: subscriptions@benthamscience.net

BENTHAM SCIENCE

CONTENTS

FOREWORD

Biotechnology will continue to be the frontline area for research and application in the 21ˢᵗ century. The potential of biotechnology is enormous, and numerous breakthroughs have benefited the humankind. Plant science research holds tremendous potential to address pressing global issues, including climate change, food insecurity and sustainability. Necessary research to generate innovative discoveries that solve urgent problems is at risk.

India is rich in bioresources but has been slow in converting them into economic wealth through appropriate technologies. Medicinal plants are active biochemical factories of a vast group of secondary metabolites (SMS), and these are indeed basic sources of various pharmaceutical drugs. It is believed that 80% of the world's population utilises herbs, and in developing nations, its percentage could be as high as 95%. The Ayurveda market in India has been valued at INR 335 billion in 2019 and is expected to reach INR > 1000 billion by 2025. There is a growing interest in the world over photomedicines and photo-chemicals. Quite frequently, unique genotypes have to be multiplied in a pure form. Also, several medicinal plants worldwide are under threat of extinction due to climate change. Clonal propagation is important to multiply elite planting materials of selected medicinal tees and many prized herbs.

Plant tissue culture has been viewed as a key technology for enhancing the capability for the production of large quantities of planting material of selected elite high-yielding varieties to boost production and productivity. This technology holds enormous potential for meeting the demands of both domestic and export markets in terms of high-quality planting material.

In this context, the present book titled "*In vitro* Propagation and Secondary Metabolite Production from Medicinal Plants: Current Trends" edited by Professor (Dr) Mohammad Anis, Former Dean, Faculty of Life Sciences, Aligarh Muslim University, is a timely one. The book will certainly appeal to postgraduate students, researchers, biotechnologists, and industry and can be used as a reference book. We must convert our biological wealth into economic wealth and job opportunities. The book will be an important step in this era.

Rajeev Varshney
Centre for Crop & Food Innovation
WA State Agricultural Biotechnology
Murdoch University
Perth, Australia

PREFACE

Plant tissue culture is one of the most important and useful areas of plant biotechnology, having both fundamental and applied significance. Secondary metabolites hold the key to many medicinal properties present in plants, which thus makes their production a commercial prospect. Optimization of various factors responsible for enhanced cell growth and production of secondary metabolites has become a pre-requisite for the use of bioreactors commercially. Plant cell culture provides a viable alternative over whole plant cultivation for the production of secondary metabolites. The discovery that these metabolites could be extracted from callus came at a time when there was a concern about dwindling plant resources. A continuous callus is used from such medicinal plants, and there would be no need to use field-grown plants to obtain secondary metabolites.

There are fluctuations in the concentrations and quantities of secondary metabolites in field-grown plants as the biosynthesis of secondary metabolites, although controlled genetically, is affected strongly by environmental influence. Moreover, very little is known about the biotransformation that takes place once the crop is harvested. To overcome these limitations biotechnologist suggested the use of plant cell and tissue culture rather than to use whole plants for the extraction of certain secondary metabolites. Plant tissue culture may very well contain metabolic pathways that have been modified and/or abbreviated from that of the plant. The impact of rapid climate changes may also have an adverse effect on wild plant species leading to the loss of useful genetic material.

In vitro cell culture and controlled environment production systems offer excellent opportunities for the selection and seasonal independent propagation of elite lines with specific, consistent levels of medicinal metabolites with minimum contamination. Additionally, the plant materials produced by *in vitro* techniques allow efficient application of emerging analytical methods. The impact of these techniques perhaps may be greatest in the improvement of medicinal plants since the resulting genetic diversity may open avenues for the discovery of new medicinal metabolites and treatments.

The continued rise in consumer demand or plant-based medicines and the expanding world population have resulted in the indiscriminate harvest of wild species of medicinal plants. The impact of rapid climate changes may also have an adverse effect on wild plant species leading to the loss of useful genetic material.

The biomass is mainly obtained through conventional methods, which pose quality issues mainly due to poor seed germination, low viability of the seeds and mainly because of environmental factors. Therefore, there is a great need to develop alternative and stable approaches by using different biotechnological approaches like cell, tissue and organ culture, which are independent of all the environmental variations and obtain uniform biomass of high quality for pharmaceutical purposes. During the last 2 decades, a large number of *in vitro* propagation procedures through direct and indirect organogenesis, somatic embryogenesis and also using synthetic seeds have been developed for the conservation aspects.

Several attempts have been made to optimize the protocol for the production of biomolecules using tissue culture and also through hairy root culture (*Agrobacterium rhizogenes* mediated transformation). These cultural techniques can be achieved by monitoring environmental conditions like media optimization, physical conditions, use of biotic and abiotic elicitors, *etc.*, where improved production of secondary metabolites for commercial scale can be achieved. With the significant information on gene regulation and the key enzymatic steps involved in the biosynthetic pathways, modulation in the production of bioactive content can be achieved to the levels required for the pharmaceutical industry. The present book will provide a comprehensive report on the research carried out in the area and will emphasize the future prospects that can be considered for the production of secondary metabolites or the development of elite germplasm with higher contents of secondary metabolites, which would benefit the mankind in an endurable way.

The purpose of this book is to provide important, state-of-the-art findings on secondary metabolite production in valuable medicinal plants. We are extremely grateful to all the contributors who warmly welcomed our invitation and agreed to contribute chapters to embellish information on the subject, thus helping in this endeavor. We also appreciate their patience and cooperation in meeting deadlines and revising their manuscripts when required. We would also like to place on record our sincere thanks to Mr. Zohaib Siddiqui for preparing the layout of the contents. As usual, my wife, Humera Anis, provided much needed morale support, and grand daughter, Haniya, provided moments of joy during a bit tiring and monotonous work.

The editors also like to acknowledge the support received from the publisher Bentham Science, Singapore.

Mohammad Anis
Plant Biotechnology Laboratory
Department of Botany
Aligarh Muslim University
Aligarh-202-002, India

&

Mehrun Nisha Khanam
Plant Biotechnology Laboratory
Department of Botany
Aligarh Muslim University
Aligarh-202-002, India

University Centre for Research & Development
Chandigarh University
Mohali-140-413
Punjab, India

List of Contributors

Ashish Gupta Department of Botany, Mahila Mahavidyalaya, Banaras Hindu University, Varanasi, India

Azra N. Kamili Centre of Research for Development, University of Kashmir, Hazratbal, Srinagar-190 006, (J&K), India

Alpana Yadav Department of Botany, Mahila Mahavidyalaya, Banaras Hindu University, Varanasi, India

Archana Prasad Department of Botany, University of Lucknow, Lucknow, Uttar Pradesh-226007, India

Anabela Romano MED – Mediterranean Institute for Agriculture, Environment and Development & CHANGE – Global Change and Sustainability Institute, Faculdade de Ciências e Tecnologia, Universidade do Algarve, Campus de Gambelas, Faro, Portugal

Abhishek Sharma Department of Biotechnology and Bioengineering, Institute of Advanced Research, Gandhinagar-382426, India
C. G. Bhakta Institute of Biotechnology, Uka Tarsadia University, Gopal-Vidyanagar, Maliba Campus, Surat-394350, India

A. Yusuf Department of Botany, University of Calicut, Kerala, India

Anil Kumar Bisht Department of Botany, Kumaun University, Nainital, India

A. Mujib Department of Botany, Jamia Hamdard, New Delhi, India

Brajesh Chandra Pandey Department of Botany, Mahila Mahavidyalaya, Banaras Hindu University, Varanasi, India

Boregowda Nandini Plant Cell Biotechnology Department, CSIR-Central Food Technological Research Institute (CFTRI), Mysuru - 570 020, Karnataka, India

Debasis Chakrabarty Academy of Scientific and Innovative Research (AcSIR), Ghaziabad, India
Biotechnology and Molecular Biology Division, CSIR-National Botanical Research Institute, Lucknow, India

Dechen Dolker Department of Biotechnology, Guru Nanak Dev University, Amritsar-143 005, Punjab, India

Fadime Karabulut Department of Biology, Firat University, Elazığ, India

Gauri Saxena Department of Botany, University of Lucknow, Lucknow, Uttar Pradesh-226007, India

Gopal W. Narkhede Department of Agricultural Botany Genetics and Plant Breeding, Vasantrao Naik Marathwada Krishi Vidyapeeth, Parbhani-431402, Maharashtra, India

Gholamreza Abdi Department of Biotechnology, Persian Gulf Research Institute, Persian Gulf University, Bushehr-7516913817, Iran

Hemant Borase C. G. Bhakta Institute of Biotechnology, Uka Tarsadia University, Gopal-Vidyanagar, Maliba Campus, Surat-394350, India

Harsh Kumar Chauhan Department of Botany, Kumaun University, Nainital, India

Inês Mansinhos	MED – Mediterranean Institute for Agriculture, Environment and Development & CHANGE – Global Change and Sustainability Institute, Faculdade de Ciências e Tecnologia, Universidade do Algarve, Campus de Gambelas, Faro, Portugal
Indra Dutt Bhatt	G.B. Pant National Institute of Himalayan Environment, Kosi-Katarmal, Almora-263643, Uttarakhand, India
Jameel M. Al-Khayri	Department of Agricultural Biotechnology, College of Agriculture and Food Sciences, King Faisal University, Hofuf, Al-Ahsa 31982, Saudi Arabia
Khushboo Chawda	Biotechnology and Molecular Biology Division, CSIR-National Botanical Research Institute, Lucknow, India Academy of Scientific and Innovative Research (AcSIR), Ghaziabad, India
Kapil D. Pandey	Department of Botany, Institute of Science, Banaras Hindu University, Varanasi, India
Krishnananda P. Ingle	Biotechnology Centre, Department of Agricultural Botany, Post Graduate Institute, Dr. Panjabrao Deshmukh Krishi Vidyapeeth, Krishi Nagar, Akola, Maharashtra, India
Kiran S. Mawale	Plant Cell Biotechnology Department, CSIR-Central Food Technological Research Institute (CFTRI), Mysuru - 570 020, Karnataka, India
Kuldeep Kaur	Department of Biotechnology, Guru Nanak Dev University, Amritsar-143 005, Punjab, India
Muneera Q. Al-Mssallem	Department of Food Science and Nutrition, College of Agriculture and Food Sciences, King Faisal University, Hofuf, Al-Ahsa-31982, Saudi Arabia
Mehrun Nisha Khanam	University Centre for Research & Development, Chandigarh University, Mohali-140-413, Punjab, India Plant Biotechnology Laboratory, Department of Botany, Aligarh Muslim University, Aligarh-202-002, India
Mohammad Anis	Plant Biotechnology Laboratory, Department of Botany, Aligarh Muslim University, Aligarh-202-002, India
Mohammad Yaseen Mir	Centre of Research for Development, University of Kashmir, Hazratbal, Srinagar-190 006, (J&K), India
Mehpara Maqsood	Govt. College for Women, M.A. Road, Srinagar, Jammu & Kashmir, India
Mir Khusrau	Government Degree College (Boys), Anantnag, Jammu and Kashmir, India
M. Raseena	Department of Botany, University of Calicut, Kerala, India
Nishi Kumari	Department of Botany, Mahila Mahavidyalaya, Banaras Hindu University, Varanasi, India
Pragya Shukla	Biotechnology and Molecular Biology Division, CSIR-National Botanical Research Institute, Lucknow, India Department of Botany, Institute of Science, Banaras Hindu University, Varanasi, India
Penna Suprasanna	Nuclear Agriculture and Biotechnology Division, Bhabha Atomic Research Centre, Trombay, Mumbai MS, India
Parvatam Giridhar	Plant Cell Biotechnology Department, CSIR-Central Food Technological Research Institute (CFTRI), Mysuru - 570 020, Karnataka, India

Panchsheela Nogia	Department of Biotechnology, Guru Nanak Dev University, Amritsar-143 005, Punjab, India
Pratap Kumar Pati	Department of Agriculture, Guru Nanak Dev University, Amritsar Punjab, India Department of Biotechnology, Guru Nanak Dev University, Amritsar-143 005, Punjab, India
Pooja Jaiswal	Department of Botany, Mahila Mahavidyalaya, Banaras Hindu University, Varanasi, India
Rajesh Arora	Department of Phyto Analytical Chemistry and Toxicology, Defence Institute of Physiology & Allied Sciences, Defence Research and Development Organization, Lucknow Road, Timarpur, Delhi- 110054, India
Sandra Gonçalves	MED – Mediterranean Institute for Agriculture, Environment and Development & CHANGE – Global Change and Sustainability Institute, Faculdade de Ciências e Tecnologia, Universidade do Algarve, Campus de Gambelas, Faro, Portugal
S. Mohan Jain	Department of Agricultural Sciences, University of Helsinki-00014, Helsinki, Finland
Sakshi Rawat	Department of Biotechnology, Guru Nanak Dev University, Amritsar-143 005, Punjab, India
Shashikanta Behera	Department of Biotechnology, Guru Nanak Dev University, Amritsar-143 005, Punjab, India
Vaishali Kumari	Department of Biotechnology, Guru Nanak Dev University, Amritsar-143 005, Punjab, India
Vyoma Mistry	C. G. Bhakta Institute of Biotechnology, Uka Tarsadia University, Gopal-Vidyanagar, Maliba Campus, Surat-394350, India
Zahoor A. Kaloo	Department of Botany, University of Kashmir, Hazratbal, Srinagar, Jammu & Kashmir, India

CHAPTER 1

Secondary Metabolite Production through Elicitation: Biotic, Abiotic, MeJA, PGRs and Stress Signaling in Improving Compounds in Select Medicinal Plants

Mehpara Maqsood[1], A. Mujib[2,*], Mir Khusrau[3] and Zahoor A. Kaloo[4]

[1] *Govt. College for Women, M.A. Road, Srinagar, Jammu & Kashmir, India*

[2] *Department of Botany, Jamia Hamdard, New Delhi, India*

[3] *Government Degree College (Boys), Anantnag, Jammu and Kashmir, India*

[4] *Department of Botany, University of Kashmir, Hazratbal, Srinagar, Jammu & Kashmir, India*

Abstract: Plants in addition to primary metabolites produce secondary metabolites which are of immense pharmaceutical importance and other industrial uses. Secondary metabolites are produced due to the stress experienced by plants in response to external triggers/agents like elicitors. Elicitation involves two types of elicitors namely biotic and abiotic. Elicitors have a vital role in plant tissue culture as these improve secondary metabolite content in cultures. Other culture conditions including volume and types of medium, duration, *etc.*, also affect the yield of alkaloids. Extensive research has been carried out for the enhanced level of alkaloids in *in vitro* cultured plants. Various common elicitors used in media are methyl jasmonate (MeJA), yeast extract (YE), fungal extract, ions from various salts like $CdCl_2$ heavy metal ions, and ionic, nonionic radiations, *etc.* The fungal cell wall components oligosaccharides and peptides have also been used as elicitors for the induction/enhancement of secondary metabolites in plant cell/organ cultures. The influence of sample representation of biotic and abiotic elicitors, *i.e.*, YE, *Aspergillus flavus*, MeJA, $CdCl_2$, $CaCl_2$, has been discussed taking a few medicinals and oil yielding plants from authors' laboratory. A direct link of stress with elicitors including plant growth regulators (PGRs) has been established showing over accumulation of proline, protein, SOD, APX and other antioxidant enzyme activity with increased levels of elicitation. Increasing demand forces researchers to conduct further investigation in this area for the production of phyto-compounds and even for viable commercial exploitation.

Keywords: Alkaloids, *Catharanthus roseus*, *Colchicum luteum*, Colchicine, Elicitor.

---

* **Corresponding author A. Mujib:** Department of Botany, Jamia Hamdard, New Delhi, India;
E-mail: amujib3@yahoo.co.in

Mohammad Anis & Mehrun Nisha Khanam (Eds.)

INTRODUCTION

The plant has been used to treat a wide range of diseases like asthma, fever, stomach ache, arthritis, menstrual disorders, toothache, migraine, insect bites and helminthiasis [1]. Plants are a rich source of metabolic products, attracting the attention of workers in amending the quantity and quality of traits. The secondary metabolites are the diverse group of organic compounds produced by plants to facilitate interaction with biotic and abiotic environments in establishing defense mechanisms [2]. These products are unique sources of pharmaceuticals, food additives, flavors and industrially important biochemicals [3]. The secondary metabolites have complex structures to be manufactured by chemical synthesis and semi-synthesis, and are frequently extracted from naturally and *in vitro* grown cultivated plants [4]. These metabolites are produced and even over-synthesized from different medicinal plants under biotic and abiotic influences [5]. Most commonly, the strategies adopted are optimization of medium component and environmental cultural conditions, the use of high producing superior cell lines, addition/feeding of precursors, overexpression of key enzymes in biosynthetic processes, and other biotechnological and cell culture techniques [6]. *In vitro* methodology may offer an alternative, promising technique for the production of phyto-compounds which can further be improved by the application of elicitors [7]. Elicitors of biotic and abiotic origin have been used extensively for the enriched synthesis of a wide variety of secondary metabolites. There are several reports of enhanced synthesis of secondary metabolites in cell cultures by using elicitors, PGRs, medium, precursor feeding and other biotechnological techniques [8]. Elicitors were used as an enhanced biomass production in different *in vitro* cultures such as *Ophiorrhiza mungos* [4], *Silybum marianum* [9], *Glycyrrhiza uralensis* [10], *Eruca sativa* [11], *Isatis tinctoria* [12] and *Centella asiatica* [13]. As an external stimuli, the elicitors are added to the medium, change cell metabolism, cause stress in culture and activate secondary metabolite synthesis [14]. Elicitors are known to activate a range of defense mechanisms including the synthesis and accumulation of diverse defensive secondary metabolites in plants [14]. The activating mechanisms of elicitors are considered to be different, complex and unpredictable at times, in relation to metabolite synthesis [15].

ELICITOR

Elicitation is an important current technique in which various elements or compounds are amended to the media for improving secondary metabolites in cultures. These molecules induce stress to cultivated cells and in response to adverse situations accumulate and synthesize improved amounts of phyto-compounds [16].

Classification of Elicitor

Elicitors can be categorized into two different types biotic and abiotic elicitors. The biotic elicitors originate from the living cells of lower/prokaryotic organisms fungi and bacteria; simple sugars, polysaccharides, chitin, glucans, pectin, cellulose, MeJA, glycoproteins or intracellular proteins and peptides in are added as external regulatory molecules which regulate a number of enzymes or ion channels through receptor binding mechanism by activating/deactivating gene expression in evoking stress response [17, 18] (Table **2**).

The abiotic elicitors, on the other hand, comprise of non-biological regulatory elements. These abiotic compounds contain a wide variety of chemicals or agents including metal ions. Various metals like Cd, Pb, Ni, Ag, Fe, Co, Al, Ca have been added to the media and are noted to be very efficient in improving the yield of alkaloids in several investigated plant materials [19, 20] (Table **1**). Abiotic elicitors like pH, extreme temperature, ultraviolet (UV) rays, X-rays, and Gamma rays have also been tested in several plants. Other signaling compounds often tried are salicylic acid, methyl jasmonates and NO_2 for enhanced synthesis and accumulation of phyto-compounds in tested samples [21].

Table 1. Various compounds (biotic, abiotic and other) and explant/ tissue used for elicitation.

Biotic Elicitor Used	Abiotic Factors Added	Explant/Tissue Used
Fungi: *Aspergillus, Pythium, Fusarium etc*; Cell wall components of fungi, sugars, pectin *etc.* Bacteria: *Pseudomonas* extract; Yeast extract; Casin hydrolysate; MeJA; Salicyclic acid; Peptides;	NaCl, KCl, $CdCl_2$, $CaCl_2$, $AlCl_2$, $AgNO_3$, $CuCl_2$, pH, temperature, UV ray, X-rays, Gamma rays.	Non-, embryogenic callus, suspension, different stages of somatic embryos, nodal stem, protoplast derived tissues, plantlets.

Table 2. Biotic and other factors' induced elicitation targeting different alkaloids: A few successful cases in medicinal plants.

Elicitor	Plant Species	Culture Type	Secondary Metabolite	References
Aspergillus flavus fungal extract	*Catharanthus roseus*	Embryogenic callus, somatic embryos	Vincristine and vinblastine	Dipti *et al.* 2016

(Table 2) cont.....

Elicitor	Plant Species	Culture Type	Secondary Metabolite	References
MeJA MeJA	*Taxus baccata,Taxus x media Coriander sativum*	Cell suspension Non-, embryogenic callus, embryos	Paclitaxel Essential oil	Sabater *et al.* 2014 Muzamil *et al.* 2020
Salicylic acid	*Gingko biloba*	Cell suspension	Bilobalide; Ginkolide a, b	Kang *et al.* 2006
Bacteria extracts	*Artemisia annua*	Hairy root	Artemisinin	Putalun *et al.* 2007
Fungal extract	*Panax ginseng*	Cell suspension	Ginsenosides	Xu 2005
Coronatine	*Glycine max*	Cell suspension	Glyceollins	Fliegmann *et al.* 2003
Chitosan and chitin	*Vitis vinifera*	Cell suspension	Stilbenes; Trans-resveratrol	Ferri *et al.* 2009
Other cell wall fragments	*Dioscorea zingiberensis*	Cell suspension	Diosgenin	Li *et al.* 2011
Cyclodextrins	*Catharanthus roseus*	Cell suspension, hairy root	Ajmalicine, Vindoline, Catharanthine and Ajmalicine	Almagro *et al.* 2011, Zhou *et al.* 2015
Yeast extract	*Catharanthus roseus*	Embryogenic callus	Vincristine and vinblastine	Mehpara and Mujib 2017

The effects of various elicitors (yeast extract, MeJA, salicylic acid, chitin, *etc.*) on the enhancement of secondary compounds production have been studied in different plant groups like *Solenostemon scutellarioides* [22], callus cultures of *Rosa hybrida* [23], hairy root cultures of soybean [24], cell suspension cultures of *Catharanthus roseus* [25] and adventitious root cultures of *Eleutherococcus koreanum* [26]. Among various elicitors, MeJA has been extensively studied in enhancing secondary compounds in a number of plants like *A. annua* for artemisinin [27]. Various medicinal plants like *Catharanthus roseus*, *Coriandrum sativum*, *Colchicum luteum*, *Taxus baccata*, *Rauwolfia serpentina*, *etc.*, have been extensively investigated in the laboratory of author for the production of secondary metabolites summarized in this present chapter.

Elicitation and Improved Yield in Some Medicinal Plants

Catharanthus roseus (L.) G. Don, a member of Apocynaceae, is an extensively investigated medicinal plant, producing over 130 alkaloids (Fig. **1a**). Vinblastine and vincristine are the two most important alkaloids showing anti-cancerous properties; ajmalicine is antihypertensive; serpentine is sedative, while others have various other properties. Beside natural synthesis from *in vivo* grown plants, these compounds are also produced chemically and semi-synthetically.

Unfortunately, the yield of these two alkaloids is very poor and is about 0.0005% dry weight basis. In *C. roseus*, different methods have been attempted for enhancing alkaloid content in tissue culture conditions. A variety of elicitors have also been tried which include methyl jasmonate [28, 29], yeast extract [7], chitosan [30], $CaCl_2$ and NaCl as abiotic salt [31, 32] (Table **1**), *Aspergillus flavus* as fungus biotic treatment [33] (Table **2**). Heavy metals like Mn, Ni and Pb [34] & Silver nanoparticles [29]. Like other fungus, yeast extract - a biotic elicitor was used and is considered to be a useful signaling compound in improving secondary compounds. Mehpara and Mujib (2017) [7] exposed protoplast-derived tissues of *Catharanthus* and vinblastine and vincristine yield was quantified (Fig. **1b**). Four different concentrations of yeast extract (T1 = 0.5, T2 = 1.0, T3 = 1.5 and T4 = 2.0 g/l) were added to the culture media which enhanced vinblastine and vincristine yield in germinating somatic embryos and in regenerated leaf tissues. Although the synthesis of alkaloid was noted to be treatment-specific the impact was maximum in T3 (1.5 mg/l) and about 22.74% increase in vinblastine and 48.49% in vincristine was reported in germinating stage of embryos. Antioxidant enzymes like SOD, CAT, APX and GR were high in yeast extract added media suggesting stress, and noted to be involved in enhanced levels of phyto-compounds. The amendment of yeast extract was noted to be efficient in enriching yield in a number of plants like *Astragalus chrysochlorus*, *Gymnema sylvestre* and other materials [35 - 37].

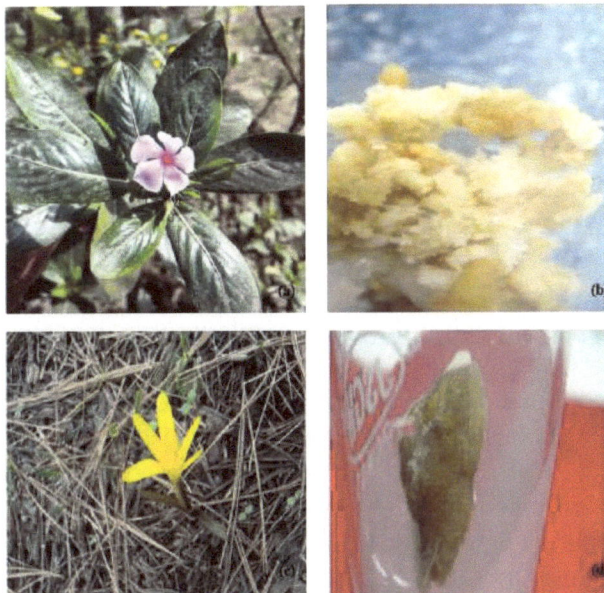

Fig. (1). (a) *Catharanthus roseus* in wild **(b)** Callus culture in *C. roseus* **(c)** *Colchicum luteum* in wild and **(d)** Callus initiation in *C. luteum.* (Bar 1a=1cm, bar 1b= 2mm, bar1c=1cm and bar 1d=2mm).

The induction of fungi/mycorrhizal fungi into the medium was noted to be efficient in inducing enhanced accumulation of ajmalicine and serpentine in *C. roseus* [38]; similar increased alkaloid accumulation was noted in other studied cases [39], Tonk *et al.* [33] investigated the influence of *Aspergillus flavus* fungus extract on alkaloid yield in *C. roseus*. Various concentrations, *i.e.*, 0.05% (T1), 0.15% (T2), 0.25% (T3), and 0.35% (T4) of fungus extract and control (T0), were incorporated into solid MS medium and the yield of vinblastine and vincristine was measured and compared in *in vitro* grown tissues. The *A. flavus* fungal extract augmented callus biomass, and improved embryogenesis with more numbers of embryos at low levels, *i.e.*, in T2. At the same low T1/T2 level, the percent germination of embryos, and the shoot and root growth of somatic embryos were noted high. Vinblastine yield was reported to be high in germinating embryo stages and the yield was improved further with addition of *A. flavus* fungus extract at 0.15%. About 7.88 and 15.50% enhancement of vinblastine and vincristine respectively was observed on *A. flavus* treated cultures. Various stress markers like antioxidant enzymes, proline, sugar levels *etc.* were checked as the amendment of fungus extract may produce stress on cultivated tissues and organs. Biochemical analyses showed higher levels of sugar, protein and proline in tested tissues including germinating embryos on *A. flavus* fungus added conditions. The mature, advanced embryos showed enhanced levels of SOD activity and with the addition of fungal extract, the enzyme activity was even higher, establishing a link of stress with elicitation on exposed tissues, resulting in enhanced accumulation of alkaloids (vinblastine and vincristine) especially at low T2/T1 levels. It has been observed that the fungus elicitors contain various oligo/polysaccharides or sugars and peptide like signaling molecules which promote the synthesis and accumulation of plant secondary products [40].

In *C. roseus*, $CaCl_2$ as an abiotic elicitor was used to improve the synthesis and accumulation of vincristine in embryogenic suspension culture [31] (Table **3**). Various levels of $CaCl_2$ namely 5, 25, 50, 75 and 100 mM were added to the MS medium along with control as an elicitor element. The suspension culture growth, *i.e.*, the dry mass, packed cell volume, and colony area, increased only up to low elicitor treatment (25 mM). HPTLC investigation of harvested embryogenic tissues and the liquid medium was conducted to detect and quantify vincristine at regular intervals. Vincristine was identified only after 20 days of elicitation in harvested suspended cells and no vincristine was detected in liquid medium in which embryogenic suspension was cultured for faster tissue growth. SOD, CAT, APX and Glutathione reductase (GR) antioxidant enzyme activities were measured in response to $CaCl_2$ exposure of tissues. All the enzymes showed increased activity with an increase in elicitor doses, the authors reported.

Table 3. Abiotic compound mediated elicitation: some examples in medicinal plants.

NaCl	*Colchicum Luteum*	Embryogenic Callus	Colchicine	Mehpara *et al.* 2020
$CaCl_2$	*C. roseus*	Embryogenic suspension	Vincristine, vinblastine	Zahid *et al.* 2012
NaCl	*C. roseus*	Embryogenic callus	Vincristine, vinblastine	Fatima *et al.* 2016
$CdCl_2$	*Rauwolfia serpentina*	Callus, embryo	Reserpine, ajmalicine	Zafar *et al.* 2020
$CdCl_2$	*Allium sativum*	Callus, different stages embryos	Alliin	Malik *et al.* 2021
$AlCl_3$	*Rauwolfia serpentina*	Callus	Reserpine, ajmalicine	Zafar *et al.* 2017

Allium sativum is a plant of the family Amaryllidaceae. Garlic shows antiviral, antimicrobial, antifungal, antioxidant, and anti-inflammatory activities [41]. It also possesses hepatoprotective, anticancerous and cardiovascular protection abilities [42]. These pharmaceutical medicinal importances are specifically due to organosulphur compounds, unique to *Allium* [43]. Over thirty different organosulphur compounds including alliin and allicin are present in garlic at high levels which produce pungent flavour while converting into diallyl thiosulfinate or allicin when cut. About one gram of raw garlic (fresh weight) contains 10 mg of alliin and this is the target point for enhancement. Moien *et al.* (2020) [44] investigated the influence of cadmium chloride ($CdCl_2$) on alliin accumulation in *A. sativum* in various cultured tissues. The *in vitro* raised tissues were exposed to various $CdCl_2$ doses *i.e.* 0.05, 0.1, 0.15 and 0.2 mM and the alliin yield was measured and compared by using high performance thin layer chromatography (HPTLC) method. It was noted that with a $CdCl_2$ dose increase, the alliin yield improved, and maximum yield was noted at 0.15 mM treatment following 4 days of elicitation treatment. Of the various *in vitro* grown tissues, the highest amount of alliin accumulation was observed in leaves, followed by somatic embryos at the same level of $CdCl_2$ treatment. In callus tissue, the alliin yield was relatively low compared to leaf tissues. In *A. sativum*, the alliin is primarily synthesized in leaves perhaps this is the reason for high alliin yield in leaves compared to other tested tissues like callus and somatic embryos [45] The catalase (CAT), superoxide dismutase (SOD) and ascorbate peroxidase (APX) antioxidant enzyme activities were monitored in different $CdCl_2$ treated tissues as the addition of elicitor to the medium causes cellular stress. It was noted that with increasing $CdCl_2$ level, the antioxidant enzyme activity also increased, with the highest enzyme activity in leaves after 6 days of treatment at 0.2 mM. Biochemical investigations of elicitated tissues indicate a higher accumulation of sugar, protein and proline in elevated levels of $CdCl_2$ all suggesting the onset and presence of stress in cultivating tissues. Increased activities of enzymes and other physiological markers may be involved in scavenging stress caused by the overproduction of reactive oxygen species (ROS) generated by $CdCl_2$.

Rauvolfia serpentina (L.) is a member of the family Apocyanaceae. This plant contains a variety of pharmaceutically important compounds like reserpine, ajmalicine, serpentine, ajmaline, and others [46]. The plant shows its impact against several ailments *i.e.* it is antidiabetic, anti-inflammatory, anti-tumoric and several other protective activities. The phyto-compounds present in this plant are primarily synthesized in roots and stem; and the content level varies from 0.7–3.0% [47]. Nadia *et al.* (2020) [48] investigated the impact of $CdCl_2$ on *Rauvolfia serpentina* alkaloid yield as the *in vitro* cultures with elicitation may overcome the limitations of low yield of important phyto-compounds. Different levels of $CdCl_2$ *i.e.* 0.05 mM (C1), 0.10 mM (C2), 0.15 mM (C3) and 0.20 mM (C4) were added to MS and various growth parameters like callus biomass and the alkaloid yield were observed. The addition of $CdCl_2$ at 0.15 mM enhanced callus biomass growth significantly. The quantification of reserpine and ajmalicine in different tissues was made through an HPTLC study. Among various tissues tested, reserpine content was maximum in the roots of regenerated plants. The yield of ajmalicine was, however, more in leaf derived callus; both the two phyto-compounds were synthesized and accumulated best at C_3 treatment. A higher $CdCl_2$ elicitor dose (0.20 mM) reduced the rate of callus proliferation and inhibited alkaloid yield in *R. serpentina*.

The use of elicitors in tissue culture medium caused cellular stress at variable intensities as was observed in several studied plant materials. In order to monitor the plant defense responses, several stress markers have been routinely monitored. Antioxidant enzyme activities like SOD, CAT and APX were assayed in $CdCl_2$-treated and non-treated tissues. The enzyme activity was high and increased almost linearly with increasing $CdCl_2$ levels suggesting stress in a culture which in turn improved the yield of reserpine and ajmalicine in *R. serpentina*. The use of $CdCl_2$ as an elicitor in promoting callus biomass, induction of stress in culture and in enriching secondary metabolites has been noted in several investigated plant systems [44, 49].

Coriandrum sativum is a spice yielding plant, used almost daily in the Indian subcontinent. The coriander seeds, tender green leaves and oil all are important in the local and global markets. The yield of oil differs with coriander genotypes and is primarily influenced by a number of external factors. In current years, several biotechnological approaches have been integrated to improve plant products. Here, Methyl jasmonate (MeJA) was added to the MS medium as it behaves as an important secondary messenger and signaling molecule in enriching compounds. MeJA concentration at T1 = 50, T2 = 100, T3 = 150 and T4 = 200 µM were prepared and added to the media and the oil yield was quantified in non-embryogenic, embryogenic and other tissues through Gas chromatography–mass spectrometry (GC–MS). All the treatments had a variable influence on oil yield the addition of 150 µM MEJA was however noted to be very effective in enriching oil in coriander.

As discussed earlier, the amendment of biotic or abiotic elicitors like MeJA generates stress in culture. The activities enzymes, *i.e.*, SOD, CAT and APX, was measured and noted to be high in treated tissues compared to the untreated control (T0). In 200 µM treatment (T4), the CAT and SOD enzyme activity was noted to be very high in maturing embryo stages. Other stress and biochemical markers such as sugar, protein and proline were high with increasing levels of MeJA treatment. The influence of MeJA effects on the enhancement of phytocompounds utilizing *in vitro* cultivated cell, tissue and organ has been investigated in different plant genera [50, 51]. The induced stress in culture was perhaps responsible for excess synthesis and accumulation of coriander oils.

Colchicum luteum Baker is a member of the family Colchicaceae (Fig. **1c**). The plant is commonly distributed in sub-alpine areas, western Himalayas, Jammu and Kashmir and other adjoining areas of an altitude of 700 and 2800 m. The primary compound present in this plant is colchicine, an alkaloid extracted from corms or tubers. The plant *C. luteum* is used against various diseases like Behcet's syndrome, rheumatism, gout, respiratory disorders, antinociceptive, antiinflammatory and exhibits anti-cancerous activity as it contains colchicine and demecolcine. Colchicine is a secondary metabolite (trade names are colcrys, mitigrare *etc.*), also produced by *Colchicum autumnale* and *Gloriosa superba*. Several analogs of colchicine namely 3-dimethyl colchicine, colchicoside, thiocolchicocide were designed and synthesized displaying improved anticancer activity in comparison to native drugs used against certain leukemic cells and solid tumours [52]. Colchicine halts polymerization of microtubules by binding to protein tubulin, required for cell division, and hence checks uncontrolled cell division. The FDA (2009) [63] approval of colchicine as a new drug had research consequences.

Elicitation has been practiced in several medicinal plants including *Colchicum* for increasing the content of secondary metabolites. Mehpara *et al.* (2020) [53] elicitated corm-callus of *Colchicum luteum* with different levels of salt (NaCl) and the colchicine yield was measured through high pressure liquid chromatography (Fig **1d**). It was noted that all the treatments improved the levels of colchicine but the yield was maximum in 100 mM salt amended medium. Mahendran *et al.* (2018) [54] investigated the influence of various elicitors like salicylic acid (SA), yeast extract (YE), casein hydrolysate (CH), and ethylene inhibitor like silver nitrate ($AgNO_3$) on the biosynthesis of colchicine and thio-colchicoside content. Colchicine was extracted and quantified through HPLC, column chromatography, HPTLC and TLC following chitosan treatment - a biotic elicitor [55]. Production of colchicine from *Colchicum autumnale* cell suspension cultures using colchicine precursors as elicitors like p-coumaric and tyramine was earlier reported [56]. Daradkeh *et al.* (2012) [57] reported colchicine production from cell suspension of another species of Colchicum, *C. hierosolymitanum* as colchicine medication is used to treat gout and other diseases like Behcet [58].

The genus Taxus is a plant of the Taxaceae family. Out of several species found, *T. brevifolia* and *T. canadensis* produce taxol (paclitaxel) - one of the important natural drugs used to treat cancers [59]. The species of *Taxus* are predominantly distributed to the Himalayan range, spread over to China, Nepal and other northeast countries like Bhutan and Myanmar. Beside anti-cancerous importance, several species of *Taxus* have been utilized in Ayurveda and traditional medicinal practices. As the taxol is immensely valuable, people have been trying to improve the content. Mujib *et al.* (2020) [54] quantified the content of taxol from callus cultured in various plant growth regulators (PGRs) amended media. PGRs especially the auxins are considered to be a strong stressor and signaling element. In 2, 4-D supplemented media, the taxol yield was maximum, the next best taxol accumulation was noted in NAA - another auxin added media and the least accumulation of taxol was noted in BAP (cytokinin) supplemented media. As to monitor the level of stress in different auxins (2,4-D and NAA) and cytokinin (BAP) added conditions SOD, APX antioxidant enzyme activities and proline level were assayed. The SOD, APX and proline levels were high in callus, cultured on 2,4-D, the next best stress condition was noted on NAA added conditions, and in BAP, the stress level was low compared to auxin supplemented media. Thus a link of stress and auxin was established which in turn stimulated taxol accumulation in cultivated tissues.

MECHANISM

The schematic pathway of an eliciting mechanism following elicitor molecule treatment is presented in Fig. (**2**). The abbreviations used are: SAR (systemic acquired response), ISR (induced systemic resistance), ROS (Reactive oxygen species), RNS (reactive nitrogen species), NADPH (nicotinamide adenine dinucleotide phosphate), SA (salicylic acid), JA (jasmonic acid), ET (ethylene).

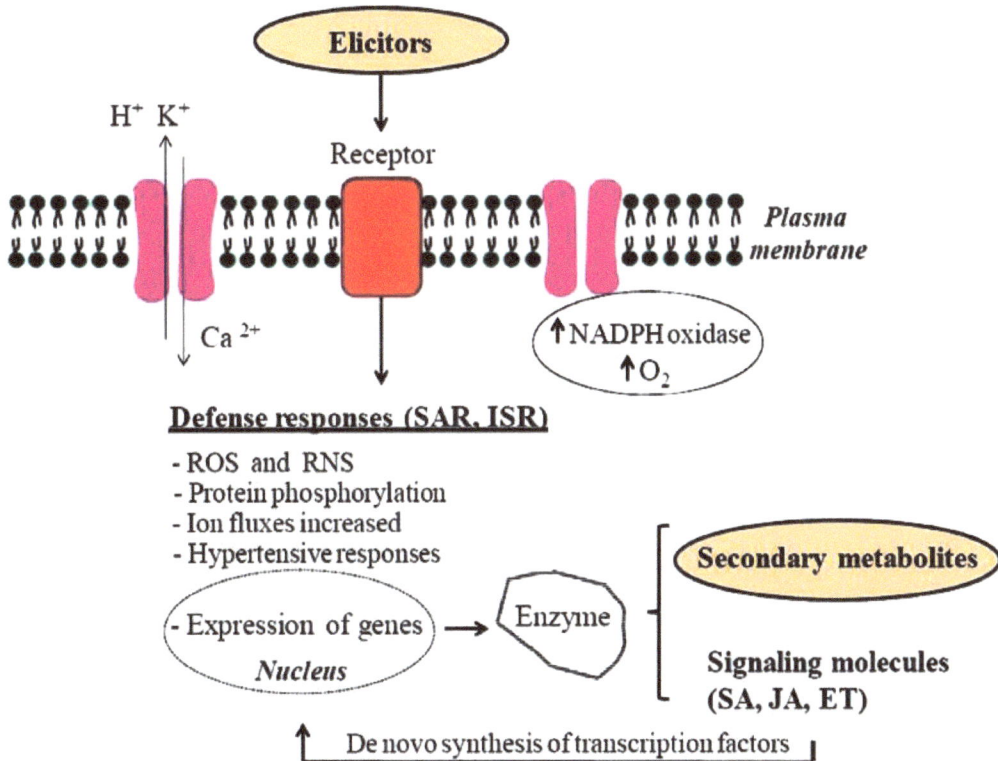

Fig. (2). Courtesy: Ferrari 2010 [60]; Nieves *et al.* 2014 [61].

CONCLUSION

Elicitation can be used as a tool for the enhancement of secondary metabolites of interest. In addition, studying elicitor-activated biosynthesis pathways with identified signaling components could be an efficient strategy for activating defense responses in plants in order to replace or reduce chemical applications to protect crops [62]. Improvement and simultaneous amendments of secondary metabolite production may help in alleviating and in preventing diseases. It is worth mentioning that the drugs and similar other plant-based formulations are easily accepted globally because of no or fewer side effects. Research in this direction may offer other alternative treatments for diseases through clinical trials.

REFERENCES

[1]   Maggi F. Feverfew *(Tanacetum parthenium (L.) Sch. Bip.).* Nonvitamin and non mineral nutritional supplements. Amsterdam: Elsevier 2019; pp. 233-5.

[2]   Wang JW, Wu JY. Effective elicitors and process strategies for enhancement of secondary metabolite production in hairy root cultures. Adv Biochem Eng Biotechnol 2013; 134: 55-89.
[http://dx.doi.org/10.1007/10_2013_183] [PMID: 23467807]

[3] Murthy HN, Lee EJ, Paek KY. Production of secondary metabolites from cell and organ cultures: Strategies and approaches for biomass improvement and metabolite accumulation. Plant Cell Tissue Organ Cult 2014; 118(1): 1-16.
[http://dx.doi.org/10.1007/s11240-014-0467-7]

[4] Deepthi S, Satheeshkumar K. Enhanced camptothecin production induced by elicitors in the cell suspension cultures of *Ophiorrhiza mungos* Linn. Plant Cell Tissue Organ Cult 2016; 124(3): 483-93.
[http://dx.doi.org/10.1007/s11240-015-0908-y]

[5] Farajpour M, Ebrahimi M, Baghizadeh A, Aalifar M. Phytochemical and yield variation among Iranian *Achillea millefolium* accessions. HortScience 2017; 52(6): 827-30.
[http://dx.doi.org/10.21273/HORTSCI11654-16]

[6] Pawar KD, Yadav AV, Shouche YS, Thengane SR. Influence of endophytic fungal elicitation on production of *inophyllum* in suspension cultures of *Calophyllum inophyllum* L. Plant Cell Tissue Organ Cult 2011; 106(2): 345-52.
[http://dx.doi.org/10.1007/s11240-011-9928-4]

[7] Maqsood M, Abdul M. Yeast extract elicitation increases vinblastine and vincristine yield in protoplast derived tissues and plantlets in *Catharanthus roseus.* Rev Bras Farmacogn 2017; 27(5): 549-56.
[http://dx.doi.org/10.1016/j.bjp.2017.05.008]

[8] Khan T, Abbasi BH, Khan MA. The interplay between light, plant growth regulators and elicitors on growth and secondary metabolism in cell cultures of *Fagonia indica.* J Photochem Photobiol B 2018; 185: 153-60.
[http://dx.doi.org/10.1016/j.jphotobiol.2018.06.002] [PMID: 29908408]

[9] Gabr AMM, Ghareeb H, El Shabrawi HM, Smetanska I, Bekheet SA. Enhancement of silymarin and phenolic compound accumulation in tissue culture of *Milk thistle* using elicitor feeding and hairy root cultures. J Genet Eng Biotechnol 2016; 14(2): 327-33.
[http://dx.doi.org/10.1016/j.jgeb.2016.10.003] [PMID: 30647631]

[10] Wang J, Li J, Wu X, Liu S, Li H, Gao W. Assessment of genetic fidelity and composition: Mixed elicitors enhance triterpenoid and flavonoid biosynthesis of *Glycyrrhiza uralensis* Fisch. tissue cultures. Biotechnol Appl Biochem 2017; 64(2): 211-7.
[http://dx.doi.org/10.1002/bab.1485] [PMID: 26872048]

[11] Kastell A, Schreiner M, Knorr D, Ulrichs C, Mewis I. Influence of nutrient supply and elicitors on glucosinolate production in *E. sativa* hairy root cultures. Plant Cell Tissue Organ Cult 2018; 132(3): 561-72.
[http://dx.doi.org/10.1007/s11240-017-1355-8]

[12] Gai QY, Jiao J, Wang X, Zang YP, Niu LL, Fu YJ. Elicitation of *Isatis tinctoria* L. hairy root cultures by salicylic acid and methyl jasmonate for the enhanced production of pharmacologically active alkaloids and flavonoids. Plant Cell Tissue Organ Cult 2019; 137(1): 77-86.
[http://dx.doi.org/10.1007/s11240-018-01553-8]

[13] Gupta S, Chaturvedi P. Enhancing secondary metabolite production in medicinal plants using endophytic elicitors: A case study of *centella asiatica* (apiaceae) and asiaticoside. Hodkinson T, Doohan F, Saunders M. Endophytes for a Growing World. Cambridge University Press 2019; pp. (pp. 310-327). Cambridge: 310-27.

[14] Zhao J, Davis LC, Verpoorte R. Elicitor signal transduction leading to production of plant secondary metabolites. Biotechnol Adv 2005; 23(4): 283-333.
[http://dx.doi.org/10.1016/j.biotechadv.2005.01.003] [PMID: 15848039]

[15] Jeong GT, Park DH. Enhancement of growth and secondary metabolite biosynthesis: Effect of elicitors derived from plants and insects. Biotechnol Bioprocess Eng 2005; 10(1): 73-7.
[http://dx.doi.org/10.1007/BF02931186]

[16] Zafar N, Mujib A, Ali M, Tonk D, Gulzar B. Aluminum chloride elicitation (amendment) improves

callus biomass growth and reserpine yield in Rauvolfia serpentina leaf callus. Plant Cell Tissue Organ Cult 2017; 130(2): 357-68.
[http://dx.doi.org/10.1007/s11240-017-1230-7]

[17]   Veeresham C. Natural products derived from plants as a source of drugs. J Adv Pharm Technol Res 2012; 3(4): 200-1.
[http://dx.doi.org/10.4103/2231-4040.104709] [PMID: 23378939]

[18]   Efferth T. Biotechnology applications of plant callus cultures. Engineering 2019; 5(1): 50-9.
[http://dx.doi.org/10.1016/j.eng.2018.11.006]

[19]   Cai Z, Kastell A, Speiser C, Smetanska I. Enhanced resveratrol production in *Vitis vinifera* cell suspension cultures by heavy metals without loss of cell viability. Appl Biochem Biotechnol 2013; 171(2): 330-40.
[http://dx.doi.org/10.1007/s12010-013-0354-4] [PMID: 23832187]

[20]   Naik PM, Al-Khayri JM. Abiotic and biotic elicitors role in secondary metabolites production through *in vitro* culture of medicinal plants. Abiotic and Biotic Stress in Plants - Recent Advances and Future Perspectives. intechopen 2016.
[http://dx.doi.org/10.5772/61442]

[21]   Ali M, Mujib A, Gulzar B, Zafar N. Essential oil yield estimation by gas chromatography-mass spectrometry (GCMS) after Methyl jasmonate (MeJA) elicitation in *in vitro* cultivated tissues of Coriandrum sativum L. 3Biotech 2019; 9: 41.
[http://dx.doi.org/10.1007/s13205-019-1936-9]

[22]   Sahu R, Gangopadhyay M, Dewanjee S. Elicitor-induced rosmarinic acid accumulation and secondary metabolism enzyme activities in *Solenostemon scutellarioides*. Acta Physiol Plant 2013; 35(5): 1473-81.
[http://dx.doi.org/10.1007/s11738-012-1188-3]

[23]   Ram M, Prasad KV, Singh SK, Hada BS, Kumar S. Influence of salicylic acid and methyl jasmonate elicitation on anthocyanin production in callus cultures of *Rosa hybrida* L. Plant Cell Tissue Organ Cult 2013; 113(3): 459-67.
[http://dx.doi.org/10.1007/s11240-013-0287-1]

[24]   Theboral J, Sivanandhan G, Subramanyam K, *et al.* Enhanced production of isoflavones by elicitation in hairy root cultures of Soybean. Plant Cell Tissue Organ Cult 2014; 117(3): 477-81.
[http://dx.doi.org/10.1007/s11240-014-0450-3]

[25]   Saiman MZ, Mustafa NR, Choi YH, Verpoorte R, Schulte AE. Metabolic alterations and distribution of five-carbon precursors in jasmonic acid-elicited *Catharanthus roseus* cell suspension cultures. Plant Cell Tissue Organ Cult 2015; 122(2): 351-62.
[http://dx.doi.org/10.1007/s11240-015-0773-8]

[26]   Lee EJ, Park SY, Paek KY. Enhancement strategies of bioactive compound production in adventitious root cultures of *Eleutherococcus koreanum* Nakai subjected to methyl jasmonate and salicylic acid elicitation through airlift bioreactors. Plant Cell Tissue Organ Cult 2015; 120(1): 1-10.
[http://dx.doi.org/10.1007/s11240-014-0567-4]

[27]   Baldi A, Dixit VK. Yield enhancement strategies for artemisinin production by suspension cultures of *Artemisia annua*. Bioresour Technol 2008; 99(11): 4609-14.
[http://dx.doi.org/10.1016/j.biortech.2007.06.061] [PMID: 17804216]

[28]   Thaler JS, Owen B, Higgins VJ. The role of the jasmonate response in plant susceptibility to diverse pathogens with a range of lifestyles. Plant Physiol 2004; 135(1): 530-8.
[http://dx.doi.org/10.1104/pp.104.041566] [PMID: 15133157]

[29]   Shahin H, de Klerk GJM, El-Hela AA. Effect of growth regulators on multiplication and alkaloid production of *Narcissus tazetta* var. *italicus* in tissue culture. Propag Ornam Plants 2018; 18: 124-30.

[30]   Pliankong P, Suka-Ard P, Wannakrairoj S. Chitosan elicitation for enhancing of vincristine and

vinblastine accumulation in cell culture of *Catharanthus roseus.* J Agric Sci 2018; 10: 287-93.

[31] Zahid SH, Mujib A. Accumulation of vincristine in calcium chloride elicitated *Catharanthus roseus* cultures. Nat Prod J 2012; 2(9): 307-15.

[32] Fatima S, Mujib A, Tonk D. NaCl amendment improves vinblastine and vincristine synthesis in *Catharanthus roseus*: a case of stress signalling as evidenced by antioxidant enzymes activities. Plant Cell Tissue Organ Cult 2015; 121(2): 445-58.
[http://dx.doi.org/10.1007/s11240-015-0715-5]

[33] Tonk D, Mujib A, Maqsood M, Ali M, Zafar N. *Aspergillus flavus* fungus elicitation improves vincristine and vinblastine yield by augmenting callus biomass growth in *Catharanthus roseus*. Plant Cell Tissue Organ Cult 2016; 126(2): 291-303.
[http://dx.doi.org/10.1007/s11240-016-0998-1]

[34] Srivastava NK, Srivastava AK. Influence of some heavy metals on growth, alkaloid content and composition in *Catharanthus roseus L.* Indian J Pharm Sci 2010; 72(6): 775-8.
[http://dx.doi.org/10.4103/0250-474X.84592] [PMID: 21969751]

[35] Cakir O, Ari S. Defensive and secondary metabolism in Astragalus chrysochlorus cell cultures, in response to yeast extract stressor. J Environ Biol 2009; 30(1): 51-5.
[PMID: 20112863]

[36] Bhat MA, Mujib A, Junaid A, Mahmooduzzafar M. *in vitro* regeneration of *Solanum nigrum* with enhanced solasodine production. Biol Plant 2010; 54(4): 757-60.
[http://dx.doi.org/10.1007/s10535-010-0136-6]

[37] Veerashree V, Anuradha CM, Kumar V. Elicitor-enhanced production of gymnemic acid in cell suspension cultures of *Gymnema sylvestre* R. Br. Plant Cell Tissue Organ Cult 2012; 108(1): 27-35.
[http://dx.doi.org/10.1007/s11240-011-0008-6]

[38] Zubek S, Mielcarek S, Turnau K. Hypericin and pseudohypericin concentrations of a valuable medicinal plant *Hypericum perforatum* L. are enhanced by arbuscular mycorrhizal fungi. Mycorrhiza 2012; 22(2): 149-56.
[http://dx.doi.org/10.1007/s00572-011-0391-1] [PMID: 21626142]

[39] Prasad A, Mathur A, Kalra A, Gupta MM, Lal RK, Mathur AK. Fungal elicitor-mediated enhancement in growth and asiaticoside content of *Centella asiatica* L. shoot cultures. Plant Growth Regul 2013; 69(3): 265-73.
[http://dx.doi.org/10.1007/s10725-012-9769-0]

[40] Liang Z, Zhang T, Zhang X, Zhang J, Zhao C. An alkaloid and a steroid from the endophytic fungus Aspergillus fumigatus. Molecules 2015; 20(1): 1424-33.
[http://dx.doi.org/10.3390/molecules20011424] [PMID: 25594349]

[41] Nile SH, Nile AS, Keum YS, Sharma K. Utilization of quercetin and quercetin glycosides from onion (*Allium cepa* L.) solid waste as an antioxidant, urease and xanthine oxidase inhibitors. Food Chem 2017; 235: 119-26.
[http://dx.doi.org/10.1016/j.foodchem.2017.05.043] [PMID: 28554615]

[42] El-Saber Batiha G, Magdy Beshbishy A, G Wasef L, *et al.* Chemical constituents and pharmacological activities of garlic (*Allium sativum* L.): A review. Nutrients 2020; 12(3): 872.
[http://dx.doi.org/10.3390/nu12030872] [PMID: 32213941]

[43] Poojary MM, Putnik P, Bursać Kovačević D, *et al.* Stability and extraction of bioactive sulfur compounds from *Allium* genus processed by traditional and innovative technologies. J Food Compos Anal 2017; 61: 28-39.
[http://dx.doi.org/10.1016/j.jfca.2017.04.007]

[44] Malik MQ, Mujib A, Gulzar B, *et al.* Enrichment of alliin in different *in vitro* grown tissues of Allium sativum through CdCl2 elicitation as revealed by high performance thin layer chromatography (HPTLC). Ind Crops Prod 2020; 158: 113007.

[http://dx.doi.org/10.1016/j.indcrop.2020.113007]

[45]   Yoshimoto N, Yabe A, Sugino Y, *et al.* Garlic Î³-glutamyl transpeptidases that catalyze deglutamylation of biosynthetic intermediate of alliin. Front Plant Sci 2015; 5: 758.
[http://dx.doi.org/10.3389/fpls.2014.00758] [PMID: 25620969]

[46]   Kumari R, Rathib B, Ranic A, Bhatnagar S. *Rauvolfia serpentine* L. Benth. ex Kurz.: phytochemical, pharmacological and therapeutic aspects. Int J Pharm Sci Rev Res 2013; 23(2): 348-55.

[47]   Pandey V, Cherian E, Patani G. Effect of growth regulators and culture conditions on direct root induction of *Rauwolfia serpentina* L. (Apocynaceae) Benth by leaf explants. Trop J Pharm Res 2010; 9(1): 27-34.
[http://dx.doi.org/10.4314/tjpr.v9i1.52031]

[48]   Zafar N, Mujib A, Ali M, *et al.* Cadmium chloride (CdCl2) elicitation improves reserpine and ajmalicine yield in Rauvolfia serpentina as revealed by high-performance thin-layer chromatography (HPTLC). 3 Biotech 2020; 10(8): 1-4.

[49]   Sivanandhan G, Arun M, Mayavan S, *et al.* Chitosan enhances withanolides production in adventitious root cultures of *Withania somnifera* (L.) Dunal. Ind Crops Prod 2012; 37(1): 124-9.
[http://dx.doi.org/10.1016/j.indcrop.2011.11.022]

[50]   Loc NH, Anh NHT, Khuyen LTM, An TNT. Effects of yeast extract and methyl jasmonate on the enhancement of solasodine biosynthesis in cell cultures of *Solanum hainanense* Hance. J Biosci Biotechnol 2014; 3(1): 1-6.

[51]   Oliveira MB, Junior ML, Grossi-de-Sá MF, Petrofeza S. Exogenous application of methyl jasmonate induces a defense response and resistance against *Sclerotinia sclerotiorum* in dry bean plants. J Plant Physiol 2015; 182(15): 13-22.
[http://dx.doi.org/10.1016/j.jplph.2015.04.006] [PMID: 26037694]

[52]   Dubey KK, Ray AR, Behera BK. Production of demethylated colchicine through microbial transformation and scale-up process development. Process Biochem 2008; 43(3): 251-7.
[http://dx.doi.org/10.1016/j.procbio.2007.12.002]

[53]   Maqsood M, Khusrau M, Kaloo ZA, Wani TA, Mujib A. Colchicine quantification in salt stress treated culture of *Colchicum luteum* Baker by high pressure liquid chromatography. European Journal of Biology 2020; 79(2): 67-74.
[http://dx.doi.org/10.26650/EurJBiol.2020.0013]

[54]   D M, P B KK, S S, P V. Enhanced biosynthesis of colchicine and thiocolchicoside contents in cell suspension cultures of Gloriosa superba L. exposed to ethylene inhibitor and elicitors. Ind Crops Prod 2018; 120: 123-30.
[http://dx.doi.org/10.1016/j.indcrop.2018.04.040]

[55]   Swapna TS, Nikhila GS. *In vitro* root induction—an improved system for production and elicitation of colchicine from Gloriosa superba L. Ind J Exp Biol 2018; 56: 519-25.

[56]   Hayashi T, Yoshida K. Cell expansion and single-cell separation induced by colchicine in suspension-cultured soybean cells. Proc Natl Acad Sci 1988; 85(8): 2618-22.
[http://dx.doi.org/10.1073/pnas.85.8.2618] [PMID: 16593925]

[57]   Daradkeh NQ, Shibli RA, Makhadmeh IM, Alali F, Al-Qudah TS. Cell suspension and *in vitro* production of colchicine in wild colchicum hierosolymitanum Feib. InThe Open Conference Proceedings Journal 2012; 3(1).
[http://dx.doi.org/10.2174/1876326X01203020052]

[58]   Shekelle PG, Newberry SJ, FitzGerald JD, *et al.* Management of gout: A systematic review in support of an american college of physicians clinical practice guideline. Ann Intern Med 2017; 166(1): 37-51.
[http://dx.doi.org/10.7326/M16-0461] [PMID: 27802478]

[59]   Zhu L, Chen L. Progress in research on paclitaxel and tumor immunotherapy. Cell Mol Biol Lett 2019; 24(1): 40.

[http://dx.doi.org/10.1186/s11658-019-0164-y] [PMID: 31223315]

[60] Ferrari S. Biological elicitors of plant secondary metabolites: mode of action and use in the production of nutraceutics. Adv Exp Med Biol 2010; 698: 152-66.
[http://dx.doi.org/10.1007/978-1-4419-7347-4_12] [PMID: 21520710]

[61] Baenas N, García-Viguera C, Moreno D. Elicitation: A tool for enriching the bioactive composition of foods. Molecules 2014; 19(9): 13541-63.
[http://dx.doi.org/10.3390/molecules190913541] [PMID: 25255755]

[62] Awang NA, Islam MR, Ismail MR, Zulkarami B, Omar D. Effectiveness of different elicitors in inducing resistance in chilli (*Capsicum annuum* L.) against pathogen infection. Sci Hortic 2013; 164: 461-5.
[http://dx.doi.org/10.1016/j.scienta.2013.08.038]

[63] FDA. Guidance for Industry: Product development under the animal rule; division of drug information. Adv Exp Med Biol 698: 152-66. Available at: http://www.fda.gov/downloads/Drugs/GuidanceCompliance

CHAPTER 2

In Vitro Multiplication and Metabolite Variations through GC-MS of a Medicinal Plant *Scaevola Taccada* (Gaertn.) Roxb.

M. Raseena[1,*] and **A. Yusuf**[1]

[1] *Department of Botany, University of Calicut, Kerala, India*

Abstract: The present study investigated the difference in the phytoconstituents in the methanolic extract of mother and tissue cultured plants of *Scaevola taccada* (Gaertn). Roxb., an important medicinal plant of the Goodiniaceae family. An efficient protocol was established to rapidly multiply *S. taccada* using nodal explants. The explants were cultured on MS medium supplemented with different concentrations of BAP (0.5 mg/l, 2.5 mg/l, 5.0 mg/l, 10.0 mg/l), IAA (1.0 mg/l), Kinetin (1.0 mg/l), ascorbic acid (100 mg/l) and citric acid (25 mg/l). The maximum number of multiple shoots were obtained in MS medium supplemented with BAP (5.0 mg/l) in combination with Kinetin (1.0 mg/l) and additives ascorbic acid (100 mg/l) and citric acid (25 mg/l). Subculturing multiple shoots at periodic intervals of every 4 weeks produced the maximum number of shoots. The *in vitro* generated shoots were rooted in half-strength MS medium supplemented with IBA (0.5,1.0,1.5,2.0,2.5) mg/l NAA (0.5,1.0,2.0,2.5) mg/l. Among these, the highest root induction was obtained in IBA (1.5 mg/l) and NAA (0.1 mg/l). The rooted plantlets were transferred to pots containing a mixture of vermiculite and perlite for acclimatization for three weeks. The plants were hardened in a greenhouse and planted in open fields. Phytochemical analysis shows the methanolic extracts of the tissue cultured plants produced more bioactive compounds having various pharmaceutical importance than the mother plant.

Keywords: Acclimatization, BAP, Gas chromatography-mass spectrometry, Growth regulators, IBA, NAA.

INTRODUCTION

Scaevola taccada (Gaertn.) Roxb is a hemi-sclerophyllous littoral shrub of the family Goodeniaceae. The name "*Scaevola*" is derived from the Greek word "Scaevus" meaning "left-handed [1], also "*Scaevola*" means "little hand" [2]. Traditionally, different parts of *S. taccada* are used for the treatment of various ailments. It has been reported to possess antiviral properties against vesicular

---

[*] **Corresponding author M. Raseena:** Department of Botany, University of Calicut, Kerala, India;
E-mails: sjkaur@rediffmail.com; irshadraseena@gmail.com

Mohammad Anis & Mehrun Nisha Khanam (Eds.)

stomatitis virus and herpes simplex virus-1 and 2 and also anti-fungal, digestive, diuretic, carminative and anti-cancer properties [3 - 5]. The fruit juice promotes menstruation and treats ringworm tinea [6]. The root extracts are employed in treating beriberi, dysentery and syphilis [7]. Due to anthropogenic pressures of deforestation activities, *S. taccada* has been classified as a species under the regionally extinct (RE) category [8]. Conventional propagation methods using stem cuttings and seed germination are rather slow and also depend on the healthy mother plants [9, 10]. Therefore, to reinforce the conservation, development and utilization of this valuable plant species, it is essential to establish a high-frequency *in vitro* regeneration protocol. Gas chromatography mass spectrometry (GC-MS) is a key technological platform for secondary metabolite profiling [11 - 13]. The present study aimed to identify the chemical components present in the leaf, stem and root of tissue culture raised plants and its comparison with the mother plant using GC-MS.

MATERIALS AND METHODS

Plant Material and Sterilization

Healthy shoots of *S. taccada* were collected from plants grown in the Botanical garden, University of Calicut, Kerala. Young shoots with 2-3 nodes were collected and cut into small pieces containing single nodes. The explants were kept in running tap water for 1 hour followed by washing with teepol (2% v/v) solution for 10 minutes followed by two or three washing with sterilized distilled water. The explants were kept in Bavistin (2%, w/v) solution for 30 minutes and then rinsed with sterile double distilled water. Surface sterilization was carried out using 0.1% (w/v) $HgCl_2$ for 5 minutes followed by washing with sterile double distilled water 7 to 8 times inside a laminar airflow cabinet. The surface sterilized explants were inoculated to MS medium containing different concentrations of growth hormones.

Culture Medium and Conditions

Murashige and Skoog's [14] medium was used for the initiation of cultures. Shoot proliferation medium was supplemented with varying concentrations of BAP (0.5mg/l-10mg/l), IAA (1.0 mg/l), Kinetin (1.0 mg/l) either singly or in combinations with additives (50 mg/l ascorbic acid and 25 mg/l citric acid). The pH of all the media was adjusted to 5.8 before autoclaving at 121 °C for 20 minutes. All cultures were incubated at 25±2 °C for 16 hr photoperiods with a light intensity of 1000 $\mu Em^{-2}S^1$. The frequency of shoot and root regeneration number and length of shoot and roots were recorded after 4 weeks from the culture initiation.

Multiplication of Shoot

For shoot induction, MS medium was supplemented with BAP (0.5mg/l-10mg/l), Kinetin (1.0 mg/l) in combination with IAA (1.0 mg/l) and additives ascorbic acid (100 mg/l), citric acid (25 mg/l). After 4 weeks, the regenerated multiple shoots were separated and transferred to a fresh medium of the same composition to and length obtain a maximum number of shoots at a periodic interval of 3 weeks. The number of shoots and roots regenerated and the length of and roots were recorded after 4 weeks from the culture initiation.

Rooting and Acclimatization

Rooting of the isolated shoots was carried out *in vitro* and *in vivo*. *In vitro* root induction was achieved in full and half strength MS medium containing IBA (0.5, 1.0, 1.5, 2.0, 2.50 mg/l) IBA (0.5, 1.0, 1.5, 2.0, 2.5 mg/l) and NAA (0.5, 1.0, 2.0, 2.5 mg/l). Plantlets with fully expanded leaflets and well developed roots were removed from the culture bottle and washed thoroughly to remove adhered agar and transferred to sterile vermiculite and perlite mixture (50:50) moistened with 1/10 MS medium. Initially, the plants were covered with perforated plastic bags to retain moisture and kept in a growth room for 4 weeks. Successfully established plantlets were subsequently transferred to field conditions.

Gas Chromatography - Mass Spectrometry

Sample Preparation

The samples for the GC-MS analysis were collected from the mother plants which were identified and authenticated. The tissue culture raised plants and *in vitro* hardened plants of 3rd, 6th and 9th month old were used for GC-MS analysis. The plant materials were washed carefully under running tap water and shade dried at room temperature and made into a powder using mortar and pestle. The dried powdered material was subjected to methanolic extraction by incubating for 24hrs on a rotary shaker. After filtering the extract, the filtrate was evaporated and concentrated by air drying. The air-dried pellet was dissolved in HPLC-grade methanol and subjected to GC-MS analysis to find out the bioactive compounds. The analysis of the methanolic extract was carried out using a gas chromatography- mass spectrometry (GC-MS) system (Shimadzu GC- 22 MS, Model Number: QP2010S) equipped with an ELITE-5MS capillary column (0.25mm Xx 30m, 0.25μm film thickness). The operating conditions were as follows: the GC temperature program consisting of 80°C for 2min, incremented at 4.25°C/min from 80°C to 260°C and held at 280°C for 2min. The injector temperature was 260°C; the sample injection volume was 1:11; and the split ratio was 100:1. Mass spectrometry conditions were: electron impact as the ion source, ionizing voltage 70 eV, source temperature 150°C, electron multiplier at 2000 eV, scan speed 1000amu/s, and scan range 50-500 amu. The constituents of the methanolic extracts were identified by comparing the retention indices and matching the recorded mass spectra of each compound with the NIST and WILEY Chemistry web book and published data [15].

RESULTS

Shoot Initiation

Surface sterilized nodal explants were transferred to a culture medium in aseptic conditions using five different concentrations of BAP (0.5mg/l-10 mg/l) (Table 1) for culture initiation. Shoot proliferation was observed within seven to ten days. The nodal explants induced a maximum number of shoots in (0.5) mg/l BAP (Table 1), (Fig. 1A-E).

Table 1. Effects of MS medium containing different concentrations of BAP on shoot induction from the nodal explants of *S. taccada*.

Sl No	BAP (mg/l)	Number of Shoots±SE	Length of Shoots±SE
1	0.5	3.33±0.66	6.33±0.33
2	1.0	2.67±0.33	5.66±0.66
3	2.5	2.67±0.33	5.66±0.33
4	5.0	2.33±0.33	5.66±0.33
5	10.0	2.33±0.33	5.33±0.33

Multiple Shoot Induction

The nodal explants cultured on MS medium supplemented with BAP (0.5 mg/l) kinetin (1.0 mg/l) ascorbic acid (100 mg/l) and citric acid (25 mg/l) induced multiple shoots. The additives in the medium enhanced the regeneration and multiplication of shoots. Among the various combinations of growth hormones used, BAP (5.0mg/l) and Kinetin (1.0 mg/l) produced better shoot multiplication within 4-5 weeks of culture. Multiplication of shoot cultures was achieved by repeated subculturing of the shoots. BAP at a higher concentration (10 mg/l) produced a lesser number of shoots with stunted growth. Shoot proliferation was also induced in the isolated nodal segments cultured on MS medium supplemented with BAP (2.5 mg/l) Kinetin (1.0 mg/l) ascorbic acid (100 mg/l) citric acid 25 mg/l) (Table 2). The best multiplication rate and growth performance of *S. taccada* were obtained in BAP (5.0 mg/l) and Kinetin (1.0 mg/l) (Table 2), (Fig. 2A-D).

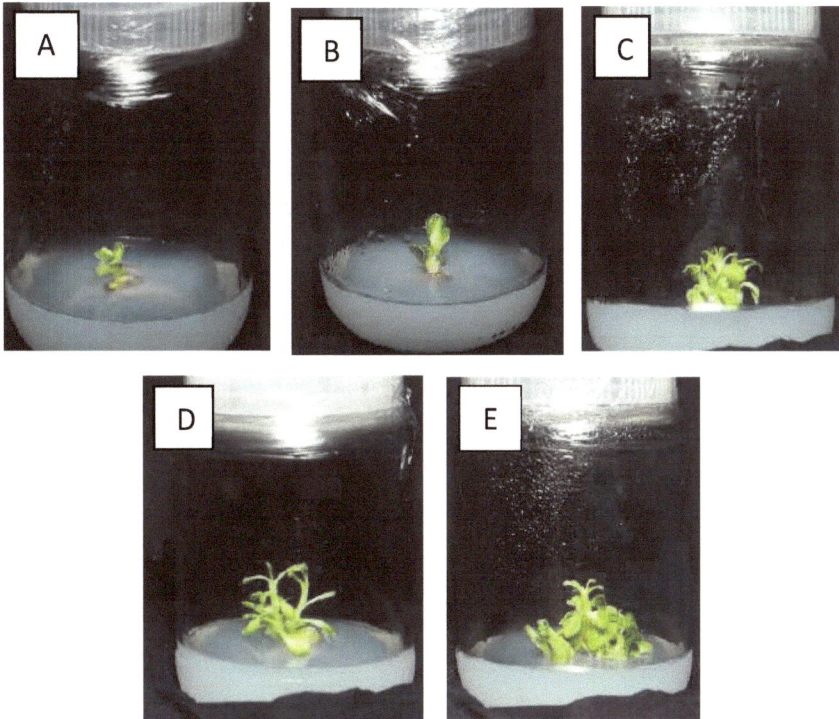

Fig. (1). Effects of different concentrations of BAP on shoot induction from the nodal explants of *S. taccada*.

Table 2. Effects of different concentrations of BAP, IAA, Kinetin and additives on multiple shoot induction in *S. taccada*.

S. No.	MS Basal Medium Containing						
	BAP (mg/l)	IAA (mg/l)	Kinetin (mg/l)	Ascorbic Acid (mg/l)	Citric Acid (mg/l)	Number of Shoots ±SE	Length of Shoots ±SE
1	-	-	-	-	-	0.00	0.00
2	0.5	1.0	-	-	-	4.33±0.33	7.66±0.33
3	1.0	1.0	-	-	-	3.67±0.33	7.33±0.66
4	2.5	1.0	-	-	-	3.33±0.33	7.33±0.33
5	5.0	1.0	-	-	-	3.33±0.66	6.66±0.66
6	10.0	1.0	-	-	-	2.67±0.66	6.66±0.33
7	0.5	-	1.0	-	-	4.67±0.33	7.66±0.33
8	1.0	-	1.0	-	-	4.67±0.33	8.33±0.66
9	2.5	-	1.0	-	-	4.33±0.33	8.33±0.33
10	5.0	-	1.0	-	-	4.33±0.66	9.33±0.33

(Table 2) cont.....

S. No.	MS Basal Medium Containing						
	BAP (mg/l)	IAA (mg/l)	Kinetin (mg/l)	Ascorbic Acid (mg/l)	Citric Acid (mg/l)	Number of Shoots ±SE	Length of Shoots ±SE
11	10.0	-	1.0	-	-	4.33±0.33	9.33±0.33
12	0.5	-	1.0	100	25	5.66±0.66	10.67±0.33
13	1.0	-	1.0	100	25	5.66±0.66	11.67±0.34
14	2.5	-	1.0	100	25	5.67±0.33	12.33±0.33
15	5.0	-	1.0	100	25	6.33±0.33	12.33±0.66
16	10.0	-	1.0	100	25	5.33±0.66	10.67±0.33

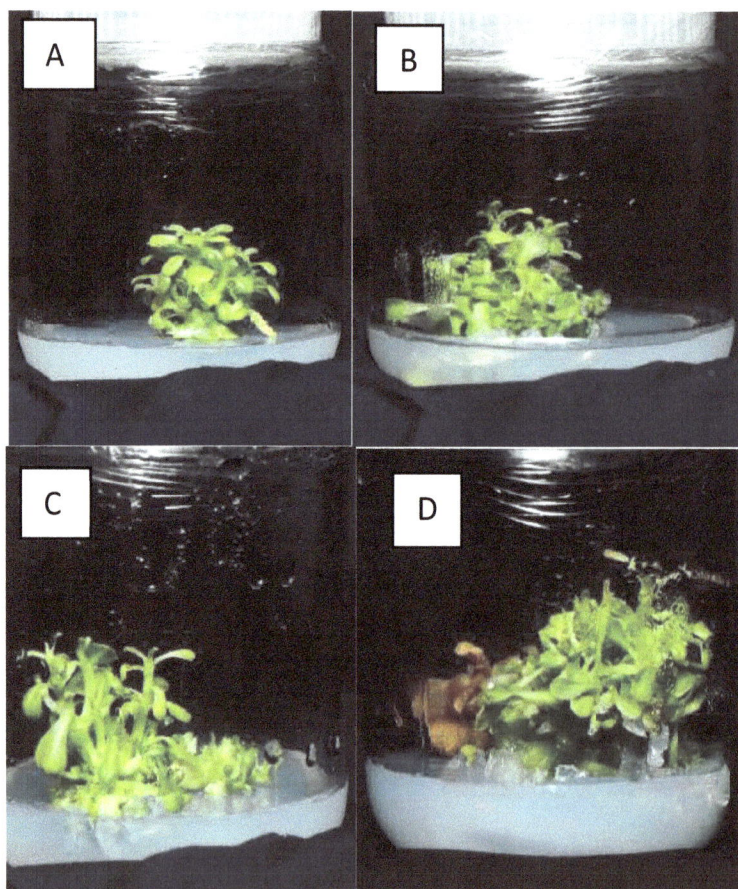

Fig. (2). Effects of different concentrations of BAP, IAA and KIN on multiple shoot induction from the nodal explants of *S. taccada* (**A**) BAP (0.5mg/l), (**B**) BAP (0.5mg/l) +IAA (1.0mg/l), (**C**) BAP (0.5mg/l) + Kinetin (1.0mg/l), (**D**) BAP (5.0mg/l) + Kinetin (1.0mg/l).

Rooting and Acclimatization

Elongated shoots were transferred to both half and full-strength MS medium containing different concentrations of IBA (0.5, 1.0, 1.5, 2.0, 2.5 mg/l) (Table 3) and half-strength MS medium supplemented with different concentrations and combinations of IBA and NAA. The highest root induction was observed on half strength MS medium supplemented with IBA (1.5 mg/l) and NAA (0.1 mg/l) (Table 3), (Fig. 3). The explants cultured on IBA (2.0 mg/l) developed a lesser number of roots.

Table 3. Effects of different concentrations of IBA and NAA on root induction from the nodal explants of *S. taccada.*

Sl No	IBA (mg/l)	Number of Roots±SE	Length of Roots±SE
1	0.5	17.33±0.33	18.66±0.33
2	1.0	17.66±0.33	19.66±0.33
3	1.5	18.33±0.33	19.66±0.66
4	2.0	18.66±0.33	20.66±0.33
5	2.5	19.33±0.66	20.66±0.33
	NAA (mg/l)		
6	0.5	18.33±0.33	20.33±0.33
7	1.0	18.33±0.66	20.66±0.33
8	1.5	19.33±0.33	20.66±0.33
9	2.0	19.66±0.66	20.66±0.66
10	2.5	19.66±0.33	21.33±0.33
	IBA (mg/l) + NAA (mg/l)		
11	0.5+0.1	24.33±0.33	21.67±0.33
12	1.0+0.1	24.33±0.66	22.33±0.33
13	1.5+0.1	24.66±0.33	23.33±0.33
14	2.0+0.1	23.33±0.33	23.67±0.33

Gas Chromatography - Mass Spectrometry

The chromatogram obtained from the methanolic extract of *S. taccada* showed several peaks, which indicate the presence of different compounds. The compounds were identified from the database of the spectrum of known components available in the GC-MS library. Various components that were detected by the GC-MS are shown in Tables **4 - 9**.

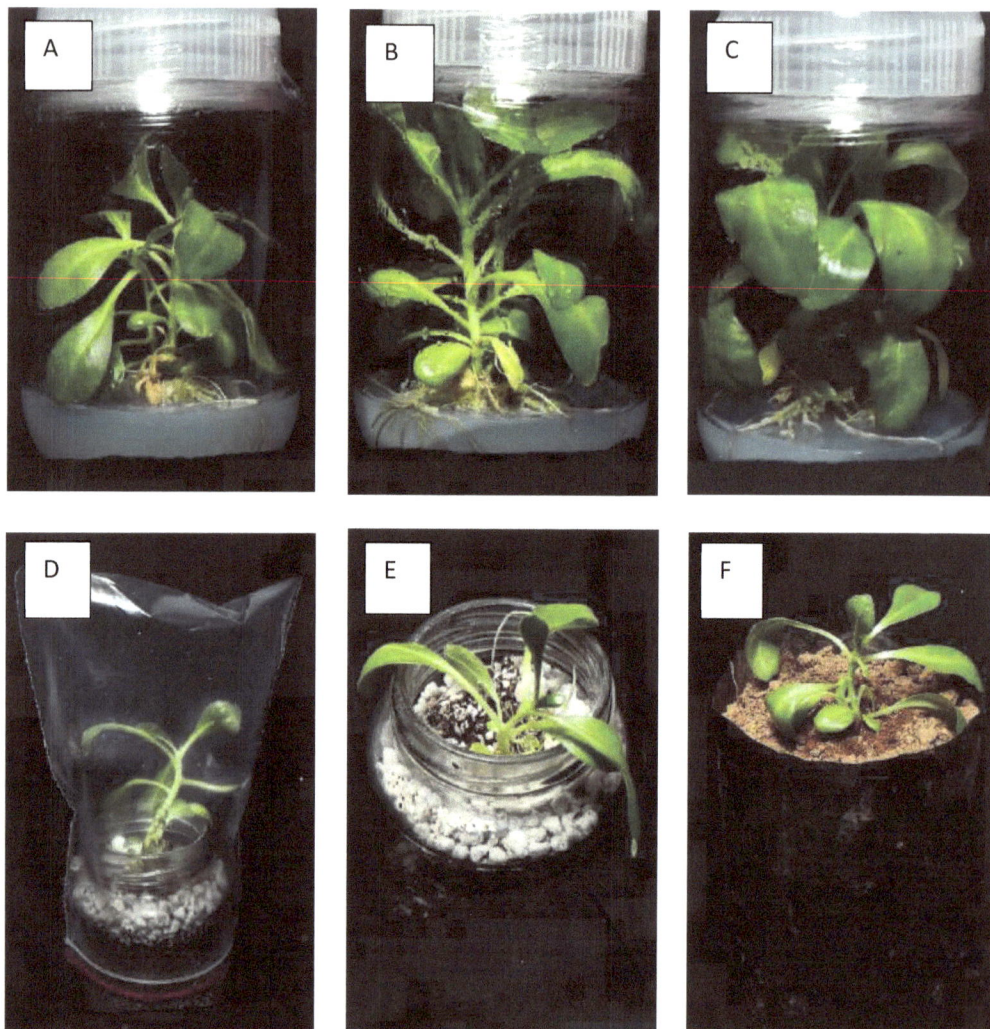

Fig. (3). Effect of different concentrations of IBA and NAA on root induction of *S. taccada* (**a**) IBA (2.5 mg/l), (**b**) NAA (2.5 mg/l), (**c**) IBA (1.5 mg/l) + NAA (0.1mg/l), (**d, e, f**) Hardening and field transfer of *in vitro* raised plantlets.

The phytochemical profile of the methanolic extracts of *S. taccada* revealed a total of 227 compounds (Tables **4-9**) belonging to phenols, flavonoids, terpenoids, alkaloids, fatty acids, *etc.* Among the mother, tissue-cultured and acclimatized plants, the highest number of compounds (113) was detected in tissue cultured plants. Seventeen compounds were found to be common in both mother and tissue cultured plants. The results indicate the occurrence of variation in the tissue cultured plant concerning the phytoconstituent's composition (Tables **4-9**). The methanolic extract of the mother plant revealed the presence of 25 compounds.

Among these 10 compounds were present in the stem, 7 in the leaf and 8 in the root respectively. The major and unique components present in the leaf, stem and root were neophytadiene, methyl margarate, methyl palmitate, linoleic acid, phytol and hexadeconic acid. The maximum number of compounds were detected in the *in vitro* cultured shoots, roots and leaves of the *S. taccada* as compared to its mother plant.

The GC-MS analysis of the stem of both tissue cultured and acclimatized plants consisted of 68 phytochemicals (Tables **4** and **5**), of these 11 compounds were common in both:octadecanal, neophytadiene, cyclohexane, cholesta-4, 6-dien-3-ol, benzoate (3-beta), docosanoic acid methyl ester, dodecanoic acid, methyl palmitate, hexadecanoic acid, hexahydrofarnesyl acetone, and linoic acid methyl ester. The number of phytoconstituents detected in the stem of *in vitro* raised plant is high during the 6th month and low in the 3rd month.

Table 4. Phytochemical constituents detected in the stem of mother (M), tissue cultured (T) and acclimatized (A) plants of *S. taccada*.

Components	Mother + Tissue Cultured	Mother + Acclimatized
3.Beta-acetoxystigmasta-4, 6,22-triene	-	+
4,8, 12,16-tetramethylheptaderan-4-olide	+	-
Cholesta-4,4, dien-3-ol, benzoate, (3 beta)	+	-
Cholesterol	+	-
Docosanoic acid, Methyl ester	+	+
Hexahydrofarnesylacetone	+	-
Methyl isostearate	+	-
Methylpalmitate	+	+
Stigmasta-4,6,22- trien-3-yl acetate	-	+

Table 5. Variations in the phytochemical constituents in the stem of mother (M), tissue cultured (T), acclimatized (A) plants.

	Components	Tissue Cultured (% Quantity)			Acclimatized (% Quantity)			Mother Plant (% Quantity)
		Month			Month			
		3rd	6th	9th	3rd	6th	9th	
1	(-) loliolide	-	1.89	-	-	-	-	-
2	(22e)-Stigmasta-4, 6, 22-trien-3-yl acetate	-	4.04	-	-	-	-	-
3	1,2 Benzenedicarboxylic acid	-	12.72	-	-	-	-	-
4	1,5-Anahydro-6-deoxyhedo-2, 3-dilulose	-	-	15.06	-	-	-	-

(Table 5) cont.....

	Components	Tissue Cultured (% Quantity) Month			Acclimatized (% Quantity) Month			Mother Plant (% Quantity)
		3rd	6th	9th	3rd	6th	9th	
5	1-Octadecanol	-	-	-	-	-	1.53	-
6	1 Heneicosanol	-	-	-	-	-	-	4.38
7	2-Hydroxy-3-(tetradecanoyloxy)propyl myristate	-	-	-	23.84	-	-	-
8	2-Methoxy-4-vinylpheol	-	-	11.2	-	-	-	-
9	2-Pentadecanone, 6, 10,14-trimethyl	6.17	-	-	-	-	-	-
10	3.Beta-acetoxystigmasta-4, 6,22-triene	-	-	-	-	1.42	-	9.24
11	4,8, 12,16-tetramethylheptaderan-4olide	-	1.90	-	-	-	-	3.36
12	4-methyl-2, 5-dimethoxybenzaldehyde	-	-	2.07	-	-	-	-
13	8-Methyl-8-azabicyclo (3,2.1) octan-3-ol	-	-	-	10.49	-	-	-
14	9,12,15-octadecatrienoic acid, (z,z,z)-	-	-	2.77	-	-	-	-
15	9-Octadecenoic acid (z)-, methyl ester	-	2.82	-	-	-	1.75	-
16	Cholesta-4, 6-dien-3-ol, (3-beta)	18.64	-	-	-	-	-	-
17	Cholesta-4,4, dien-3-ol, benzoate, 3(beta)	-	-	-	-	6.81	4.87	17.93
18	Cholesta-4, 6-dien-3-ol, benzoate, (e beta).	-	17.93	-	-	-	-	-
19	Cholesta-4,6-dien-3-ol, benzoate, (3 beta)-(22e)-	-	-	-	-	-	2.26	-
20	Cholesterol	-	-	1.21	-	-	-	8.61
21	Cis-13-octadecenoic acid	-	-	-	-	1.71	-	-
22	Cyclohexane, Eicosyl-	-	1.56	-	-	1.34	-	-
23	Docosanoic acid, Methyl ester	-	1.49	-	-	3.44	-	3.40
24	Dodecanoic acid	-	-	1.80	-	2.73	-	-
25	E-Phytol	-	1.30	-	-	-	-	-
26	Gamma-sitosterol	-		-	-	-	52.73	-
27	Heptadecanoic acid	-	-	-	-	-	1.90	-
28	Hexadecanal	-	1.22	-	-	-	-	-
29	Hexadecanoic acid	-	-	16.57	-	29.21	4.57	-
30	Hexahydrofarnesyl acetone	-	3.65	-	-	-	3.19	2.24
31	Linoleic acid, methyl ester	-	-	2.63	-	-	1.65	-
32	Linolsaeure	-	-	-	-	3.63	-	-
33	L-Proline, 5-oxo, methyl ester	-	-	9.25	-	-	-	-
34	Methyl arachate	-	1.24	-	-	-	-	-

(Table 5) cont.....

	Components	Tissue Cultured (% Quantity)			Acclimatized (% Quantity)			Mother Plant (% Quantity)
		Month			Month			
		3rd	6th	9th	3rd	6th	9th	
35	Methyl isostearate	6.74	-	-	-	-	-	3.18
36	Methyl octadecea-9, 12- Dienoate	-	1.73	5.88	-	-	-	-
37	Methyl stearate	-	-	-	-	-	2.16	-
38	Methylpalmitate	28.39	15.17	4.59	-	-	6.89	5.82
39	Neophytadiene	-	2.80	1.25	-	3.44	2.28	-
40	Octadec-9-enoic acid	-	-	-	-	5.44	-	-
41	Octadecanal	-	1.74	-	-	1.18	-	-
42	Octadecanamide	-	1.51	-	-	-	-	-
43	Octadecane, 1, 1-Dimethoxy-	-	1.88	-	-	-	-	-
44	Octadecanoic acid	-	-	-	-	8.78	-	-
45	Octadecanoic acid, methyl ester	-	4.81	-	-	-	-	-
46	Oxacycloheptadec-8-en-2one	-	-	8.21	-	-	-	-
47	Palmitic acid vinyl ester	-	-	-	65.67	-	-	-
48	Phytol	-	1.15	1.49	-	-	1.25	-
49	Stigmasta-4,6,22- trien-3-yl acetate	-	-	-	-	-	1.41	41.83
50	Tetradecanoic acid	-	--	-	-	2.11	-	-

The GC-MS analysis of the leaf methanolic extract cocnsists of 40 and 26 phytochemicals (Tables **6** and **7**) in the tissue cultured and acclimatized plants. Out of these, 3,7,11,15, - tetramethyl-2- hexadecen-1-ol, 9,12,15, - octadecatrienoic acid, 6-octen-1-ol, 3,7-dimethyl - propanoate, linoleic acid methyl ester, linolenic acid methyl ester, methyl palmitate, neophytadiene and phytol are common in both tissue cultured and acclimatized plants. Among the different aged tissue cultured plants, a greater number of phytochemicals were present during the 9th month whereas, in the case of acclimatized plants more phytochemicals were seen in the 6th month. The tissue cultured and acclimatized plants showed more numbers of compounds compared to the field grown mother plant.

Table 6. Phytochemical constituents detected in the leaf of mother (M), tissue cultured (T) and acclimatized (A) plants.

Components	Mother + Tissue Cultured	Mother + Acclimatized
3,7,11,15, -Tetramethyl-2-Hexadecen-1-ol	+	+

(Table 6) cont.....

Components	Mother + Tissue Cultured	Mother + Acclimatized
2-Tridecen1-ol	+	-
6-Octen-1-ol, 3,7-dimethyl, - propanoate	+	-
Neophytadine	+	+
Phthalic acid, Cyclobutyl triedcyl ester	+	-

Table 7. Variations in the phytochemical constituents in the leaf of mother (M), tissue cultured (T) and acclimatized (A) plants.

	Components	Tissue Cultured (% Quantity)			Acclimatized (% Quantity)			Mother Plant (% Quantity)
		Month			Month			
		3rd	6th	9th	3rd	6th	9th	
1	(-) Loliolide	-	-	-	-	-	5.04	-
2	(-) -.Beta.-caryophyllene	-	-	5.14	-	-	-	-
3	1- Hexyne, 5-methyl-	-	4.92	-	-	-	-	-
4	2,3-anhytro-d-gactosa	-	-	6.83	-	-	-	-
5	2-Tridecen1-ol	1.44	-	-	-	-	-	2.56
6	3,7,11,15-Tetramethyl-2-Hexadecen-1-ol	-	38.19	4.25	-	4.0	4.32	47.23
7	3-Cyclopentylpropionic acid, 2-Dimethylaminoethyl ester	-	-	-	-	-	9.64	-
8	4-Amino-5-methyl-2(1h)-pyrimidinethione	-	-	2.12	-	-	-	-
9	4-Methyl-2,3-hexadien-1-ol	-	-	2.07	-	-	-	-
10	6 (e), 9(z), 13(e), Pendectriene	-	-	-	-	-	-	4.57
11	6,9-Pentadecadien-4-ol, 3-Bromo-, [s-r,s-(z,z)]]	-	3.65	-	-	-	-	-
12	6-Octen-1-ol, 3,7-dimethyl, - propanoate	3.24	-	4.60	-	-	-	5.55
13	8-Azabicyclo (3.2.1) octan-3-ol, methyl	31.94	-	-	-	-	-	-
14	9, 12, 15-Octadecatrienal	6.24	8.78	-	-	-	-	-
15	9,12, octadecadienoic acid methyl ester	-	-	-	-	11.85	-	-
16	9, 12, 15-Octadecatrienoc acid methyl ester (Z,Z,Z)	-	-	-	-	5.36	-	-
17	9,12,15-octadecatrienoic acid, (z,z,z)	-	-	8.58	-	2.63	-	-
18	Alpha.-amyrin	-	-	5.45	-	-	-	-
19	Alpha.-d-galactopyranose, 6-o-(trimethylcily-)-,cyclic 1,2:3,4-bis(butylboronate) Bis(butylboronate)	-	-	2.44	-	-	-	-
20	Alpha.-tocopheryl acetate	-	-	2.48	-	-	-	-
21	A-neogammacer-22(29)-ene	-	-	-	50.65	-	-	-

(Table 7) cont.....

	Components	Tissue Cultured (% Quantity)			Acclimatized (% Quantity)			Mother Plant (% Quantity)
		Month			Month			
		3rd	6th	9th	3rd	6th	9th	
22	Beta.-indolylacetic acid methyl ester	-	-	4.88	-	-	-	-
23	Beta-friedelinol	-	-	-	5.12	-	-	-
24	Cis-thujan-10-oic acid methyl ester	-	-	3.78	-	-	-	-
25	Cyclopropanecarboxylic acid, 3-(3-butenyl2-2-dimethyl-	-	-	8.07	-	-	-	-
26	Diethylene glycol dibenzoate	-	4.92	-	-	-	-	-
27	Friedelan-3-one	-	-	-	4.59	-	-	-
28	Gamma-sitosterol		-	-	18.17	-	-	-
29	Hexadecanoic acid	-	-	-	-	3.51	-	-
30	Isophyto acetate	-	-	-	-	13.0	-	-
31	Linoleic acid, Methyl ester	-	-	-	1.61	-	12.29	-
32	Linolenic acid, methyl ester	-	-	1.81	-	-	19.23	-
33	Loliolide	-	-	3.01	-	-	-	-
34	Lupeol	-	-	-	7.23	-	-	-
35	Methyl 12-methylteradecanoate	-	-	-	-	-	-	5.85
36	Methyl margarate	4.62	5.85	-	-	-	-	-
37	Methyl stearate	-	-	-	-	3.75	-	-
38	Methylpalmitate	-	-	-	3.79	18.98	10.52	-
39	Neocurdione	-	-	3.89	-	-	-	-
40	Neophytadiene	16.49	23.73	10.83	1.64	36.93	13.37	29.88
41	Noruns-12-ene	-	7.37	-	-	-	-	-
42	Octadecanoic acid, 2-(2-hydroxyethoxy) ethyl ester	-	-	2.15	-	-	-	-
43	Oleyl alcohol, trifluroacetate	-	-	2.36	-	-	-	-
44	Pentanal, 2- Methyl-	-	3.35	-	-	-	-	-
45	Phthalic acid, cyclobutyl tridecyl ester	2.74	2.90	-	-	-	-	4.35
46	Phytol	33.28	5.53	-	1.78	-	20.82	-
47	Phytol,acetate	-	-	-	2.26	-	-	-
48	Spiropentane, butyl-	-	4.02	-	-	-	-	-

In comparison to the leaf and root extract, the highest number of secondary metabolites was observed in the stem extract of the 9-month-old tissue culture raised plant followed by the leaf and root of the 6-month-old tissue culture raised plant.

The GC-MS analysis of the secondary metabolites revealed marked differences between the tissue cultured and field grown mother plant, while there was no significant difference between the stem, leaf and roots of plants regenerated *in vitro*. The difference in the chemical constituents of tissue cultured, field grown tissue cultured plant and mother plant could be the result of different environmental conditions and receiving an optimum supply of nutrients. In the present study, individual plant parts produced different types of secondary metabolites, for instance, the leaf showed lupeol but was not represented in the stem. Whole plant can be a better source of phytoconstituents with specific pharmaceutical importance. It is observed that the phytoconstituent during the 6th month is comparatively high when compared to the 3rd and 9th month, that could be the result of different developmental stages of plants. Secondary metabolite production can be influenced by the exogenous supply of PGRs, culturing period and external stress applied during different micropropagation stages. Therefore, under defined culture conditions, it is possible to produce plants with higher bioactive contents in a shorter period. Similar components were identified from the methanolic extract of the mother plant and tissue cultured plants even though, there is a marked difference in the percentage of the occurrence.

DISCUSSION

Tissue culture offers an effective and potential alternative to metabolite production because the number of secondary metabolites produced in tissue culture can be even higher than in parent plants [16]. For *in vitro* propagation, the shoot tip and nodal explants are the better source material for the large-scale production of plants [17]. Metabolite profiling is a powerful technique used for the identification of phenotype diagnosis and plant analysis [18, 19]. Growth regulators like BAP and KIN are used individually or in combination as they have proven morphogenetic proliferation in plants. The combination of BAP (0.5 mg/L) and KIN (1.0 mg/L) produced a maximum number of multiple shoots. The results are in agreement with earlier findings as observed in *Mentha viridis* [20] *Bacopa monneiri* [21] *Lobelia nicotianifolia* [22] and *Solanum nigrum* [23], where BAP and KIN resulted in a marked increase in shoot multiplication. Higher concentrations of BAP reduced shoot multiplication rate as reported in other species [24, 25]. The effectiveness of BAP on the induction of bud break and shoot proliferation has been reported in *Vigna radiate* [26]. The present study showed that a lower concentration of BAP (0.5 mg/L) was sufficient for shoot multiplication. The combination of IAA with cytokinins (BAP or KIN) promoted shoot formation in various plant species [27 - 29] and the best shoot induction was achieved in the medium containing IAA and BAP. In the shoot cultures of *S. taccada*, growth regulators (PGRs) facilitated metabolite synthesis which supported the earlier findings that PGRs in the medium affected the synthesis of metabolites *in vitro* [30]. The primary effects of BAP in inducing multiple shoots have been reported [31, 32]. The results corroborate with the earlier reports in other plants [33, 34] that the hormones supplied exogenously during tissue culture not only influenced shoot proliferation but also *in vitro* bioactive secondary metabolites production.

Tissue culture raised plants may vary from the mother plant in yield of phytoconstituents. GC-MS analysis revealed 25 different chemical compounds in the mother plant and 202 compounds in the tissue cultured plants. This is in corroboration with the previous report showing variations in the constituents of *in vivo* and *in vitro* plants are influenced by various non-genetic and genetic factors [35]. Seventeen compounds were common in both mother and tissue cultured plants. This result indicated that the dissimilarity arises in the tissue cultured plants due to variations in the biosynthetic pathways of secondary metabolites that are genetically controlled [36]. It was also observed that the occurrence of more components is an advantage, but the disappearance of a few compounds (Piperidine and phytol acetate) in tissue cultured plants may be due to either loss in genetic ability or repression of the relevant genes under culture conditions [37]. In different parts of medicinal plants, the secondary metabolites may be synthesized through special regulatory pathways in certain organs and tissues [38]. Similar reports were observed in the present study, as the individual plant parts produced different types of secondary metabolites. The bioactive component production during the 6th month is comparatively high when compared to the 3rd and 9th months, that could be the result of the different developmental stages of the plants. This observation is contradictory to the report that different parts of the medicinal plants may possess different medicinal properties during developmental stages [39].

The phytochemical compounds identified from the roots of tissue cultured and acclimatized plants showed different patterns (Tables **8** and **9**). Compounds such as neophytadiene, methyl palmitate, methyl stearate, phytol, 2-methoxy-4-vinylphenol, Pyranone and 6-octen-1-ol, 3,7-dimethyl-, m propanoate, 9,12-octadecadienoic acid methyl ester and lupeol were common in both tissue cultured and acclimatized plants.

Table 8. Phytochemical constituents detected in the root of mother (M), tissue cultured (T) and acclimatized (A) plants.

Components	Mother + Tissue Cultured	Mother + Acclimatized
3,7,11,15-Tetramethyl-2-hexadecen-1-ol	+	-
Hexadecanoic Acid	-	+
Linoleic acid, methyl ester	+	-
Methylpalmitate	+	+
Methyl Stearate	+	+
Neophytadiene	+	+

Table 9. Variations in the phytochemical constituents in the root of mother (M), tissue cultured (T) and acclimatized (A) plants.

	Components	Tissue Cultured (% Quantity) Month			Acclimatized (% Quantity) Month			Mother Plant (% Quantity)
		3rd	6th	9th	3rd	6th	9th	
1	(+)-Alpha-tocopherol	-	4.47	-	-	-	-	-
2	(9e)-9-dodecen-1-ol	-	1.89	-	-	-	-	-
3	1,2-benzenedicarboxylic acid, dibutyl ester	-	-	-	13	-	-	-
4	1,7 Octadiene Diepoxide	-	-	3.55	-	-	-	-
5	1-cyclopropylethanol	-	4.19	-	-	-	-	-
6	1-Undecyme	-	-	-	3.75	-	-	-
7	2-methoxy-4-vinylphenol	18.98	-	-	-	-	17.46	-
8	2-Methylamalonodiamide	4.0	-	-	-	-	-	-
9	2-Pyrrrolidinemethanol, 1-methyl-	-	-	4.0	-	-	-	-
10	3', 5'-Dimethodyacetophenone	-	-	-	-	-	3.74	-
11	3,7,11,15-Tetramethyl-2-hexadecen-1-ol	-	-	6.46	-	-	-	1.49
12	3,7-dihydropurine-2, 6-dione, 7-(--dimethylaminoethyl)-3-methyl	-	4.48	-	-	-	-	-
13	3-Isoprophyl-4-methyl-1-decen-4-ol	-	-	1.87	-	-	-	-
14	3-Nonynoic acid	-	7.93	-	-	-	-	-
15	4-vinyl-2-methoxy-phenol	-	-	-	4.0	-	-	-
16	6(e), 9(z), 13(e), Pendectriene	3.75	-	-	-	-	-	-
17	6-octen,1—ol, 3,7 dimethyl, propanoate	-	2.66	-	11.85	-	-	-
18	9,12-Octadecadienoic Acid, Methyl Ester	-	-	26.16	-	6.78	26.16	-
19	Alpha- Amyrin Acetate	-	-	-	-	31.93	-	-

(Table 9) cont.....

	Components	Tissue Cultured (% Quantity)			Acclimatized (% Quantity)			Mother Plant (% Quantity)
		Month			Month			
		3rd	6th	9th	3rd	6th	9th	
20	Alpha-Linolenic Acid Methyl Ester	-	-	-	-	3.04	-	-
21	Benzene,1-Chloro-2-Methody-	-	-	7.08	-	-	-	-
22	Cholesterol	-	-	-	-	-	2.36	-
23	Cyclohexaneethanamine,N,Alpha-Dimethyl	-	14.01	-	-	-	-	-
24	Cyclopentane, (1-methylethyl)-	3.51	-	-	-	-	-	-
27	Dimethyl-2-(methoxymethylene) malonate]	-	-	-	18.98	-	-	-
28	Diploptene	-	-	-	-	15.73	-	-
29	Formic acid, 2-ethylbutyl ester	2.63	-	-	-	-	-	-
30	Friedelan-3-One	-	-	-	-	2.37	-	-
31	Gamma-Sitosterol	-	-	-	-	9.37	-	-
32	Guanosine	-	-	-	3.51	-	-	-
33	Hexadecanoic Acid	-	-	-	-	3.50	16.42	25.25
34	Hexanenitirile	-	-	-	2.63	-	-	-
35	Limonene diodixe 2	-	5.64	-	-	-	-	-
36	Linolenic acid, methyl ester	-	11.8	-	-	-	-	10.57
37	L-Proline, 5-Oxo, Methyl ester	-	-	-	-	5.24	-	-
38	Lupeol	-	2.66	-	-	6.66	-	-
39	Methyl 11,14-Eicosadienoate	-	-	11.65	-	-	-	-
40	Methyl Linolenate	-	-	7.38	-	-	-	-
41	Methyl margarate	11.85	4.47	-	-	-	-	-
42	Methyl octadeca-9, 12-dienoate	-	-	-	-	-	-	20.71
43	Methyl stearate	-	-	2.54	-	-	2.54	12.32
44	Methylpalmitate	-	-	9.14	-	7.87	11.99	10.83
45	Neophytadiene	-	11.07	9.17	-	1.30	2.28	4.57
46	Phthalic acid, cyclobutyl isobutyl ester	-	2.14	-	-	-	-	-
47	Phthalic acid, cyclobutyl tridecyl ester	5.36	-	-	-	-	-	-
48	Phytol	-	17.19	-	-	2.40	3.30	-
49	Phytol, acetate	-	-	-	-	-	-	1.92
50	Piperidine, 1-(1-Cyclopenten-1-Yl)-	-	-	-	-	-	1.64	-
51	Piperidine, 2-Pentyl-	-	-	-	-	3.79	-	-
52	Pyranone	36.93	-	32.53	36.93	-	-	-

(Table 9) cont.....

	Components	Tissue Cultured (% Quantity)			Acclimatized (% Quantity)			Mother Plant (% Quantity)
		Month			Month			
		3rd	6th	9th	3rd	6th	9th	
53	Spiropentane,butyl- 6(e), 9(z), 13(e),	13.0	-	-	-	-	-	-
54	Spiropentante, butyl-	-	5.03	-	-	-	-	-
55	Tetradecanoic acid, 12-methyl-, meth,yl ester	-	-	-	5.36	-	-	

3, 7, 11, 15-tetramethyl-2-hexadecen-1-ol also called phytol is an important diterpene identified from the methanolic extract of tissue cultured and acclimatized plant which possesses antimicrobial, antioxidant, and anticancer activities [40]. Hexadecanoic acid was detected in the stem, leaf and root of tissue cultured plants and is known to exhibit strong antimicrobial and anti-inflammatory activity [41, 42]. The leaf of the *in vitro* regenerated plant is an excellent source of 9, 12, 15-octadecatrienal and linoleic acid which has anti-inflammatory, hypocholesterolemic, cancer preventive hepatoprotective, nematicide, insectifuge, antihistaminic, antieczemic, antiacne, 5-alpha-reductase inhibitor, anti-androgenic, antiarthritic, anti-coronary and insecticidal activity [43 - 45]. The present study suggests that the whole plants of *S. taccada* can be used as a source of neophytadiene and can be recommended as a good analgesic, antipyretic, anti-inflammatory, antimicrobial, and antioxidant compound [22]. The compound α-Amyrin known to possess antidiabetic, anti-inflammatory, antiarthritic, and anticancer activities, obtained from the leaves of tissue culture raised 9th-month-old plants [24]. Lupeol is a prominent compound obtained from the tissue cultured leaf and root and it exhibits antioxidant, antiflu, antihyperglycemic, antitumor, antiviral, cytotoxic, anti-inflammatory and anticancer properties [46, 47]. The phytoconstituents present in the tissue cultured plants of *S. taccada* exhibit a number of biological activities, hence having important applications in the pharmaceutical industry. Somaclonal variations which are basically encountered in tissue culture would lead to a change in the genetic properties of the plant culture. This would lead to increased biomass yield and production of secondary metabolites. In addition to the exogenous supply of PGRs used during micropropagation can also influence the level of secondary metabolites [48].

CONCLUSION

Plants are natural reservoirs of phytonutrients and compounds, which are essential for life in general. An efficient regeneration protocol has been established, which can help in the mass propagation as well as conservation of this medicinally important plant. The presence of various bioactive compounds in *S. taccada* proved its pharmaceutical importance. In the present investigation, the tissue culture raised plants are capable of producing additional secondary metabolites in comparison mother plants and thus they can be used for harnessing important metabolites as an alternative to its mother plant. The comparative analysis of the mother and *in vitro* derived plants exhibited differences in phytochemical composition and biological activity. The secondary metabolite in medicinal plants varied with changes in growth stages, stress conditions and metabolic pathways in different organs, which can provide suitable information about secondary metabolite production at different developmental stages and the use of different plant parts. In the phytochemical evaluation, the increase in the percentage of components proved as a valuable tool to substantiate the use of modern techniques like tissue culture for obtaining quantitatively and qualitatively superior plants. The plant extract in tissue culture derived plants confirms the superior phytochemical and biological efficiency.

REFERENCES

[1]   Wagner WL, Herbst DR, Sohmer SH. Manual of the flowering plants of hawai'i. University of Hawai'i and Bishop Museum Press. 1999; 1-2.

[2]   Carolin RC. Goodeniaceae. Flora of Australia 1992; 35: 147-281.

[3]   Ruangrungsi N, Mangkhla KT. Thai herbs. Bangkok: B Healthy 2004.

[4]   Chandran A, Arunachalam G. Evaluation of *in vivo* anticancer activity of *Scaevola taccada* Roxb against Ehrlich ascites carcinoma in Swiss albino mice. Journal of Pharmaceutical Sciences and Research 2015; 7(9): 626.

[5]   Locher CP, Witvrouw M, De Béthune MP, *et al.* Antiviral activity of Hawaiian medicinal plants against human immunodeficiency Virus Type-1 (HIV-1). Phytomedicine 1996; 2(3): 259-64.
      [http://dx.doi.org/10.1016/S0944-7113(96)80052-3] [PMID: 23194626]

[6]   Khare CP. Indian medicinal plants: an illustrated dictionary. Springer Science & Business Media 2008.

[7]   Tan BYJ. Fan flowers in horticulture. Aust Plants 1997; 19: 112-7.

[8]   Alam J, Ali SI. Contribution to the red list of the plants of Pakistan. Pak J Bot 2010; 42(5): 2967-71.

[9]   Satake Y, Hara H, Watari S, Tominari T. *Wild flowers of Japan*. Heibonsha. 1989.

[10] Wrigley RJ, Fagg M. Australian native plants. Australia: Reed Books 1998; pp. 16-20.

[11] Robertson DG. Metabonomics in toxicology: A review. Toxicol Sci 2005; 85(2): 809-22.
      [http://dx.doi.org/10.1093/toxsci/kfi102] [PMID: 15689416]

[12] Fernie AR, Trethewey RN, Krotzky AJ, Willmitzer L. Metabolite profiling: From diagnostics to systems biology. Nat Rev Mol Cell Biol 2004; 5(9): 763-9.
      [http://dx.doi.org/10.1038/nrm1451] [PMID: 15340383]

[13] Kell DB, Brown M, Davey HM, Dunn WB, Spasic I, Oliver SG. Metabolic footprinting and systems biology: The medium is the message. Nat Rev Microbiol 2005; 3(7): 557-65.
      [http://dx.doi.org/10.1038/nrmicro1177] [PMID: 15953932]

[14] Murashige T, Skoog F. A revised medium for rapid growth and bio assays with tobacco tissue cultures. Physiol Plant 1962; 15(3): 473-97.
      [http://dx.doi.org/10.1111/j.1399-3054.1962.tb08052.x]

[15] Adams PD, Afonine PV, Bunkóczi G, *et al. PHENIX* : A comprehensive Python-based system for

macromolecular structure solution. Acta Crystallogr D Biol Crystallogr 2010; 66(2): 213-21.
[http://dx.doi.org/10.1107/S0907444909052925] [PMID: 20124702]

[16]   Ramachandra Rao S, Ravishankar GA. Plant cell cultures: Chemical factories of secondary metabolites. Biotechnol Adv 2002; 20(2): 101-53.
[http://dx.doi.org/10.1016/S0734-9750(02)00007-1] [PMID: 14538059]

[17]   Sen J, Sharma AK. Micropropagation of *Withania somnifera* from germinating seeds and shoot tips. Plant Cell Tissue Organ Cult 1991; 26(2): 71-3.
[http://dx.doi.org/10.1007/BF00036108]

[18]   Krishnan P, Kruger NJ, Ratcliffe RG. Metabolite fingerprinting and profiling in plants using NMR. J Exp Bot 2004; 56(410): 255-65.
[http://dx.doi.org/10.1093/jxb/eri010] [PMID: 15520026]

[19]   Schauer N, Semel Y, Roessner U, *et al.* Comprehensive metabolic profiling and phenotyping of interspecific introgression lines for tomato improvement. Nat Biotechnol 2006; 24(4): 447-54.
[http://dx.doi.org/10.1038/nbt1192] [PMID: 16531992]

[20]   Rahman MM, Ankhi UR, Biswas A. Micropropagation of *Mentha viridis* L.: An aromatic medicinal plant. Int J Pharmacy & Life Sciences 2013; 4(9).

[21]   Gurnani C, Kumar V, Mukhija S, Dhingra A, Rajpurohit S, Narula P. *In vitro* regeneration of brahmi (*Bacopa monneiri* (l.) penn.)-a threatened medicinal plant. *Kathmandu University Journal of Science. Engineering and Technology* 2012; 8(1): 97-9.

[22]   Ganesan CM, Paulsamy S. Mass propagation of an economically important medicinal plant, *Lobelia nicotianefolia* Heyne. using *in vitro* culture technique. Natural Prod Indian J 2012; 8(1): 35-40.

[23]   Bhat MA, Mujib A, Junaid A, Mahmooduzzafar M. *In vitro* regeneration of *Solanum nigrum* with enhanced solasodine production. Biol Plant 2010; 54(4): 757-60.
[http://dx.doi.org/10.1007/s10535-010-0136-6]

[24]   Pal A, Das D, Panda P, Rath M, Sharma T, Das D. GC-MS analysis of bioactive compounds in the methanol extract of *Clerodendrum viscosum* leaves. Pharmacognosy Res 2015; 7(1): 110-3.
[http://dx.doi.org/10.4103/0974-8490.147223] [PMID: 25598644]

[25]   Waman AA, Sathyanarayana BN, Umesha K, *et al.* Optimization of growth regulators and explant source for micropropagation and cost effective ex vitro rooting in Poshita Winter Cherry (Withania somnifera L.). J Appl Hortic 2011; 13(2): 150-3.
[http://dx.doi.org/10.37855/jah.2011.v13i02.34]

[26]   Saini R, Jaiwal PK. *In vitro* multiplication of Peganum harmala--an important medicinal plant. Indian J Exp Biol 2000; 38(5): 499-503.
[PMID: 11272417]

[27]   Yasmeen AZRA, Rao SRINATH. Regeneration of multiple shoots from cotyledons of *Vigna radiata* (L.) Wilczek. J Indian Bot Soc 2005; 84: 141-3.

[28]   Guo B, Gao M, Liu CZ. *In vitro* propagation of an endangered medicinal plant Saussurea involucrata Kar. et Kir. Plant Cell Rep 2007; 26(3): 261-5.
[http://dx.doi.org/10.1007/s00299-006-0230-6] [PMID: 16988830]

[29]   Jawahar M, Ravipaul S, Jeyaseelan M. *In vitro* regeneration of *Vitex negundo* L.-a multipurpose woody aromatic medicinal shrub. Plant Tissue Cult Biotechnol 1970; 18(1): 37-42.
[http://dx.doi.org/10.3329/ptcb.v18i1.3263]

[30]   Dörnenburg H, Knorr D. Strategies for the improvement of secondary metabolite production in plant cell cultures. Enzyme Microb Technol 1995; 17(8): 674-84.
[http://dx.doi.org/10.1016/0141-0229(94)00108-4]

[31]   Chen CC, Chen SJ, Sagare AP, Tsay HS. Adventitious shoot regeneration from stem internode explants of *Adenophora triphylla* (Thunb.) A. DC. (Campanulaceae)-an important medicinal herb. Bot

Bull Acad Sin 2001; 42.

[32]   Huang Z, Li H. Control of oxidative stress by a combination of PBU, BAP and DMTU enhances adventitious shoot formation in *Eucalyptus urophylla*. Plant Cell Tissue Organ Cult 2020; 141(3): 533-41.
[http://dx.doi.org/10.1007/s11240-020-01812-7]

[33]   Kumar Bhardwaj A, Naryal A, Bhardwaj P, *et al.* High efficiency *in vitro* plant regeneration and secondary metabolite quantification from leaf explants of *Rhodiola imbricata*. Pharmacogn J 2018; 10(3): 470-5.
[http://dx.doi.org/10.5530/pj.2018.3.77]

[34]   Karuppusamy S. A review on trends in production of secondary metabolites from higher plants by *in vitro* tissue, organ and cell cultures. J Med Plants Res 2009; 3(13): 1222-39.

[35]   Cardoso JC, Oliveira MEBS, Cardoso FCI. Advances and challenges on the *in vitro* production of secondary metabolites from medicinal plants. Hortic Bras 2019; 37(2): 124-32.
[http://dx.doi.org/10.1590/s0102-053620190201]

[36]   Hefendehl F, Murray M. Monoterpene composition of a chemotype of *Mentha piperita* having high limonene. Planta Med 1973; 23(2): 101-9.
[http://dx.doi.org/10.1055/s-0028-1099419] [PMID: 4705788]

[37]   Brown JT, Charlwood BV. The accumulation of essential oils by tissue cultures of *Pelargonium fragrans* (Willd.). FEBS Lett 1986; 204(1): 117-20.
[http://dx.doi.org/10.1016/0014-5793(86)81397-7]

[38]   Belkheir AK, Gaid M, Liu B, Hänsch R, Beerhues L. Benzophenone synthase and chalcone synthase accumulate in the mesophyll of *Hypericum perforatum* leaves at different developmental stages. Front Plant Sci 2016; 7: 921.
[http://dx.doi.org/10.3389/fpls.2016.00921] [PMID: 27446151]

[39]   Bartwal A, Mall R, Lohani P, Guru SK, Arora S. Role of secondary metabolites and brassinosteroids in plant defense against environmental stresses. J Plant Growth Regul 2013; 32(1): 216-32.
[http://dx.doi.org/10.1007/s00344-012-9272-x]

[40]   Papitha R, Ravi L, Selvaraj CI. Phytochemical studies and GC-MS analysis of Spermadictyon suaveolens Roxb. Int J Pharm Pharm Sci 2017; 9(3): 143-9.
[http://dx.doi.org/10.22159/ijpps.2017v9i3.16059]

[41]   Swamy M, Sinniah U. A comprehensive review on the phytochemical constituents and pharmacological activities of *Pogostemon cablin* Benth: An aromatic medicinal plant of industrial importance. Molecules 2015; 20(5): 8521-47.
[http://dx.doi.org/10.3390/molecules20058521] [PMID: 25985355]

[42]   Amarowicz R, Estrella I, Hernández T, *et al.* Antioxidant activity of a red lentil extract and its fractions. Int J Mol Sci 2009; 10(12): 5513-27.
[http://dx.doi.org/10.3390/ijms10125513] [PMID: 20054484]

[43]   Sermakkani M, Thangapandian V. GC-MS analysis of *Cassia italica* leaf methanol extract. Asian J Pharm Clin Res 2012; 5(2): 90-4.

[44]   Kumar A, Singh S, Jain S, Kumar P. Synthesis, antimicrobial evaluation, QSAR and *in Silico* ADMET studies of decanoic acid derivatives. Acta Pol Pharm 2011; 68(2): 191-204.
[PMID: 21485292]

[45]   Raja Rajeswari N. GC-MS analysis of bioactive components from the ethanolic leaf extract of *Canthium dicoccum* (Gaertn.) Teijsm & Binn. J Chem Pharm Res 2011; 3(3): 7928.

[46]   Ardiansyah , Yamaguchi E, Shirakawa H, *et al.* Lupeol supplementation improves blood pressure and lipid metabolism parameters in stroke-prone spontaneously hypertensive rats. Biosci Biotechnol Biochem 2012; 76(1): 183-5.
[http://dx.doi.org/10.1271/bbb.110559] [PMID: 22232260]

[47] Saleem M, Maddodi N, Abu Zaid M, *et al.* Lupeol inhibits growth of highly aggressive human metastatic melanoma cells *in vitro* and *in vivo* by inducing apoptosis. Clin Cancer Res 2008; 14(7): 2119-27.
[http://dx.doi.org/10.1158/1078-0432.CCR-07-4413] [PMID: 18381953]

[48] Aremu AO, Bairu MW, Szücová L, Doležal K, Finnie JF, Van Staden J. Assessment of the role of meta-topolins on *in vitro* produced phenolics and acclimatization competence of micropropagated 'Williams' banana. Acta Physiol Plant 2012; 34(6): 2265-73.
[http://dx.doi.org/10.1007/s11738-012-1027-6]

CHAPTER 3

Metabolic Engineering & Synthetic Biology of Monoterpenoid Indole Alkaloids Pathway in *Catharanthus Roseus*

Vyoma Mistry[1], Hemant Borase[1], Abhishek Sharma[1,3,*] and Rajesh Arora[2]

[1] *C. G. Bhakta Institute of Biotechnology, Uka Tarsadia University, Gopal-Vidyanagar, Maliba Campus, Surat-394350, India*

[2] *Department of Phyto Analytical Chemistry and Toxicology, Defence Institute of Physiology & Allied Sciences, Defence Research and Development Organization, Lucknow Road, Timarpur, Delhi-110054, India*

[3] *Department of Biotechnology and Bioengineering, Institute of Advanced Research, Gandhinagar-382426, India*

Abstract: The anti-neoplastic herb, *Catharanthus roseus* (L.) G. Don (Apocynaceae), is a high-value, low-volume medicinal herb, which is the focus of global attention in view of being the source of terpenoid indole alkaloids (MIAs). MIAs are one of the largest classes of phyto-alkaloids, and many of them are sources of important pharmaceutical products. *C. roseus* is known to harbour more than 130 different bioactive MIAs that make it an interesting plant, finding use in several traditional and modern medical therapies. The remarkable presence of cellular and subcellular compartmentations for the synthesis and storage of MIAs allows the accumulation of these medicinally important MIAs in leaves (viz. vindoline, catharanthine, vinblastine, vincristine) and stem and roots (viz. tabersonine, ajmalicine, reserpine, serpentine, vindoline, catharanthine, horhammericine, leurosine, lochnerine). Out of them, any medicinally active MIAs found in *Catharanthus roseus*, vinblastine and vincristine are special since they possess anticancerous properties, along with ajmalicine and serpentine, which possess antihypertensive properties. However, the low plant yield and nonavailability of alternative chemical synthesis methods have increased their demand and market cost. In the research era of more than three decades, a plethora of studies have been carried out on *C. roseus* to explore, understand, explain, improve and enhance the *Homo/Heterologous* biosynthesis of MIAs. Metabolic engineering (ME) and synthetic biology are two powerful tools that have played and contributed majorly to MIAs studies. This chapter concentrates mainly on the efforts made through metabolic engineering and synthetic biology of MIAs in plant and microbial factories in the last three decades.

---
* Corresponding author Abhishek Sharma: C. G. Bhakta Institute of Biotechnology, Uka Tarsadia University, Gopal-Vidyanagar, Maliba Campus, Surat-394350, India; & Department of Biotechnology and Bioengineering, Institute of Advanced Research, Gandhinagar-382426, India;
E-mails: sjkaur@rediffmail.com; abhi19ind@gmail.com

Mohammad Anis & Mehrun Nisha Khanam (Eds.)

Keywords: *Catharanthus roseus*, Monoterpenoid indole alkaloids, Metabolic engineering, Synthetic biology.

INTRODUCTION

Alkaloids are a structurally assorted class of low molecular weight nitrogenous compounds that comprise 15.6% of all known natural products, but they account for more than 50% of the annual total sales of clinically used plant-based drugs (4-5 billion US $) [1]. Plants include self-defense mechanisms against insects and other herbivores. However, the biological activities of plant alkaloids may range from antihypertensive to anti-neoplastic, analgesic, CNS stimulant, vasodilatory, hypnotic, sedative, antihepatotoxic, mydriatic, cholinergic, antispasmodic, narcotic and antirheumatic. Around 53 plant alkaloids are currently used as drugs in different pharmaceutical preparations [2]. Monoterpenoid indole alkaloids (MIAs) are one of the major classes of alkaloids with over 3000 natural products containing a residue of tryptophan or tryptamine (*i.e.,* indole part) and terpenoid building blocks derived from secologanin [3]. MIAs majorly protect plants from pests and pathogens, and MIAs derivatives are also used as medicinally important phytomolecules acting as anticancer, antihypertensive, antimalarial, and antiarrhythmic agents (Table **1**). The well-known and well-studied plants producing MIAs are *Catharanthus roseus*, *Tabernaemontana divericata,* and *Rauwolfia serpentina.* However, *C. roseus* always attracts attention for remaining the only available source of anticancer phytomolecules, vinblastine, and vincristine. A large and diverse number of MIAs are biosynthesized in *C. roseus.* Being secondary metabolites, MIAs have very low plant yield (>3% of dry weight) [8]. For instance, extraction of 1 gm vinblastine and 1 kg of Paclitaxel requires 500 kg of dried Catharanthus leaves [9] and 10,000 kg of dry bark of taxol, respectively [10]. Therefore, the bark of 2-3 fully grown taxol trees is required to treat the cancer patient through paclitaxel. Being the only source of anticancer phytomolecules, vinblastine, and vincristine, *C. roseus* has been extensively studied. The extremely low (0.0001-0.0005% leaf dry weight) *in-plant* yields of vinblastine and vincristine makes their extraction difficult and exorbitantly expensive. Moreover, the extraction of vinblastine and vincristine from plant sources is extremely variable depending upon the environmental conditions and location of grown plants and harvest season. Also, the complex chirality of vinblastine and vincristine makes their chemical extraction very difficult and economically nonviable [11].

Table 1. Some important plant-derived alkaloids are under clinical use as drugs and phytomedicines.

Alkaloids	Alkaloid Class	Plant Source	Clinical Applications
Aconitine	MIA	*Aconitum variegatum*	Rheumatism, neuralgia, sciatica
Ajmalicine	MIA	*C. roseus, Rauwolfia* spp.	Vascular disorders
Ajmaline	MIA	*Rauwolfia serpentina*	Antiarrhythmic agent
Atropine	Tropane	*Atropa belladonna*	Antispasmodic, anti-Parkinson, cycloplegic drug
Berberine	BIA	*Berberis spp.*	Eye irritations, AIDS, hepatitis
Boldine	Aporphine	*Lindera aggregate*	Cholelithiasis, vomiting, constipation
Caffeine	Purine	*Coffea arabica,*	Neonatal apnea, atopic dermatitis
Camptothecin	MIA	*Camptotheca acuminate*	Antineoplastic
Canescine	MIA	*Rauwolfia spp.*	Antihypertensive agent
Cinchonidine	BIA	*Cinchona officinalis*	Increases reflexes, epileptiform convulsions
Cocaine	Tropane	*Erythroxylumnovogranatense*	Local anesthetic
Codeine	BIA	*Papaver somniferum*	Antitussive, analgesic
Colchicine	Tropane	*Colchicum autumnale*	Amyloidosis treatment, acute gout
Emetine	MIA	*Carapicheaipecacuanha*	Intestinal amoebiasis, expectorant drug
Ephedrine	Cathinon	*Ephedra sinica*	Nasal decongestant, bronchodilator
Ergometrine	Ergot	*Clavicepspurpurea*	Postpartum/postabortalhemorrhage
Ergotamine	Ergot	*C. purpurea*	Migraine treatment
Eserine	Tropane	*Physostigmavenenos*	Ophthalmology, antidote/poisoning
Galanthamine	Tropane	*Galanthus spp.*	Muscle relaxant, Alzheimer's
Hydrastine	BIA	*Hydrastis canadensis*	Gastrointestinal disorders
Hyoscine	Tropane	*Hyoscyamus niger*	Motion sickness
Hyoscyamine	Tropane	*Hyoscyamus niger*	Antispasmodic, antiparkinson, cycloplegic drug
Morphine	BIA	*Papaver somniferum*	Pain relief, diarrhoea
Narceine	BIA	*Papaver somniferum*	Cough suppressant
Nicotine	Tropane	*Nicotiana spp.*	Anti-smoking
Noscapine	BIA	*Papaver somniferum*	Cough suppressant
Papaverine	BIA	*Papaver somniferum*	Vasodilator, gastrointestinal disorders
Pilocarpine	Isopilocarpine	*Pilocarpus microphyllus*	Miotic in treatment of glaucoma, leprosy
Quinidine	MIA	*Cinchona spp.*	Ventricular arrhythmias, malaria, cramping

(Table 1) cont.....

Alkaloids	Alkaloid Class	Plant Source	Clinical Applications
Quinine	MIA	*Cinchona spp.*	Malaria, babesiosis, myotonic disorders
Rescinnamine	MIA	*R. serpentina*	Hypertension
Reserpine	MIA	*R. vomitoria*	Hypertension, psychoses
Sanguinarine	BIA	*Sanguinaria canadensis*	Antiplaque agent
Sparteine	BIA	*Cytisus scoparius*	Uterine contractions, cardiac arrhythmias
Strychnine	MIA	*Strychnosnuxvomica*	Eye disorders
Synephrine	MIA	*Citrus spp.*	Vasoconstrictor, conjunctival decongestant
Taxol	DIA	*Taxus brevifolia*	Mamma and ovary carcinoma
Theobromine	Purine	*Theobroma cacao*	Asthma, diuretic agent
Theophylline	Purine	*Theobroma cacao*	Asthma, bronchospasms
Vinblastine	MIA	*C. roseus*	Hodgkin's disease, testicular cancer
Vincristine	MIA	*C. roseus*	Burkitt's lymphoma
Vincamine	MIA	*Vinca minor*	Vasodilator
Yohimbine	MIA	*Pausinystalia yohimbe*	Aphrodisiac, urinary incontinence

BIA- Benzylisoquinoline alkaloid; MIA- Monoterpenoid Indole Alkaloid; DIA- Diterpenoid Indole Alkaloid; Source [4 - 7]"

To bridge the gap between demand and supply, plant tissue culture-based *in vitro* phytomolecule production systems (viz. elicitation and gene expression) have been investigated. The production of these MIAs is highly complex and regulated through co-ordinately regulated networks of enzymes and intermediate compounds in different cellular and subcellular compartmentations. Studies have shown that biosynthesis of MIAs required complex cellular and subcellular organization of at least four different cells (laticifers, epidermis, idioblasts, and internal phloem associated parenchyma) and five sub-cellular compartmentations (chloroplast, nucleus, vacuoles, cytosol, endoplasmic reticulum) [12, 13]. In addition to this, the active selective transport protein also plays a major role as a rate-determining factor [12, 14]. The last three decades of extensive research in the areas of enzyme chemistry, metabolite profiling, and gene expression biology in *C. roseus* have made the MIAs pathway one of the best-understood and elucidated metabolic routes in plants today. Better insight into the architecture of the MIAs biosynthetic pathway, spatio-temporal complexities related to MIAs pathway gene expression and diverse facades of its developmental and genetic regulation have provided enormous opportunities to contrive diverse biosynthetic pathway engineering options in *C. roseus*.

THE MIAs BIOSYNTHETIC PATHWAY

Recently, the complete MIAs biosynthetic pathway (Fig. **1**) is completely discovered and explained as a network of more than 35 known enzymatic steps and pathway intermediates [15 - 17]. The synthesis of a vast diverse class of MIAs in *C. roseus* strictosidine, formed by joininig of tryptamine and secologanin, works as a central intermediate. The Shikimate pathway produced tryptamine and Isopentenyl to derive secologanin [3].

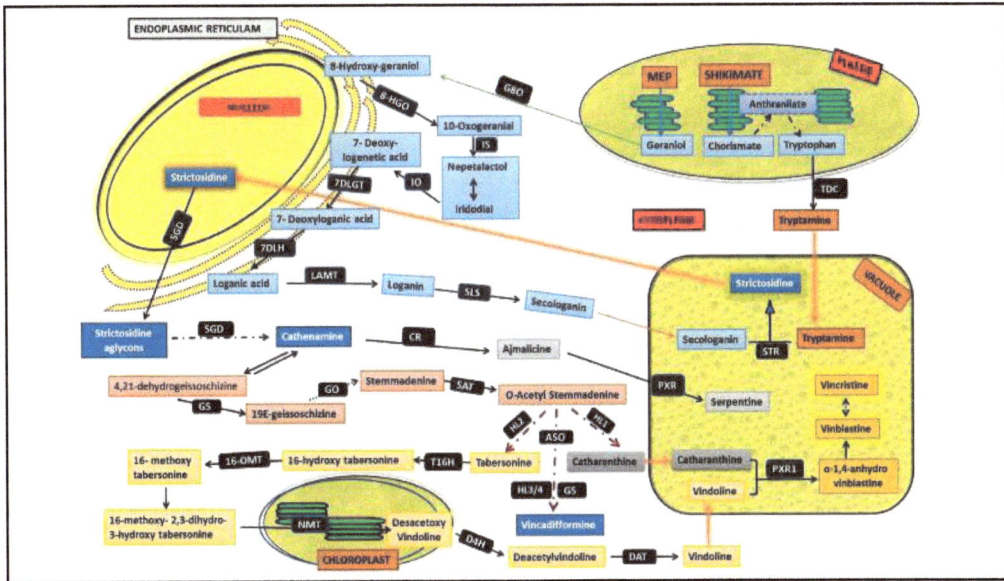

Fig. (1). (Credit: Sharma *et al.* 2020 [7]): MIAs biosynthesis pathway in *Catharanthus roseus*- schematic representation. *G8O* geraniol 8-oxidase, *8-HGO* 8-hydroxygeraniol oxidoreductase, *IO* iridoid oxidase, IRIDOID synthase, *7-DLGT* 7-deoxyloganetic acid glucosyltransferase, *LAMT* loganic acid O-methyltransferase, *TDC* tryptophan decarboxylase, *SLS* secologanin synthase, *STR* strictosidine synthase, *SGD* strictosidine-β-D-glucosidase, *CR* cathenamine reductase, *GS* geissoschizine synthase, *GO* grissoschizine oxidase, *SAT* stemmadenine-*O*-acetyltransferase, ASO acetylestemmadenine oxidase, *HL1, HL2, HL3, HL4 α/β* hydrolase type enzymes, *T16H*tabersonine 16 hydroxylase, *16-OMT* 16-methoxytabersonin, *NMT* N-methyltransferase, *DAT* desacetoxyvindoline-4-*O*-acetyltransferase, *D4H* desacetoxyvindolene-4-hydroxylase, *DAT* desacetoxyvindoline-4-*O*-acetyltransferase, *PRX1* α-3',4' anhydrovinblastine synthase, *PRX* peroxidase. *Arrows: Highlighted straight arrow- molecule transport; straight arrow: direct enzymatic reaction; broken arrow: enzymatic reaction with stable/unstable intermediates.*

The inclusive route of the MIAs biosynthetic pathway can be divided into four realms:

a) Secologanin synthesizing the primary metabolic pathway methyl erythritol 4-phosphate (MEP) and seco(iridoid) pathway.

b) Tryptophan synthesizing the Shikimate pathway leading the synthesis of the indole moiety tryptamine.

c) Joining of secologanin and tryptamine to derive the central MIAs precursor strictosidine, further leading to the synthesis of vindoline and catharanthine.

d) Final coupling of catharanthine and vindoline to produce dimeric MIAs Vinblastine.

METABOLIC ENGINEERING AND SYNTHETIC BIOLOGY: OPERATIONAL CONSTRAINTS AND KEYS

Catharanthus is the source of vinblastine and vincristine, and the very low *implant* yields of these compounds, coupled with the nonavailability of alternative chemical synthesis, have prompted researchers to go for metabolic engineering and synthetic biology to enhance the production of *C. roseus* MIAs in Homologous/Heterologous systems. In the last four decades, several studies were carried out for the same purpose and it was observed that four conditions must be satisfied in a plant (cell) before attempting metabolic and synthetic biology approaches aiming for a significant increment in the yield of the desired metabolite. These are:

(i) Optimal induction of genes/enzymes of an intended pathway at the right time and right place;

(ii) Assured availability of starting precursor(s) and/or limiting intermediates, particularly those that lie at the interface of primary and secondary metabolisms and;

(iii) Availability of a suitable sink to store the synthesized product and;

(iv) Ability to respond to the associated elicitation and signal transduction mechanisms by up-or down-regulating an intended pathway *in vivo* as well as *in vitro*.

[3, 18, 19]. It is now becoming gradually apparent that the majority of plant bioactive secondary metabolites are cytotoxic to cell viability and need to be compartmentalized to minimize their adverse effects on cell growth. Therefore, whenever an attempt is made to overexpress a pathway in a cultured cell/tissue, the cell must be engineered to bear this extra load of metabolite(s) that may offer no additional advantage to the cell in terms of its growth. Overlooking this important consideration was probably the main reason why the high-yielding cell lines selected in many earlier studies failed to sustain their growth and productivity level in due course of time during their *in vitro* cultivation [20]. They might have got sequentially eliminated during sub-culturing because of their slow growth on account of metabolite burden in comparison to fast multiplying less productive cells. In addition, studies concerning phytomolecules production in cultured cells and tissues must not only focus on manipulating the synthesis part of the desired metabolite. Post-biosynthetic steps of catabolism of this product like enzymatic modification/conversions, transport, storage, and degradation that usually decide the final outcome were overlooked and should be studied with equal importance. Based on the knowledge gained over the last four decades, more holistic approaches to metabolic engineering are now forthcoming. Therefore, better insight into the controlling steps of the pathway and its spatial and temporal regulation are being gathered to devise better modulatory controls in *C. roseus* [7].

It was in most of these contemporary developments when the term "Metabolic Engineering" was first coined by Bailey in 1991 [21]. Abstractly, metabolic engineering accounts for the identification of major building blocks and control points in metabolic pathways at the molecular level and the concomitant removal of these confines with cellular engineering intrusions [18, 22 - 24]. The majority of pathway upregulation attempts in the past were mainly aimed to "push" the metabolic flux of a pathway towards the desired end product by overexpressing the enzymatic steps located upstream in the biogenetic route. However, it has been observed in many cases now that such manipulations do not normally result in better channelization of the flux in the expected direction, as the native regulatory mechanism of a cell always tries to neutralize the effect of a hyper-expressed gene. An alternative approach now being advocated is to 'pull' the flux toward a targeted product by upregulating the terminal step of the pathway located downstream in the sequence of a biochemical route [25, 26].

Profound understanding gathered of *C. roseus* MIAs biosynthetic pathway rate-limiting steps and spatio-temporal regulation was used to formulate improved modulatory control over MIAs metabolic flux. Conceptually, the metabolic flux of a metabolite is considered as a summation of metabolic pathway regulatory factors viz.,(a) Inactivity/lower activity of rate-limiting enzymes, (b) feedback inhibition of rate-limiting enzymes, (c) Participation of inducible enzyme(s), (d) diverse affinity of enzymes at overlapping routes branch points, (e) very low expression of competitive pathways sharing similar intermediates or precursor, (f) cellular capacity to hold and store the desired metabolites [7, 27]. Therefore, to overcome these metabolite flux glitches and to divert metabolite flux into the desired route, different experimental methods are developed: (a) Developing mutants that can produce target enzyme with less sensitivity to feedback inhibition; (b) overexpression of enzyme by inserting a gene that codes for an enzyme with similar function in the combination of the constitutive promoter; (c)

By applying gene silencing approach to target enzyme competitive pathway; (d) Introduction of the enzyme with higher affinity to the shared substrate that opens a new mini-pathway; (e) Targeting enzyme with transport proteins to directly at cellular location [12, 16, 28 - 31]. Previously, the majority of MIAs pathway metabolic regulation studies were attempted by aiming 'push' the metabolic flux toward the end products by overexpressing the genes of the indole and terpenoid pathways along with condensation reactions [viz. anthranilate synthase α/β (ASα, Asβ, ASα + β); tryptophan decarboxylase (TDC); 3-hydroxy-3-methylglutaryl reductase (HMGR), 2-C methyl-D-erythritol 2,4-cyclodiphosphate synthase (MECS), 1-deoxy-D-xylulose 5-phosphate (DXS),geraniol 8-hydroxylase (G8H/G10H) and strictosidine synthase (STR)]. Parallelly, an alternative pathway flux 'pull' approach is also used to divert the pathway flux towards a targeted product through up-regulating terminal steps of vindoline and downstream pathways [viz. monovincine 19-*O*-acetyltransferase (MAT), tabersonine-3-epoxidase (T3O), tabersonine-19-hydroxylase (T16H), tabersonine-3-reductase (T3R), 16-methoxytarbersonin (16OMT), deacetylvindoline-4-*O*-acetyltransferase (DAT), deacetylvindoline-4 hydrolase (D4H), and peroxidase (PRX)] [25, 26].

In the presence of advanced genomics and metabolomics tools, improved recombinant DNA technology used for gene silencing, overexpression, and disruption of metabolic pathways provides incredible possibilities for metabolic engineering. These tremendous approaches of both metabolic engineering and synthetic biology were fantastically used in MIAs pathway engineering in both homologous and heterologous systems. Due to the recalcitrant nature of *C. roseus*, transgenic plant developments through metabolic engineering are not routine, and hence the majority of metabolic engineering efforts were executed with hairy roots and cell suspension culture [7, 32, 33]. Recent studies have also demonstrated the possibility of synthetic biology to use the microbial platform and microbial cell factories by expressing the MIAs pathway steps in heterologous microbial cells for seeking them as an alternative MIAs production system [15, 17, 23, 34, 35]. This microbial cell heterologous MIAs expression was carried out with the intent to:

(a) Identification of previously unidentified MIAs pathway, genes, and linked transcription factors,

(b) Identification of rate-limiting MIAs pathway steps,

(c) Enhancing the production of MIAs in plant tissue culture systems,

(d) Accommodating MIAs biosynthetic pathway steps in the microbial system.

MIAs 'Pathway Genes' and 'Transcriptional Factors Metabolic Engineering'

The recalcitrant nature of *C. roseus* restricts the transgenic plant development for metabolic engineering strategies and therefore, the majority of MIAs metabolic engineering efforts were executed through the expression of metabolic pathway genes that regulate different branches of MIAs biosynthesis (viz. indole, terpenoid, methylerythritol 4-phosphate, iridoid, condensation of STR and vindoline pathway) along with transcription factors in the homologous hairy root, callus and cell suspension systems (Table **2**).

Table 2. Substantial impact on MIAs production in *C. roseus*via metabolic engineering of 'pathway genes' and 'transcriptional factors.

Culture	Transgenes	Effect on MIAs Accumulation	References
HR	HMGR	Serpentine↑, ajmalicine↓	[40]
HR	TDC	Serpentine↑	[41]
HR	ASα + TDC	Tryptamine↑	[41]
HR	ASα +TDC	Tryptophan↑, tryptamine↑	[42]
HR	DAT	Horhammericine↑	[45]
HR	ORCA3	Lochnericine↓, tabersonine↓, horhammericine↓	[46]
HR	ORCA3	Catharanthine↑	[47]
HR	ORCA3 + G10H	Catharanthine↑	[48]
HR	ORCA2	Catharanthine↑, vindoline↑	[49]
HR	DXS + G10H	Ajmalicine↑, lochnericine↑, tabersonine↑	[50]
HR	DXS + Asα	Lochnericine↑, tabersonine↑, horhammericine↑	[50]
HR	CrPRX1	Serpentine↑, ajmalicine↑	[51]
HR	ORCA2	Strictosidine↓, secologenine↓, serpentine↑, tabersonine↓↓	[52]
HR	DXR/STR/MECS	Ajmalicine↑	[53]
HR	ORCA3/ ORCA3 + SGD	Serpentine↑, ajmalicine↑, catharanthine↑, tabersonine↑	[54]
HR	T16H/16OMT	16-Hydroxytabersoni↑, 16-methoxytabersonin↑, lochnericine↓, horhammericine↓, 19-hydroxytabersonin↓	[55]
CS	ORCA3	Tryptophan↑, tryptamine↑	[56]
CS	CYP76B6	10-Hydroxy geraniol↑	[39]

(Table 2) cont.....

Culture	Transgenes	Effect on MIAs Accumulation	References
CS	TDC + STR	TIA accumulation↑	[37,38,57]
CS	ORCA3	Catharanthine↑↑, vindoline↑	[58]
CS	WRKY1	Serpentine↑, catharanthine↑, tabersonine↓	[59]
CS	WRKY2	Serpentine↑, tabersonine↑	[59]
CS	BIS2	MEP pathway↑	[60]
CS	GES	Valine↑,Leucine↑, Phenylalanine↑, Tyrosine↑	[61]
CL CS	TDC + STR	Strictosidine↑, ajmalicine↑, serpentine↑, catharanthine↑, tabersonine↑	[36]
CL	TDC + STR	TIA accumulation↑	[44]
CL	TDC + STR	Catharanthine, vindoline↑	[32]
LF	TDC + STR	TIA accumulation↑	[43]
LF	TDC + STR	Catharanthine↑, vindoline↑, vinblastine↑	[32]
PT	MYC2 + ORCA/ BISI/ORCA3	Iridoid pathway↑	[62]
SL	GATA1	Vindoline↑	[63]
SL	ORCA2/ZCT1	STR promoter activity↑	[64]
ST	DAT	Vindoline↑	[65]
ST	ORCA3 + G10H	Strictosidine↑, ajmalicine↑, vindoline↑, catharanthine↑	[66]
ST	TDC + STR	Tryptamine↑, secologenine↑, catharanthine↑, vindoline↑, vinblastine↑	[33]
ST	GGPS + GES	3,4-Anhydrovinblastine↑	[67]
ST	GGPS	Vinblastine↑	[67]

HR hairy roots, CS cell *suspension,* PT *petal*, CL *callus*, SL *seedlings*, ST *multiple shoots.*

MIAs pathway engineering is carried out at all important pathway points viz. indole pathway, terpenoid pathway, and tryptamine and secologanin condensation to synthesize strictosidine. TDC conversion of tryptophan to tryptamine and condensation of tryptamine and secologanin through STR were targeted by Canel *et al* . [36] by expressing TDC and STR in cell suspension and callus culture. This overexpression resulted in the increased accumulation of strictosidine, ajmalicine, catharanthine, serpentine, and tabersonine with the enhanced tenfold activity of STR, but, the expression of TDC is lowered. Whitmer *et al* . [37, 38] reported the long-term instability of TDC and STR activity in these suspension cell lines. When fed with secologanin and loganin, TDC overexpressing cell lines accumulated strictosidine and catharanthine. Collu *et al* . [39] identified and cloned G10H and studied the homologous expression of G10H inserted in a plasmid CaMV35S-CYP76B6 gene in cell suspension culture that resulted in enhanced CYP76B6 and G10H transcript levels. The role of the HMGR gene in MIAs biosynthesis is also elucidated. When overexpression in hairy roots, HMGR enhanced the accumulation of serpentine with the lower accumulation of ajmalicine, and no catharanthine was detected [40]. Hughes *et al* . [41] explained the role of glucocorticoid inducible TDC promoter with and without feedback-resistant GENE. TDC+A/B-SUBUNITS expressing transgenic hairy roots demonstrated high feedback resistance with higher tryptophan levels, whereas 129% enhanced the accumulation of serpentine in TDC-expressing lines [42]. Furthermore, the first transient expression of TDC and STR genes in *Catharanthus* leaves was achieved [43]. This study showed improved MIAs accumulation and detected recombinant STR and TDC in vacuoles, cytosol, and chloroplast. Taha *et al* . [44] and Sharma *et al* . [32] attempted a similar experiment with transient expression of TDC and STR gene expression on callus culture and *in vitro* grown leaves. As a result, better MIAs accumulation and higher vindoline, vinblastine, and catharanthine production were observed.

Magnotta *et al* . [45] worked with newly identified DAT genes and examined their role in the transformed hairy root DAT genes where vindoline synthesis was not observed. Results suggested that DAT cross-talked with MAT in transformed roots that inhibited 19-*O*-acetyl-horhammecine and enhanced horhammericine accumulation. The role of the primary metabolic pathway genes DXS + G10H and DXS + AS was studied by Peebles *et al* . [46]. DXS + G10H expression increases the production of ajmalicine, serpentine, and lochnericine, however, decreases the production of horhammericine and tabersonine. Enhanced ajmalicine production was recorded in similar studies with transgenic lines expressing DXR + STR and MECS + STR [47]. Sun *et al* . [48] attempted the engineering of the vindoline pathway with the expression of T16H and 16OMT. T16H and 16OMT expression enhanced the expression of 16-hydroxytabersonin and 17-methoxytabersonin. But, reduced root-specific alkaloids like lochnericine, horhammericine, and 19-hydroxytabersonin. Saiman *et al* . [49] performed plastidial or cytosolic expression of GES in non-MIAs producing *C. roseus* cell lines, where engineered cells failed to synthesize MIAs till not elicited by jasmonic acid. Results advised the involvement of discrete inducible pathway genes in MIAs biosynthesis. Jaggi *et al* . [50] studied the role of the lower pathway gene peroxidase. Transgenic hairy roots, one expressing PRX and another with RNAi-blocked PRX, were developed. PRX expression enhanced ajmalicine and serpentine production, whereas RNAi-suppressed transgenic lines showed lower MIAs pathway transcript levels. As the regeneration of transgenic plants from recalcitrant plants like *Catharanthus roseus* is not easily feasible, therefore, the actual worth of

MIAs pathway engineering needs to be valued. Verma and Mathur [51] presented the first report of the development of a complete *Agrobacterium tumefaciens* strain-LBA4404 (with PbI121 plasmid + Gus + nptII gene interrupted with p35SGUS-INT) mediated transgenic plant in *C. roseus*. Pan *et al* . [52] figured out the effect of expressing ORCA3 alone (OR line) and with G10H (GO line) through whole plant transgenics. Transgenic plants reported increased AS, TDC, STR, and D4H transcript level, without affecting the CRMYC2 G10H transcript. Transgenic lines also synthesized higher levels of strictosidine, ajmalicine, catharanthine, and vindoline. One more *Catharanthus* regeneration protocol developed from hypocotyls and over-expressing DAT resulted in more than the double accumulation of vindoline [53]. Pathway 'push' approach to increase the pathway flux to MIAs secologanin and pathway intermediate strictosidine were developed also developed [33, 54]. Sarma *et al* . [54] expressed Geranylgeraniol pyrophosphate synthase (GGPS) with and without GES transiently in *C. roseus* leaves to dazed the restraint of MIAs pathway flux on the way to terpene moiety precursor of initial MIAs pathway. GGPS expression when expressed with and without GES resulted in enhanced biosynthesis of secologanin and ajmalicine, whereas vinblastine was detected only in GGPS-expressing lines along with increased PRX transcript levels. Sharma *et al* . [33] developed whole-plant transgenics co-expressing the TDC and STR genes. Transgenic lines reported enhanced transcript levels of TDC, STR, SGD, T30, T3R, DAT, D4H, and PRX that resulted in enhanced accumulation of total alkaloid content along with vindoline, catharanthine, and vinblastine.

Like pathway genes, transcriptional factors also play an important role in MIAs manipulation (by triggering or suppressing the pathway and/or related genes). Therefore, transcriptional factors viz. ORCA2, ORCA3, ORCA4, ORCA5, WRKY1, WRKY2, GATA, PIF, BISI/BIS2, and ZCT1 were also engineered in *C. roseus* to chase their effect over MIAs biosynthesis [52, 55 - 65]. Van der Fits and Memelink [61] made the first transcription factors engineering by expressing ORCA3 in cell suspension that improved tryptophan and tryptamine accumulation with the enhanced level of AS, DXS, TDC, STR, CRP, and D4H pathway genes. Obtained results specified the role of ORCA3 as the central MIAs regulator. Peeble *et al* . [55] also engineered ORCA3 with Jasmonic acid as elicited hairy roots that exhibited ORCA3 levels enhanced 170-fold with no effect over enhanced MIAs accumulation. In a separate study, ORCA3 under the control of glucocorticoid inducible promoter also showed the same results [60]. However, the production of ajmalicine, catharanthine, tabersonine, horhammericine, and lochnericine improved when co-expressed with SGD. In a similar study, Zhou *et al* . [56] obtained decreased catharanthine accumulation in ORCA3 expressing hairy roots. Wang *et al* . [57] developed transgenic hairy root lines expressing G10H and ORCA3 + G10H that resulted in more than 6.5-fold higher catharanthine accumulated. Similarly, expression of ORCA3 in cell suspensions accumulated increased catharanthine by more than twofold and vindoline by fourfold [62]. When ORCA3 + G10H is expressed at the whole plant level, the transgenic plant accumulated improved strictosidine, ajmalicine, catharanthine, and vindoline with no effect on 3,4-anhydrovinblastine. The expression of ORCA2 also resulted in the accumulation of more than twofold increased catharanthine and more than threefold increased vindoline production with high transcript levels of MIAs regulatory genes [58, 59]. Suttipanta *et al*. [66] engineered WRKY1 and WRKY2 in cell suspension cultures that enhanced catharanthine, tabersonine, and serpentine. Specific helix-loop-helix (bHLH) transcription factors BIS1 and BIS2areidentified to play an important role in the expression and activation of iridoid synthesis and pathway promoters (60). BIS2 homodimerizes and/or heterodimerizes with BIS1. When tested in cell suspension and transiently in petal limbs, BIS2 improved MEP and iridoid pathway gene transcript levels with no effect on other MIAs pathway genes [63]. Schweizer *et al*. [63] suggested the limited role of the transcription factor MYC2-ORCA on the iridoid pathway. When transiently over-expressed in petals, depressed MYC2 (MYC2^{D126N}) activated key iridoid pathway genes. But, when engineered with BIS1 and/or ORCA3, it failed to alter the vindoline pathway genes. Liu *et al*. [65] recently identified a (leucine-leucine-methionine domain) transcription factor GATA1 that facilitates promoter activation and expression of T16H$_2$, T3O, T3R, D4H, and DAT genes of light-induced vindoline pathway and vindoline accumulation. However, VIGS-mediated silencing led to the repression of important vindoline pathway genes and hence was considered to regulate vindoline biosynthesis [65]. In a study, using a transient expression system with ORCA2 as a transcription activator enhanced STR promoter expression nine-fold, whereas ZCT1 as a repressor failed to develop STR promoter activity [67].

MIAs Synthetic Biology of Plant and Microbial Cell Factories

In the last two decades of *C. roseus* research, several synthetic biology approaches were developed and experimented with for tailoring a broad range of MIAs, including vinblastine and vincristine. Like metabolic engineering, synthetic biology can also suffer from the high possibility of unbalanced and unnatural modifications in parental metabolic pathway products. However, unnatural variations can impart novel bioactivity to the parent natural product. Developments in synthetic biology through engineering microbial factories have permitted phytomolecules synthesis and their analogs in heterologous systems like *E. coli* and yeast. The engineering of plant biosynthetic pathways in homologous plants to yield particular phytomolecules has been found inadequate, especially when compared to the results obtained in heterologous engineering of plant biosynthetic pathways in microbial factories [69]. The past period has perceived the engineering of *Escherichia coli* and *Saccharomyces cerevisiae* for the synthesis of high-valued *C. roseus* MIAs. Majorly, the synthetic biology approach for phytomolecules production has been targeted exclusively in microbial systems, as the organizational complexity and genetically intractable nature of plants prevented the scientist to use plant systems for metabolic pathway engineering using synthetic biology approaches. As per the studies, Runguphan [68, 69] described the following strategies while using the system biology approach in homologous plants:

(a) Introduction and expression of a biosynthetic enzyme with redesigned substrate specificity in plants: this strategy will result in the development of transgenic plants, in the presence of an enzyme specifically redesigned substrate, biosynthesize several unnatural alkaloids.

(b) Allowing autonomous *in situ* synthesis of precursor analogs in transgenic plants developed as per point (a): Viz. Insertion of naturally unavailable halogenation machinery of the prokaryotic system in plant cells, which later can be shuttled to MIAs metabolism to produce halogenated alkaloids.

(c) RNAi-mediated silencing of MIAs biosynthesis: Developed RNAi-suppressed transgenic plants can synthesize unnatural fluorinated alkaloids in the presence of fluorinated initial substrate; however, this will not lead to the production of natural MIAs.

(d) Chemical functionalization of halogenated MIAs: After chemical derivatization of halogenated MIAs using specific palladium-catalyzed Suzuki-Miyaura cross-coupling reactions robustly afforded aryl and heteroaryl analogs of MIAs.

Altogether, these strategies define the flexibility of medicinal plants for synthetic biology, however, this will always result in the production of unnatural alkaloids. Therefore, microbial cells are actually preferred over plant cells for metabolic pathway engineering using synthetic biology approaches.

Synthetic biology is an interdisciplinary science that is emerging as the centerpiece of crucial plant metabolite engineering [70]. Metabolic engineering is a direct modification of the metabolic pathways in living organisms, whereas synthetic biology encompasses engineering approaches with the intention to (re)design and produce biological systems that do not exist naturally. Metabolic engineering is one such approach that is widely used for synthetic biology interventions. As discussed earlier, the organizational complexity and genetically intractable nature of plants prevented scientists to use plant systems for metabolic pathway engineering using synthetic biology approaches, and hence, the major synthetic biology tactic of phytomolecules biosynthesis has been embattled exclusively in microbial systems. Targeted introduction of a metabolic partial/complete pathway for secondary metabolite production in heterologous systems like microbial cells (viz. *E. coli* and *S. cerevisiae*) is, therefore, a promising approach [7, 35] (Table **3**).

Table 3. Summary of MIAs synthetic biology efforts in plant and microbial cells.

TIAs Gene	Transformed Host	Purpose and Result	References
CrTPT2	*S. cerevisiae*	Heterologous expression of the CrTPT2 gene facilitated the export of catharanthine from yeast cells to the culture media	[34]
8-HGO, IO, 7-DLGT, 7-DLH	*S. cerevisiae*	Successfully identified the four enzymes and chased the last missing step of the (seco)iridoid pathway	[15]
8-HGO, IO, DLGT, 7-DLD, GPPS, GES, IS, G8O/G10H, LMAT, SLS	*N. benthamiana*	Successfully expressed MIAs pathway from IPP upto strictosidine	[15]
TDC + STR	*V. minor*	Achieved vincamine production in rol gene integrated transgenic cell lines	[72]
T16H,T19H, NMT, T3O,T3R, D4H, DAT	*S. cerevisiae*	Reconstructed entire seven step tabersonine into vindoline pathway	Qu *et al*. (2015)
GPPS2, GES, G8H, GOR, IS, IO, 7-DLGT, 7-DLH, LMAT,SLS,TDC, STR, CYB5, CPR, CYPADH	*S. cerevisiae*	*De novo* synthesis of complete (seco)iridoid pathway (expressing 14 MIAs biosynthesis pathway genes) from geraniol to strictosidine)	[23]
TDC + STR	*B. monnieri*	TDC expression facilitated the conversion of tryptophan into tryptamine	[32]
MAT	*S. cerevisiae*	MAT failed to transform the 19-hydroxylated tabersonine into its acetylated product.	[17]
ASO	*N. benthamiana*	ASO converted to vincadifformine in the presence of H3/H4 and GS	[24]

Later they used agroinfiltration to express the MIAs pathway from IPP to MIAs central intermediate strictosidine (by expressing IO, 8-HGO, 7-DLGT, 7-DLH, GPPS, GES, IS, G8H/G10H, LAMT, SLS) in *Nicotiana benthamiana* plant system. In continuation with the above molecular and biochemical characterization of missing MIAs pathway genes, the genes responsible for geraniol to secologanin formation, viz. UGT8 [71], 8-HGO, IO, 7-DLGT, 7-DLH [72], THAS [73], T3O and T3R [34, 74]. In the series of MIAs microbial biosynthesis, the major achievement was achieved by Brown *et al*. [35] where they successively expressed 14 genes leading to the completion of the entire (seco)iridoid pathway under *de novo* condition in recombinant yeast strain modified for providing the crucial MIAs precursors and metabolic cofactors. This experiment achieved 0.5mg/L strictosidine biosynthesis in a microbial synthetic system. Identification and molecular/biochemical characterization of T3O and T3R genes were also achieved as a major exploration of the MIAs biosynthetic pathway [23]. Identification of T3O and T3R led to the complete identification of 7 steps of conversion of tabersonine to vindoline. Later, the entire 7-step tabersonine to vindoline pathway was engineered in yeast that consecutively attained 1.1mg/L/12h conversion of tabersonine to vindorosine and vindoline, and 2.7 mg/L/12h conversion of 16-methoxytabersonine into vindoline.

The availability of several advanced and recombinant genetic modification tools, along with a short life span and generation time, has made *E. coli and S. cerevisiae* the first choice to be used for heterologous plant metabolite production in microbial systems. However, *S. cerevisiae-based* microbial production system plays a more important role in plant-based metabolite production and helps in the identification of bottlenecks and the discovery of new biosynthetic pathway genes [7]. Yu and De Luca (34) carried out the very first MIAs pathway engineering attempt in yeast to understand the catharanthine transportation mechanism and expressed a typical full ABC transporter (CrTPT2) in eight major ABC transporter genes lacking yeast strain AD12345678. This CrTPT2 expression facilitated the export of catharanthine from yeast cells to culture media. However, when suppressed using the VIGS approach in *C. roseus,* it suppresses the catharanthine transportation toward the leaf surface, including increased dimeric MIAs synthesis [16, 34]. Miettinen *et al* . [15] used proteomics and integrated transcriptome tactics and carried out the first successful attempt for MIAs biosynthesis in yeast, recognized four enzymes, and chased the last missing step of the (seco)iridoid pathway.

The metabolic engineering and synthetic biology approaches developed using microbial and plant systems have helped in the missing MIAs step characterization along with the synthesis of complex MIAS and their derivatives. In these studies, major attempts were done for the identification and characterization of leaf-associated MIAs and only two root-associated genes, T19H and MAT, were identified. T19H is found to carry out the hydroxylation of tabersonine [75], whereas MAT enables the acetylation reaction for 9-*O*-acetylhorhammericine and echitovenine synthesis [76]. When studied *in planta* activity of mat was found very low, however, it is synthetic engineering into yeast resulted in futile and did not convert 19-hydroxylated tabersonine into its acetylated product. This happened due to the participation of an additional root-associated BHAD acetyltransferase, which was later identified as tabersonine 19-

O-acetyltransferase (TAT) (acetylating 19-hydroxytabersonin derivatives monovincine and horhammericine), which is confirmed following expressing in yeast [17].

Along with microbial cells, heterologous plant cells are also used for the synthetic biology engineering of MIAs. Already transformed with the rol gene, *Vinca minor* cell suspensions were again engineered to express *C. roseus* TDC and STR genes [77, 78]. This co-expression resulted in the formation of PVG1, PVG2, and PVG3, three cell lines, out of which PVG3 accumulated double alkaloid content and accumulated vincamine on bioreactor upscaling with more than sevenfold TDC and STR transcript levels. Similarly, the expression of TDC and STR gene constructs engineered in *Bacopa monnieri* resulted in tryptamine accumulation due to inserted TDC activity [32]. Very recently, the discovery of one more enzyme acetylstemmadenine oxidase- ASO (Like BBE like oxygenase family) from the tabersonine and catharanthine pathway was discovered [24]. ASO was found responsible for the conversion of O-acetylstemmadenine (OAS) into unstable intermediates that finally convert to the new product vincadifformine with the help of H3/H4 and GS. When tested for OAS conversion, recombinant ASO purified from tobacco failed to convert it further, however, OAS was found to disappear from the reaction. This study revealed that the formation of catharanthine, tabersonine, and vincadifformine from OAS requires a concerted reaction involving ASO, GS, and H1-4, respectively. The transient VIGS-mediated silencing of ASO accumulated OAS and reduced catharanthine by 60% and vindoline levels by 26%. Thus, synthetic biology approaches enable the elucidation of this canonical pathway and will be very helpful for dimeric antineoplastic vinblastine and vincristine production.

CONCLUSION

The availability of advanced genomic, proteomic, and metabolomic approaches, amended recombinant DNA technologies designed for metabolic pathway modulation*via* overexpression, repression, gene silencing, *etc.*, provides implausible opportunities for synthetic biology and metabolic engineering, especially in medicinal important plants like *C. roseus*. However, the synthetic biology approach using metabolic engineering suffers from the high possibilities of unbalanced and unnatural modifications in the native metabolic pathways, but still, these variations can impart novel bioactivities to the natural phytomolecules. Metabolic engineering efforts of biosynthetic pathways in homologous plant systems to yield particular phytomolecules have been found inadequate, specifically equated to heterologous engineering plant biosynthetic pathways in microbial cells. Therefore, enormous opportunities are left, and future scopes for metabolic pathway modulation using synthetic biology and metabolic engineering should be explored.

REFERENCES

[1]   Heinrich M, Barnes J, Gibbons S, Williamson EM. Fundamentals of Pharmacognosy and phytotherapy. Edinburgh: Churchill Livingstone 2012.

[2]   Heinrich M, Lee Teoh H. Galanthamine from snowdrop—the development of a modern drug against alzheimer's disease from local caucasian knowledge. J Ethnopharmacol 2004; 92(2-3): 147-62.
[http://dx.doi.org/10.1016/j.jep.2004.02.012] [PMID: 15137996]

[3]   Zhao L, Sander GW, Shanks JV. Perspectives of the metabolic engineering of terpenoid indole alkaloids in *Catharanthus roseus* hairy roots. Biotechnology of Hairy Root Systems. Berlin, Heidelberg: Springer 2013; pp. 23-54.
[http://dx.doi.org/10.1007/10_2013_182]

[4]   Cordell GA. Introduction to alkaloids: A biogenetic approach. New York: Wiley 1981; p. 587.

[5]   Buckingham J, Baggaley KH, Roberts AD, Szabo LF, Eds. Dictionary of alkaloids with CD-ROM. CRC press 2010.
[http://dx.doi.org/10.1201/EBK1420077698]

[6]   Amirkia V, Heinrich M. Alkaloids as drug leads : A predictive structural and biodiversity-based analysis. Phytochem Lett 2014; 10: xlviii-liii.
[http://dx.doi.org/10.1016/j.phytol.2014.06.015]

[7]   Sharma A, Amin D, Sankaranarayanan A, Arora R, Mathur AK. Present status of *Catharanthus roseus* monoterpenoid indole alkaloids engineering in homo- and hetero-logous systems. Biotechnol Lett 2020; 42(1): 11-23.
[http://dx.doi.org/10.1007/s10529-019-02757-4] [PMID: 31729591]

[8]   Roberts SC. Production and engineering of terpenoids in plant cell culture. Nat Chem Biol 2007; 3(7): 387-95.
[http://dx.doi.org/10.1038/nchembio.2007.8] [PMID: 17576426]

[9]   Noble RL. The discovery of the vinca alkaloids—chemotherapeutic agents against cancer. Biochem Cell Biol 1990; 68(12): 1344-51.
[http://dx.doi.org/10.1139/o90-197] [PMID: 2085431]

[10]   Kingston DGI. Taxol: The chemistry and structure-activity relationships of a novel anticancer agent. Trends Biotechnol 1994; 12(6): 222-7.
[http://dx.doi.org/10.1016/0167-7799(94)90120-1] [PMID: 7765351]

[11]   Hughes EH, Shanks JV. Metabolic engineering of plants for alkaloid production. Metab Eng 2002; 4(1): 41-8.
[http://dx.doi.org/10.1006/mben.2001.0205] [PMID: 11800573]

[12]   Pan Q, Mustafa NR, Tang K, Choi YH, Verpoorte R. Monoterpenoid indole alkaloids biosynthesis and its regulation in *Catharanthus roseus*: a literature review from genes to metabolites. Phytochem Rev 2016; 15(2): 221-50.
[http://dx.doi.org/10.1007/s11101-015-9406-4]

[13]   Sharma A, Mathur AK, Ganpathy J, Joshi B, Patel P. Effect of abiotic elicitation and pathway precursors feeding over terpenoid indole alkaloids production in multiple shoot and callus cultures of *Catharanthus roseus*. Biologia 2019; 74(5): 543-53.
[http://dx.doi.org/10.2478/s11756-019-00202-5]

[14]   Courdavault V, Papon N, Clastre M, Giglioli-Guivarc'h N, St-Pierre B, Burlat V. A look inside an alkaloid multisite plant: The catharanthus logistics. Curr Opin Plant Biol 2014; 19: 43-50.
[http://dx.doi.org/10.1016/j.pbi.2014.03.010] [PMID: 24727073]

[15] Miettinen K, Dong L, Navrot N, *et al.* The seco-iridoid pathway from *Catharanthus roseus.* Nat Commun 2014; 5(1): 3606.
[http://dx.doi.org/10.1038/ncomms4606] [PMID: 24710322]

[16] Thamm AMK, Qu Y, De Luca V. Discovery and metabolic engineering of iridoid/secoiridoid and monoterpenoid indole alkaloid biosynthesis. Phytochem Rev 2016; 15(3): 339-61.
[http://dx.doi.org/10.1007/s11101-016-9468-y]

[17] Carqueijeiro I, Dugé de Bernonville T, Lanoue A, *et al.* A BAHD acyltransferase catalyzing 19- *O* - acetylation of tabersonine derivatives in roots of *Catharanthus roseus* enables combinatorial synthesis of monoterpene indole alkaloids. Plant J 2018; 94(3): 469-84.
[http://dx.doi.org/10.1111/tpj.13868] [PMID: 29438577]

[18] Abiri R, Valdiani A, Maziah M, *et al.* A critical review of the concept of transgenic plants: Insights into pharmaceutical biotechnology and molecular farming. Curr Issues Mol Biol 2016; 18: 21-42.
[PMID: 25944541]

[19] Farré G, Twyman RM, Christou P, Capell T, Zhu C. Knowledge-driven approaches for engineering complex metabolic pathways in plants. Curr Opin Biotechnol 2015; 32: 54-60.
[http://dx.doi.org/10.1016/j.copbio.2014.11.004] [PMID: 25448233]

[20] Benedito VA, Modulo LV. Introduction to metabolic genetic engineering for the production of valuable secondary metabolites in *in vivo* and *in vitro* plant systems. Rec Pat Biotechnol 2013.
[http://dx.doi.org/10.2174/1872208307666131218125801]

[21] Bailey JE. Toward a science of metabolic engineering. Science 1991; 252(5013): 1668-75.
[http://dx.doi.org/10.1126/science.2047876] [PMID: 2047876]

[22] Verpoorte R, Alfermann AW. Metabolic engineering of plant secondary metabolism. In: Verpoorte R, Alfermann AW, Eds. Kluwer Academic Publishers. Dordrecht 2000.
[http://dx.doi.org/10.1007/978-94-015-9423-3]

[23] Qu Y, Easson MLAE, Froese J, Simionescu R, Hudlicky T, De Luca V. Completion of the seven-step pathway from tabersonine to the anticancer drug precursor vindoline and its assembly in yeast. Proc Natl Acad Sci 2015; 112(19): 6224-9.
[http://dx.doi.org/10.1073/pnas.1501821112] [PMID: 25918424]

[24] Qu Y, Safonova O, De Luca V. Completion of the canonical pathway for assembly of anticancer drugs vincristine/vinblastine in *Catharanthus roseus.* Plant J 2019; 97(2): 257-66.
[http://dx.doi.org/10.1111/tpj.14111] [PMID: 30256480]

[25] Charlwood BV, Pletsch M. Manipulation of natural product accumulation in plants through genetic engineering. J Herbs Spices Med Plants 2002; 9(2-3): 139-51.
[http://dx.doi.org/10.1300/J044v09n02_20]

[26] Julsing KM, Quax JW, Oliver K. The engineering of medicinal plants: prospects and limitations of medicinal plant biotechnology. In: Kayser O, Quax WJ, Eds. Medicinal Plant Biotechnology. Weinheim: Wiley 2007; pp. 3-8.

[27] Mathur AK, Mathur A, Seth R, Verma P, Vyas D. Biotechnological interventions in designing specialty medicinal herbs for twenty first century: Some emerging trends in pathway modulation through metabolic engineering. Herbal drugs: A twenty first century perspective. New Delhi: Jaypee Brothers Medical Publishers 2006; pp. 83-94.

[28] Schwender J. Metabolic flux analysis as a tool in metabolic engineering of plants. Curr Opin Biotechnol 2008; 19(2): 131-7.
[http://dx.doi.org/10.1016/j.copbio.2008.02.006] [PMID: 18378441]

[29] Wilson SA, Roberts SC. Metabolic engineering approaches for production of biochemicals in food and medicinal plants. Curr Opin Biotechnol 2014; 26: 174-82.
[http://dx.doi.org/10.1016/j.copbio.2014.01.006] [PMID: 24556196]

[30]   Verma P, Sharma A, Khan SA, Mathur AK, Shanker K. Morphogenetic and chemical stability of long-term maintained *Agrobacterium* -mediated transgenic *Catharanthus roseus* plants. Nat Prod Res 2015; 29(4): 315-20.
[http://dx.doi.org/10.1080/14786419.2014.940348] [PMID: 25102992]

[31]   Verma P, Mathur AK, Khan SA, Verma N, Sharma A. Transgenic studies for modulating terpenoid indole alkaloids pathway in *Catharanthus roseus*: Present status and future options. Phytochem Rev 2017; 16(1): 19-54.
[http://dx.doi.org/10.1007/s11101-015-9447-8]

[32]   Sharma A, Verma N, Verma P, Verma RK, Mathur A, Mathur AK. Optimization of a Bacopa monnieri-based genetic transformation model for testing the expression efficiency of pathway gene constructs of medicinal crops. *In Vitro* Cell Dev Biol Plant 2017; 53: 22-32.

[33]   Sharma A, Verma P, Mathur A, Mathur AK. Overexpression of tryptophan decarboxylase and strictosidine synthase enhanced terpenoid indole alkaloid pathway activity and antineoplastic vinblastine biosynthesis in *Catharanthus roseus*. Protoplasma 2018; 255(5): 1281-94.
[http://dx.doi.org/10.1007/s00709-018-1233-1] [PMID: 29508069]

[34]   Yu F, De Luca V. ATP-binding cassette transporter controls leaf surface secretion of anticancer drug components in *Catharanthus roseus*. Proc Natl Acad Sci 2013; 110(39): 15830-5.
[http://dx.doi.org/10.1073/pnas.1307504110] [PMID: 24019465]

[35]   Brown S, Clastre M, Courdavault V, O'Connor SE. *De novo* production of the plant-derived alkaloid strictosidine in yeast. Proc Natl Acad Sci 2015; 112(11): 3205-10.
[http://dx.doi.org/10.1073/pnas.1423555112] [PMID: 25675512]

[36]   Canel C, Lopes-Cardoso MI, Whitmer S, *et al.* Effects of over-expression of strictosidine synthase and tryptophan decarboxylase on alkaloid production by cell cultures of *Catharanthus roseus*. Planta 1998; 205(3): 414-9.
[http://dx.doi.org/10.1007/s004250050338] [PMID: 9640666]

[37]   Whitmer S, van der Heijden R, Verpoorte R. Effect of precursor feeding on alkaloid accumulation by a strictosidine synthase over-expressing transgenic cell line S1 of *Catharanthus roseus*. Plant Cell Tissue Organ Cult 2002; 69(1): 85-93.
[http://dx.doi.org/10.1023/A:1015090224398]

[38]   Whitmer S, van der Heijden R, Verpoorte R. Effect of precursor feeding on alkaloid accumulation by a tryptophan decarboxylase over-expressing transgenic cell line T22 of *Catharanthus roseus*. J Biotechnol 2002; 96(2): 193-203.
[http://dx.doi.org/10.1016/S0168-1656(02)00027-5] [PMID: 12039535]

[39]   Collu G, Unver N, Peltenburg-Looman AMG, van der Heijden R, Verpoorte R, Memelink J. Geraniol 10-hydroxylase [1], a cytochrome P450 enzyme involved in terpenoid indole alkaloid biosynthesis. FEBS Lett 2001; 508(2): 215-20.
[http://dx.doi.org/10.1016/S0014-5793(01)03045-9] [PMID: 11718718]

[40]   Ayora-Talavera T, Chappell J, Lozoya-Gloria E, Loyola-Vargas VM. Overexpression in *Catharanthus roseus* hairy roots of a truncated hamster 3-hydroxy-3-methylglutaryl-CoA reductase gene. Appl Biochem Biotechnol 2002; 97(2): 135-46.
[http://dx.doi.org/10.1385/ABAB:97:2:135] [PMID: 11996224]

[41]   Hughes EH, Hong SB, Gibson SI, Shanks JV, San KY. Metabolic engineering of the indole pathway in *Catharanthus roseus* hairy roots and increased accumulation of tryptamine and serpentine. Metab Eng 2004; 6(4): 268-76.
[http://dx.doi.org/10.1016/j.ymben.2004.03.002] [PMID: 15491856]

[42]   Hong SB, Peebles CAM, Shanks JV, San KY, Gibson SI. Expression of the Arabidopsis feedback-insensitive anthranilate synthase holoenzyme and tryptophan decarboxylase genes in *Catharanthus roseus* hairy roots. J Biotechnol 2006; 122(1): 28-38.
[http://dx.doi.org/10.1016/j.jbiotec.2005.08.008] [PMID: 16188339]

[43]   Di Fiore S, Hoppmann V, Fischer R, Schillberg S. Transient gene expression of recombinant terpenoid indole alkaloid enzymes in *Catharanthus roseus* leaves. Plant Mol Biol Report 2004; 22(1): 15-22.
[http://dx.doi.org/10.1007/BF02773344]

[44]   Taha HS, El-Bahr MK, Seif-El-Nasr MM. *in vitro* studies on Egyptian *Catharanthus roseus* (L.) G. Don.: 1-Calli production, direct shootlets regeneration and alkaloids determination. J Appl Sci Res 2008; 4: 1017-22.

[45]   Magnotta M, Murata J, Chen J, De Luca V. Expression of deacetylvindoline-4-O-acetyltransferase in *Catharanthus roseus* hairy roots. Phytochemistry 2007; 68(14): 1922-31.
[http://dx.doi.org/10.1016/j.phytochem.2007.04.037] [PMID: 17574634]

[46]   Peebles CAM, Sander GW, Hughes EH, Peacock R, Shanks JV, San KY. The expression of 1-deoxy-D-xylulose synthase and geraniol-10-hydroxylase or anthranilate synthase increases terpenoid indole alkaloid accumulation in *Catharanthus roseus* hairy roots. Metab Eng 2011; 13(2): 234-40.
[http://dx.doi.org/10.1016/j.ymben.2010.11.005] [PMID: 21144909]

[47]   Chang K, Qiu F, Chen M, *et al.* Engineering the MEP pathway enhanced ajmalicine biosynthesis. Biotechnol Appl Biochem 2014; 61(3): n/a.
[http://dx.doi.org/10.1002/bab.1176] [PMID: 24237015]

[48]   Sun J, Zhao L, Shao Z, Shanks J, Peebles CAM. Expression of tabersonine 16-hydroxylase and 16-hydroxytabersonine-O-methyltransferase in *Catharanthus roseus* hairy roots. Biotechnol Bioeng 2018; 115(3): 673-83.
[http://dx.doi.org/10.1002/bit.26487] [PMID: 29105731]

[49]   Saiman MZ, Miettinen K, Mustafa NR, Choi YH, Verpoorte R, Schulte AE. Metabolic alteration of *Catharanthus roseus* cell suspension cultures overexpressing *geraniol synthase* in the plastids or cytosol. Plant Cell Tissue Organ Cult 2018; 134(1): 41-53.
[http://dx.doi.org/10.1007/s11240-018-1398-5] [PMID: 31007320]

[50]   Jaggi M, Kumar S, Sinha AK. Overexpression of an apoplastic peroxidase gene CrPrx in transgenic hairy root lines of *Catharanthus roseus*. Appl Microbiol Biotechnol 2011; 90(3): 1005-16.
[http://dx.doi.org/10.1007/s00253-011-3131-8] [PMID: 21318361]

[51]   Verma P, Mathur AK. Agrobacterium tumefaciens-mediated transgenic plant production *via* direct shoot bud organogenesis from pre-plasmolyzed leaf explants of *Catharanthus roseus.* Biotechnol Lett 2011; 33(5): 1053-60.
[http://dx.doi.org/10.1007/s10529-010-0515-2] [PMID: 21207108]

[52]   Pan Q, Wang Q, Yuan F, *et al.* Overexpression of ORCA3 and G10H in *Catharanthus roseus* plants regulated alkaloid biosynthesis and metabolism revealed by NMR-metabolomics. PLoS One 2012; 7(8): e43038.
[http://dx.doi.org/10.1371/journal.pone.0043038] [PMID: 22916202]

[53]   Wang Q, Xing S, Pan Q, *et al.* Development of efficient *catharanthus roseus* regeneration and transformation system using agrobacterium tumefaciens and hypocotyls as explants. BMC Biotechnol 2012; 12(1): 34.
[http://dx.doi.org/10.1186/1472-6750-12-34] [PMID: 22748182]

[54]   Sarma RK, Shilpashree HB, Nagegowda DA. Engineering overexpression of ORCA3 and strictosidine glucosidase in *Catharanthus roseus* hairy roots increases alkaloid production. Protoplasma 2018; 253: 1255-64.

[55]   Peebles CAM, Hughes EH, Shanks JV, San KY. Transcriptional response of the terpenoid indole alkaloid pathway to the overexpression of ORCA3 along with jasmonic acid elicitation of *Catharanthus roseus* hairy roots over time. Metab Eng 2009; 11(2): 76-86.
[http://dx.doi.org/10.1016/j.ymben.2008.09.002] [PMID: 18955153]

[56]   Zhou ML, Zhu XM, Shao JR, Wu YM, Tang YX. Transcriptional response of the catharanthine biosynthesis pathway to methyl jasmonate/nitric oxide elicitation in *Catharanthus roseus* hairy root

culture. Appl Microbiol Biotechnol 2010; 88(3): 737-50.
[http://dx.doi.org/10.1007/s00253-010-2822-x] [PMID: 20714717]

[57] Wang CT, Liu H, Gao XS, Zhang HX. Overexpression of G10H and ORCA3 in the hairy roots of *Catharanthus roseus* improves catharanthine production. Plant Cell Rep 2010; 29(8): 887-94.
[http://dx.doi.org/10.1007/s00299-010-0874-0] [PMID: 20535474]

[58] Dong Hui L, Wei Wei R, Li Jie C, Li Da Z, Xiao Fen S, Ke Xuan T. Enhanced accumulation of catharanthine and vindoline in *Catharanthus roseus* hairy roots by overexpression of transcriptional factor ORCA2. Afr J Biotechnol 2011; 10(17): 3260-8.
[http://dx.doi.org/10.5897/AJB10.1556]

[59] Li CY, Leopold AL, Sander GW, Shanks JV, Zhao L, Gibson SI. The ORCA2 transcription factor plays a key role in regulation of the terpenoid indole alkaloid pathway. BMC Plant Biol 2013; 13(1): 155.
[http://dx.doi.org/10.1186/1471-2229-13-155] [PMID: 24099172]

[60] Sun J, Peebles CAM. Engineering overexpression of ORCA3 and strictosidine glucosidase in *Catharanthus roseus* hairy roots increases alkaloid production. Protoplasma 2016; 253(5): 1255-64.
[http://dx.doi.org/10.1007/s00709-015-0881-7] [PMID: 26351111]

[61] van der Fits L, Memelink J. ORCA3, a jasmonate-responsive transcriptional regulator of plant primary and secondary metabolism. Science 2000; 289(5477): 295-7.
[http://dx.doi.org/10.1126/science.289.5477.295] [PMID: 10894776]

[62] Tang KX, Liu DH, Wang YL, Cui LJ, Ren WW, Sun XF. Overexpression of transcriptional factor ORCA3 increases the accumulation of catharanthine and vindoline in *Catharanthus roseus* hairy roots. Russ J Plant Physiol 2011; 58(3): 415-22.
[http://dx.doi.org/10.1134/S1021443711030125]

[63] Van Moerkercke A, Steensma P, Gariboldi I, *et al.* The basic helix-loop-helix transcription factor BIS2 is essential for monoterpenoid indole alkaloid production in the medicinal plant *Catharanthus roseus*. Plant J 2016; 88(1): 3-12.
[http://dx.doi.org/10.1111/tpj.13230] [PMID: 27342401]

[64] Schweizer F, Colinas M, Pollier J, *et al.* An engineered combinatorial module of transcription factors boosts production of monoterpenoid indole alkaloids in *Catharanthus roseus*. Metab Eng 2018; 48: 150-62.
[http://dx.doi.org/10.1016/j.ymben.2018.05.016] [PMID: 29852273]

[65] Liu Y, Patra B, Pattanaik S, Wang Y, Yuan L. GATA and phytochrome interacting factor transcription factors regulate light-induced vindoline biosynthesis in *Catharanthus roseus*. Plant Physiol 2019; 180(3): 1336-50.
[http://dx.doi.org/10.1104/pp.19.00489] [PMID: 31123092]

[66] Suttipanta N, Pattanaik S, Kulshrestha M, Patra B, Singh SK, Yuan L. The transcription factor CrWRKY1 positively regulates the terpenoid indole alkaloid biosynthesis in *Catharanthus roseus*. Plant Physiol 2011; 157(4): 2081-93.
[http://dx.doi.org/10.1104/pp.111.181834] [PMID: 21988879]

[67] Mortensen S, Bernal-Franco D, Cole LF, Sathitloetsakun S, Cram EJ, Lee-Parsons CWT. EASI transformation: An efficient transient expression method for analyzing gene function in *Catharanthus roseus* seedlings. Front Plant Sci 2019; 10: 755.
[http://dx.doi.org/10.3389/fpls.2019.00755] [PMID: 31263474]

[68] Runguphan W. Agrobacterium tumefaciens-mediated transgenic plant production *via* direct shoot bud organogenesis from pre-plasmolyzed leaf explants of *Catharanthus roseus*. Biotechnology letters 2011; 33: 1053-60.

[69] Runguphan W, Maresh JJ, O'Connor SE. Silencing of tryptamine biosynthesis for production of nonnatural alkaloids in plant culture. Proc Natl Acad Sci 2009; 106(33): 13673-8.
[http://dx.doi.org/10.1073/pnas.0903393106] [PMID: 19666570]

[70]   Moses T, Mehrshahi P, Smith AG, Goossens A. Synthetic biology approaches for the production of plant metabolites in unicellular organisms. J Exp Bot 2017; 68(15): 4057-74.
[http://dx.doi.org/10.1093/jxb/erx119] [PMID: 28449101]

[71]   Asada K, Salim V, Masada-Atsumi S, *et al.* A 7-deoxyloganetic acid glucosyltransferase contributes a key step in secologanin biosynthesis in Madagascar periwinkle. Plant Cell 2013; 25(10): 4123-34.
[http://dx.doi.org/10.1105/tpc.113.115154] [PMID: 24104568]

[72]   Salim V, Wiens B, Masada-Atsumi S, Yu F, De Luca V. 7-Deoxyloganetic acid synthase catalyzes a key 3 step oxidation to form 7-deoxyloganetic acid in *Catharanthus roseus* iridoid biosynthesis. Phytochemistry 2014; 101: 23-31.
[http://dx.doi.org/10.1016/j.phytochem.2014.02.009] [PMID: 24594312]

[73]   Stavrinides A, Tatsis EC, Foureau E, *et al.* Unlocking the diversity of alkaloids in *Catharanthus roseus*: Nuclear localization suggests metabolic channeling in secondary metabolism. Chem Biol 2015; 22(3): 336-41.
[http://dx.doi.org/10.1016/j.chembiol.2015.02.006] [PMID: 25772467]

[74]   Kellner F, Kim J, Clavijo BJ, *et al.* Genome-guided investigation of plant natural product biosynthesis. Plant J 2015; 82(4): 680-92.
[http://dx.doi.org/10.1111/tpj.12827] [PMID: 25759247]

[75]   Giddings LA, Liscombe DK, Hamilton JP, *et al.* A stereoselective hydroxylation step of alkaloid biosynthesis by a unique cytochrome P450 in *Catharanthus roseus*. J Biol Chem 2011; 286(19): 16751-7.
[http://dx.doi.org/10.1074/jbc.M111.225383] [PMID: 21454651]

[76]   Laflamme P, St-Pierre B, De Luca V. Molecular and biochemical analysis of a Madagascar periwinkle root-specific minovincinine-19-hydroxy-O-acetyltransferase. Plant Physiol 2001; 125(1): 189-98.
[http://dx.doi.org/10.1104/pp.125.1.189] [PMID: 11154328]

[77]   Verma P, Sharma A, Khan SA, Shanker K, Mathur AK. Over-expression of *Catharanthus roseus* tryptophan decarboxylase and strictosidine synthase in rol gene integrated transgenic cell suspensions of Vinca minor. Protoplasma 2015; 252(1): 373-81.
[http://dx.doi.org/10.1007/s00709-014-0685-1] [PMID: 25106473]

[78]   Whitmer S, Canel C, van der Heijden R, Verpoorte R. Long-term instability of alkaloid production by stably transformed cell lines of *Catharanthus roseus*. Plant Cell Tissue Organ Cult 2003; 74(1): 73-80.
[http://dx.doi.org/10.1023/A:1023368309831]

CHAPTER 4

Impact of Abiotic Stresses on *In Vitro* Production of Secondary Metabolites

Inês Mansinhos[1], **Sandra Gonçalves**[1] and **Anabela Romano**[1,*]

[1] MED – Mediterranean Institute for Agriculture, Environment and Development & CHANGE – Global Change and Sustainability Institute, Faculdade de Ciências e Tecnologia, Universidade do Algarve, Campus de Gambelas, Faro, Portugal

Abstract: Climate change conditions affect plant growth, net primary productivity, photosynthetic capability, and other biochemical functions that are essential for normal metabolism. The stimulation of biosynthesis of secondary metabolites is an important strategy developed by plants to cope with adverse environmental conditions. Many of these metabolites display a wide array of biological and pharmacological properties (*e.g.*, antioxidant, anti-inflammatory, antiproliferative, anti-allergic, antiviral, and antibacterial) and, thus, have valuable applications as pharmaceuticals, agrochemicals, cosmetics, fragrances, and food additives. The aim of this review is to present an overview of the impact of abiotic stress factors in the biosynthesis of secondary metabolites by *in vitro* cultures. Our literature survey showed that plant tissue culture has been an effective tool to understand plant response to abiotic stresses, such as drought, salinity, temperature, nutrient deficiency, or exposure to ultraviolet radiation, which is of particular interest in the actual scenario of climate change conditions. Furthermore, this technique appears as an environmentally friendly alternative for the production of high-value secondary metabolites for many applications.

Keywords: Drought, Environmental changes, *In vitro* cultures, Phenolics, Secondary metabolites, Temperature.

INTRODUCTION

Resisting adverse environmental conditions, which are now being exacerbated by climate change, is one of the major threats faced by plants. Climate change may occur due to natural processes or anthropogenic activities, and an increased incidence of coastal floods associated with sea-level rise and long-term droughts related to rainfall variations is expected. Also, by the end of the twenty-first cen-

* **Corresponding author Anabela Romano:** MED – Mediterranean Institute for Agriculture, Environment and Development & CHANGE – Global Change and Sustainability Institute, Faculdade de Ciências e Tecnologia, Universidade do Algarve, Campus de Gambelas, Faro, Portugal; E-mail: aromano@ualg.pt

Mohammad Anis & Mehrun Nisha Khanam (Eds.)

tury, global mean temperatures rising at least 5°C os expected [1, 2]. These extreme alterations expose plants to stressful abiotic factors that are outside of their physiological limits, negatively affecting plant growth and forcing them to adapt. Some plants have a great capacity to recognize environmental changes and adapt quickly, minimizing the adverse effects of these alterations. The accumulation of secondary metabolites (SM) is an example of an adaptive response by plants in coping with abiotic stress conditions [3, 4]. The changes in SM biosynthesis in plants under stress may be due to the "passive shift" mechanism, which occurs by the cell over-reduced status and the "active" mechanism, involving enzyme up-regulation [5]. SM like phenolics, alkaloids, and terpenes play an essential role in the interaction between the plant and its environment and are considered crucial defense compounds to scavenge reactive oxygen species (ROS) produced in response to environmental stresses, such as drought, salinity, ultraviolet (UV) radiation, extreme temperatures, nutrients deficiency, or heavy metals [5]. Many of these metabolites display a broad range of biological properties, namely antioxidant, anti-inflammatory, antitumoral, anti-allergic, antiviral, and antibacterial [6], and became useful compounds in several sectors, such as pharmaceutical, agrochemical, cosmetic, and food industries [7]. This is of particular relevance in the current context of increasing interest in natural products for industrial applications [8]. In some cases, natural supply is limited or chemical synthesis is unviable to produce SM, and, in this way, plant tissue culture (PTC) techniques emerge as a good alternative [9]. PTC techniques, besides providing a way to protect endangered species [7], allow the application of several strategies to improve or modify the production of SM of interest, such as the optimization of culture medium composition, changing environmental conditions, or inducting the SM pathways by elicitation and metabolic engineering, among other strategies. PTC techniques have been used in the last years to understand plant responses to several abiotic stresses. Hence, this chapter aims to make an overview of the last twenty years of literature about the impact of abiotic stress factors – drought, salinity, nutrient deficiency, UV radiation, and temperature – in the production of SM by *in vitro* plant cultures.

SECONDARY METABOLITES OF PLANTS

Higher plants synthesize a broad variety of low molecular weight SM derived from primary metabolites [10]. Contrary to the primary metabolism, which comprises all metabolic pathways that are essential to plants' growth and development, secondary metabolism is not essential for plants' life but is required for their survival [6, 11, 12]. SM serve as signals to attract pollinators and seed dispersers or protection against other abiotic and biotic stresses. Moreover, they can also contribute to the specific colors, odors, and tastes in plants [6, 10]. The accumulation of SM occurs in specific tissues, such as specialized glands, vacuoles, and trichomes. Though most of these metabolites are genus and species-specific [11], there is a high chemical diversity with an estimated 200,000 compounds, being terpenoids, alkaloids, and phenolics the most diverse groups [12]. Terpenoids derive directly from the glycolysis of glucose *via* the methylerythritol phosphate (MEP) pathway or the mevalonic acid (MVA) pathway. Most alkaloids are originated from amino acid precursors and phenolic compounds from shikimic acid [13]. The production of these compounds depends on several factors (*e.g.*, plant species, physiology, developmental stages, or environmental conditions) and is generally stimulated by exposure to potential stress conditions [9, 14] (Fig. **1**).

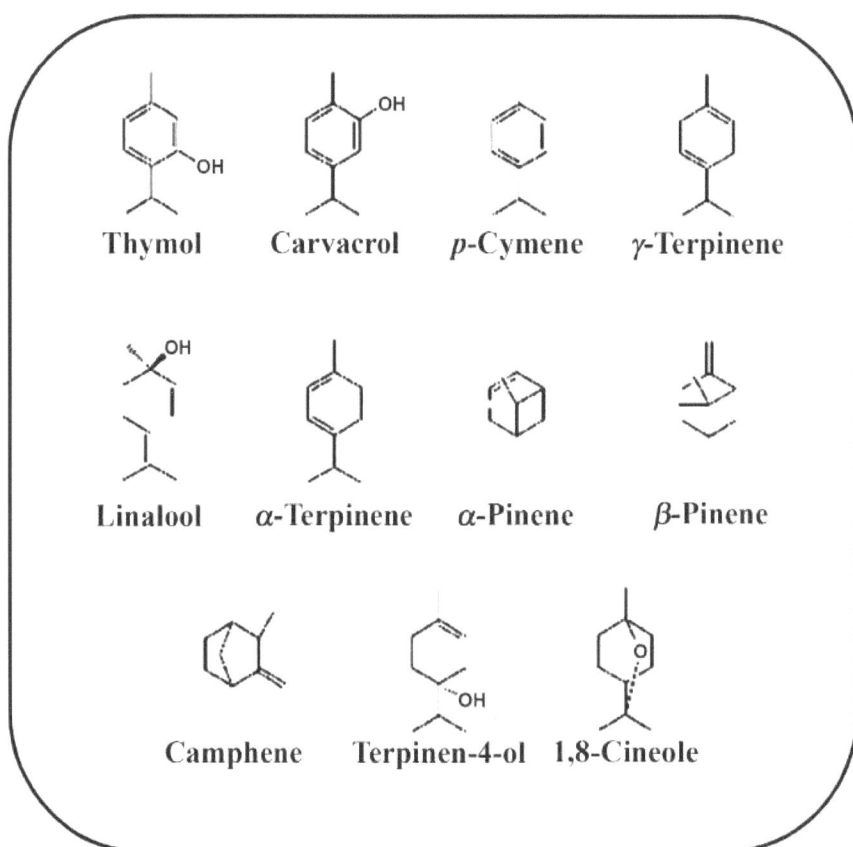

Fig. (1). Chemical structures of the most importante monoterpenes present in *Thymus* plants. Adapted from Li *et al.*(2019).

Presently there is a growing interest in products from natural sources to reduce the use of synthetic chemical substances with potentially toxic consequences [9].

Plant SM are applied in several industries, namely pharmaceutical, agriculture, cosmetic, nutraceutical, and food, with high economic impact [12, 15]. These compounds can display various beneficial effects for human health, exhibiting a wide array of biological and pharmacological properties (*e.g.*, antioxidant, anti-inflammatory, antiproliferative, anti-allergic, antiviral, and antibacterial, *etc.*) [6]. Some important SM have already revealed significant therapeutic benefits on cardiovascular [16], oncologic [17], and neurodegenerative [18] diseases. Artemisinin, for example, is the most important metabolite produced by *Artemisia*, which is well known due to its high efficiency to treat malaria. Besides that, this sesquiterpene lactone has protective effects against cancer and antiviral properties [15]. Other examples are the plant-derived anticancer compounds camptothecin, podophyllotoxin, taxol, vinblastine, or vincristine [19, 20]. Interestingly, around 60% of anticancer drugs are derived from plants [21], highlighting the importance of plant SM in drug discovery. In the cosmetic industry, extracts of polyphenols have been used in many products due to their antioxidant, anti-aging, anti-inflammatory, and antimicrobial properties. Moreover, phenolic compounds have chromophores in their structure able to absorb UV radiation, providing them with solar photoprotection abilities. Apigenin, caffeic acid, and kaempferol are some examples of phenolics that stand out due to their high UV-B protection with sun protection factor values of 28.8, 28.0, and 24.9, respectively [22]. Plant essential oils are other widely explored plant products in the cosmetic industry. Due to their pleasing odor and preserving characteristics, essential oils are mainly incorporated in perfumes, cosmetics, and household products [23, 24]. In the food sector, phenolic compounds and essential oils have gained great interest as a natural promising alternative to conventional preservatives to improve microbial safety and inactivate spoilage and pathogenic microorganisms [24 - 26].

BENEFITS OF USING PLANT TISSUE CULTURE FOR SECONDARY METABOLITES PRODUCTION

Despite being possible to synthesize some important metabolites *via* chemical synthesis, some of them (with complex structures) are difficult to produce (*e.g.*, alkaloids) because their structure remains unclear or their cost outweighs their commercial availability [7, 9, 27]. For these reasons, many of the promising pharmaceutical compounds are still extracted from their natural plant sources. For example, taxol production still depends on biomass derived from the *Taxus brevifolia* Nutt. because its synthesis remains inefficient [28, 29], and there are still some gaps, namely in the understanding of the biosynthetic pathway, regulatory mechanisms, and catalytic enzymes involved in this process [30]. Essential oils are another example that cannot be chemically synthesized because they are complex mixtures of compounds that are exclusively produced by glandular trichomes and other secretory structures of plants [31]. Nevertheless, in some cases, it is difficult to obtain plant SM of interest using conventional cultivation systems because some species are difficult to propagate by traditional techniques or take several years to grow [9]. Moreover, commercial production can be limited by regional and environmental restrictions [27]. PTC techniques emerge as a good alternative to chemical synthesis or conventional cultivation methods to efficiently produce SM within a short time [8]. The first attempt to use PTC techniques for SM production occurred in 1950, and over time the scale-up systems allowed the development of SM production methods with a high impact at commercial and functional levels [32]. These techniques, besides allowing the mass production of plant material [32], also offer other advantages, namely the faster production of pathogen-free material, the production under controlled conditions independent of geographical and seasonal variations, and the prevention of the use of pesticides and herbicides [7, 32]. The simplicity of metabolite extraction from *in vitro*-produced tissues is a further benefit making the technique more appellative for commercial use [9]. Moreover, it is possible to use traditional or metabolic engineering strategies to alter the production of desired compounds [9, 12]. *In vitro* culture also provides an alternative to overcome problems associated with species conservation [7, 32]. Due to their various benefits, PTC has been applied as a major system for SM production [8].

Generally, the most used methodologies to obtain SM *in vitro* are organized structures like shoots or roots, undifferentiated calli, or cell suspension cultures. In special cases, some SM are only synthesized in specialized plant tissues (*e.g.*, essential oils), and, therefore, production is only possible in organized structures [9]. Among organized structures, hairy root cultures are the furthermost promising alternative system to produce compounds synthesized in plant roots [8]. This system seems to be more appropriate to produce SM than cell or callus cultures due to its high biomass, long-time production capacity, and genetic stability [33]. Several SM such as ginsenosides [34], anthraquinones [35], artemisinin [36], withanolide [37], and camptothecin [38] have been produced using this culture system. However, it is difficult to cultivate hairy roots at an industrial scale, which limits its commercial application. Contrary, cell suspension cultures (CSC) overcomes large-scale production obstacles, being a simple and cost-effective method [27]. Growing plant cell cultures in bioreactors allows the large-scale production of SM [7], and the use of biosynthetic precursors (biotransformation) may even allow the production of new products not usually produced by the native plant [39, 40]. In this way, CSC has more potential than tissue/organ cultures for commercial application [9]. Several high-value natural compounds, including taxol [41, 42], taraxerol and taraxasterol [42], resveratrol [43], kaempferol [44], and flavonolignan [45] have been produced using CSC.

Different strategies can be used to increase SM production *in vitro* [7]. Regarding traditional methods, many factors can be optimized, namely culture medium composition and pH, inoculum density, agitation and aeration, and environment conditions (*e.g.*, temperature, light intensity, and quality), among others [8]. Elicitation is a strategy that could control biochemical and molecular cellular events, upregulating specific genes, improving SM production [9]. The use of elicitors (biotic or abiotic) triggers secondary metabolic pathways, stimulating plant defense mechanisms [7, 46]. Biotic elicitors are derived from biological sources and can be exogenous or endogenous. Exogenous elicitors are microbial cell wall (chitin, chitosan) or plant cell wall constituents (polysaccharides or oligosaccharides), while endogenous elicitors are produced by the plant in reaction to determined stress (*e.g.*, polysaccharides, salicylic acid, or methyl jasmonate) [8]. Abiotic elicitors are constituents of nonbiological sources, such as metal ions, salts of heavy metals, metal oxides, temperature, radiation, drought, salinity, *etc.* [8, 9, 46]. Immobilization, which uses calcium alginate, gelatin, agarose, polyacrylamide, and carrageenan as matrices, is another approach for increasing the production of SM in plant cell systems [9]. This strategy is mainly used to overcome problems of cell aggregation and low shear resistance [9], and increases the viability of cells for a longer time, providing SM stability [47]. Finally, metabolic engineering is the most advanced strategy to enhance the SM productivity of plant cell cultures. Its principle is based on the manipulation/optimization of genetic and regulatory processes within cells to increase the synthesis of a desired metabolite [48]. Nevertheless, the overexpression of some genes may not always improve production [9].

IMPACT OF ABIOTIC STRESS ON *IN VITRO* PRODUCTION OF SECONDARY METABOLITES

Drought, salinity, soil nutrient limitation, ultraviolet radiation, and temperature are some examples of abiotic stresses that plants face every day and that have been exacerbated by climate change. In this sense, many studies at physiological, biochemical, and metabolic levels, have been performed to understand plant responses to these stress factors and to stimulate the production of SM for many potential applications. In this section, an update on studies about metabolic responses of *in vitro* cultures to the five abovementioned abiotic stresses is provided.

Drought

Drought is one of the most significant stresses [10] that affects plant growth and development, photosynthesis, cellular dehydration, and other metabolic processes [14]. This abiotic stress is characterized by water deficit, usually accompanied by solar radiation and high temperatures [10]. Among other osmotic agents (*e.g.*, sorbitol and mannitol) used *in vitro* to induce drought stress, polyethylene glycol (PEG) is the most applied (Table **1**). PEG is an inert, non-ionic, and non-toxic chemical available in a wide range of molecular weights (*e.g.*, 4000, 6000, 8000). In contrast to sorbitol and mannitol (penetrating non-ionic agents) [49], PEG is cell impermeable due to its high molecular weight and, therefore, does not cause permanent damage to cell walls. Moreover, this compound is known to cause severe water potential effects [50] and, thus, is used by many authors to study the physiological, biochemical, and metabolic responses of plants to drought stress. In many recent reports, this osmotic agent caused a positive outcome on SM accumulation (Table **1**). It induced higher total phenolic contents, in comparison with the controls, in *Stevia rebaudiana* Bertoni [51], *Lathyrus sativus* L [52], *Thymus vulgaris* L [53], *Carum copticum* L. [54], and *Allium hirtifolium* Boiss [55]. An improvement of allicin [55] and artemisinin [56] production was also obtained in *A. hirtifolium* and *Artemisia aucheri* Boiss shoot cultures, respectively. Using CSC, PEG also improved phenylethanoid glycosides production *Cistanche deserticola* Y. C. Ma [57], the biosynthesis of taxol in *Taxus chinensis* Rehder [58], and the accumulation of steviol glycosides in *S. rebaudiana* [59]. The concentration of rebaudioside A and stevioside in *S. rebaudiana* shoot cultures that experienced drought (PEG 6000 4%) for four weeks was twice that obtained in the control without PEG [51]. Contrarily, in another report using the same species and culture type, these steviol glycosides had a drastic reduction in their production after 21 days of PEG 6000 stress (2.5, 5, 7 and 10%) [4].

It has been found that the PEG concentration greatly affects SM production. The PEG percentage of 5% provoked the highest increase of SM production in callus cultures of *S. rebaudiana* (7-fold increase of rebaudioside A and stevioside) [59], *Pilocarpus microphyllus* Stapf ex Wardleworth (3-fold increase of pilocarpine) [60], *Trigonella foenum-graecum* L. (2-fold increase of trigonelline) [61], and *Salvia leriifolia* Benth (4-fold increase of caffeic acid and salvianolic acid B) [62]. In callus cultures of *Taxus baccata* L., the highest contents (2.5 times more than in the control) of taxol and 10-deacetylbaccatin III were obtained with 3% and 2% PEG, respectively [63]. Additionally, PEG effects also vary with treatment duration. The production of hypericin and pseudohypericin in seedlings of *Hypericum adenotrichum* Spach increased after 15 days of treatment with 10 g/L PEG, but when the treatment duration increased to 30 days the hypericin levels were negatively affected [64].

Table 1. Effect of drought on secondary metabolites production in *in vitro* cultures of several species.

Drought Agent	Culture Type	Plant Species	Changes in Secondary Metabolites Accumulation	References
Polyethylene glycol	Callus culture	*Carum copticum* L.	Thymol, ρ-cymene ↑; carvacrol, β-caryophyllene, β-pinene, sabinene, γ-terpinene ↓	[54]
		Pilocarpus microphyllus Stapf ex Wardleworth	Pilocarpine ↑	[60]
		Salvia leriifolia Benth	Rosmarinic and caffeic acids, salvianolic acid B ↑	[62]
		Stevia rebaudiana Bertoni	Rebaudioside A, stevioside ↑	[59]
		Taxus baccata L.	10-Deacetylbaccatin III, taxol ↑	[63]
		Thymus vulgaris L.	γ-Terpinene, ρ-cymene and geraniol ↑; thymol, carvacrol ↓	[53]
		Trachyspermum ammi (L.) Sprague	ρ-Cymene, α-thujene, α and β-pinene, α-terpinene, γ-terpinene, β-phellandrene ↑; sabinene ↓	[65]
		Trigonella foenum-graecum L.	Trigonelline ↑	[61]
	Cell suspension culture	*Cistanche deserticola* Y. C. Ma	Phenylethanoid glycosides ↑	[57]
		Taxus chinensis Rehder	Taxol ↑	[58]
	Seed culture	*Hypericum adenotrichum* Spach	Hypericin, pseudohypericin ↑	[64]
		Verbascum sinuatum L.	Anthocyanins ↑	[69]
		Zea mays L.	Phenolics ↓	[70]
	Shoot culture	*Allium hirtifolium* Boiss.	Allicin ↑	[55]
		Artemisia aucheri Boiss.	Artemisinin ↑	[56]
		Lathyrus sativus L.	Phenolics ↑	[52]
		Stevia rebaudiana Bertoni	Rebaudioside A, stevioside ↑	[51]
		Stevia rebaudiana Bertoni	Rebaudioside A, stevioside, steviol, α and β-pinene, sabinene, α-terpinolene, limonene, α-terpinolene, 3-heptanol, 3-hexen-1-ol, 7-octen-4-ol, 1-octen-3-ol, ʟ-linalool, α-bergamotene, β-caryophyllene, *trans*-β-farnesene, *cis*-α-bisabolene, junipene, (+)-calarene, α-humulene, cadinene, β-cubebene, α-cadinol ↓	[4]
Mannitol	Seed culture	*Silybum marianum* L.	Phenolics, flavonoids ↑	[66]

(Table 1) cont.....

Drought Agent	Culture Type	Plant Species	Changes in Secondary Metabolites Accumulation	References
Mannitol and sorbitol	Callus culture	*Taxus baccata* L.	10-Deacetylbaccatin III, taxol ↑	[68]
Sorbitol	Hairy root culture	*Salvia miltiorrhiza* Bunge	Tanshinones ↑	[67]

↑: increase, ↓: decrease

Regarding essential oils, there is contradictory information in the literature about their accumulation and constituents under drought stress. PEG treatment showed a positive effect on the essential oil yield of *Trachyspermum ammi* (L.) Sprague (α-thujene, α and β-pinene, and γ-terpinene) [65], *T. vulgaris* (ρ-cymene, geraniol, and γ-terpinene) [53] and *C. copticum* (thymol and ρ-cymene) [54]. On the other hand, drought had a negative impact in essential oils production of *S. rebaudiana* (α and β-pinene, sabinene, α-terpinolene, limonene, α-terpinolene, 3-heptanol, 3-hexen-1-ol, 7-octen-4-ol, 1-octen-3-ol, L-linalool, α-bergamotene, β-caryophyllene, *trans*-β-farnesene, *cis*-α-bisabolene, junipene, (+)-calarene, α-humulene, cadinene, β-cubebene, α-cadinol) [4], *T. vulgaris* (thymol and carvacrol) [53] and *C. copticum* (carvacrol, β-caryophyllene, β-pinene, sabinene, γ-terpinene) [54].

Regarding other osmotic agents, it was observed that mannitol increased the phenolic and flavonoid accumulation in seed cultures of *Silybum marianum* L [66]. and sorbitol enhanced the yield of tanshinone in hairy root cultures of *Salvia miltiorrhiza* Bunge [67]. Both individual uses of mannitol and sorbitol boosted the production of 10-deacetylbaccatin III and taxol in callus cultures of *T. baccata* [68]. Phenylalanine ammonia lyase (PAL), a key enzyme in the synthesis of phenolic compounds, is considered a biochemical marker of plant defense against abiotic stresses, and its activity was significantly improved by increasing drought intensity [68].

In most of the reported cases, the increase in SM accumulation is accompanied by a decrease in plant growth and development [4, 52, 53]. When plants are exposed to stress conditions, they usually accumulate cellular osmolytes (*e.g.*, proline, glycine betaine, polyols, sugar alcohols) to help cells keep the turgor pressure and soluble sugars (mannitol, sorbitol, sucrose, glutamate, oligosaccharides, *etc.*) in their cytosol [3, 53 - 56, 62, 68 - 70]. Some authors have shown that the antioxidant activity of the extracts increased in plants exposed to water stress [53, 66], likewise the activity of antioxidant enzymes [52, 54, 55, 62, 63, 65, 66]. This antioxidant status is indicative of possible oxidative stress occurring in the cells, which is also evidenced by the enhanced levels of membrane lipid peroxidation and hydrogen peroxide (H_2O_2) that occurs in cultures submitted to drought conditions [52, 53, 55, 61 - 63, 68]. Drought stress also changes the pigment concentration in several species. A reduction in chlorophyll content was reported in *L. sativus* [52], *T. vulgaris* [53], *C. copticum* [54], *Zea mays* L [70], and *A. hirtifolium* [55].

Salinity

Salt stress is a great obstacle to plant growth around the world. The problem of this stress arises due to inorganic salt excess and poor quality of irrigation water. The high salt concentration changes the soil texture, decreasing porosity, aeration, and water conductance [5]. Besides inducing osmotic stress, salinity generates ionic toxicity associated with excessive Cl^- and Na^+ uptake, which leads to Ca^{2+}, K^+, and NO_3^- deficiency and other nutrient imbalances. Moreover, excess accumulation of Cl^- and Na^+ ions causes a higher generation of ROS and, consequently, higher oxidative damage [5, 52]. One of the primary ROS compounds generated under oxidative stress is H_2O_2 and, generally, extra amounts of ROS enhance lipid peroxidation, resulting in higher contents of malondialdehyde (MDA), an indicator of lipid peroxidation. Many authors have reported the highest accumulation of H_2O_2 and MDA in salt-stressed plants [71 - 74]. Antioxidant enzymes are crucial to neutralize produced ROS in stressed plants, whereby higher enzymatic activities indicate superior ROS detoxification and higher capability to survive. Several authors have demonstrated higher enzymatic antioxidant activities in plants exposed to salinity [73 - 77]. Also, the antioxidant capacity dropped in plants grown at higher concentrations of NaCl [52, 71, 72, 78 - 80]. Overall, at lower NaCl concentrations, it is possible to increase SM production without substantial cellular damage [75]. Similarly to drought, salinity leads to plants' poor growth and development [4, 52, 74, 81], reduction in chlorophyll contents [49, 52, 73, 82] and accumulation of a diversity of osmoprotectants [72 - 74, 82].

The accumulation of SM in response to NaCl was reported by several authors (Table **2**). The highest levels of phenolic compounds were recorded in cultures of several species grown on a medium with NaCl [71, 72, 77, 78, 80, 82, 83]. The maximum accumulation of 20-hydroxyecdysone in shoot cultures of *Spinacia oleracea* L [74]. and of solasodine in callus cultures of *Solanum nigrum* L [84]. was obtained in a medium with 200 mM and 150 mM NaCl, respectively. Using 100 mM NaCl [79], achieved the highest amount of rebaudioside A and stevioside in shoot cultures of *S. rebaudiana*. The largest levels of glucosinolates were also obtained in seed cultures under 100 mM NaCl treatment [80, 85]. With a lower NaCl amount (25 mM) [4, 76, 60] obtained the greatest contents of steviol in *S. rebaudiana*, vincristine in *Catharanthus roseus* L. (G), and pilocarpine in *P. microphyllus*, respectively. On the other hand, the same NaCl amount induced a decrease in rebaudioside A and stevioside levels in *S. rebaudiana* [4]. Chalcone synthase is a key enzyme of the phenylpropanoid route, which plays an important role in the production of SM. The highest expression of the chalcone synthase gene in the tissues of *in vitro* propagated *Coelogyne ovalis* Lindl was observed at 100 μM of NaCl treatment [83].

Table 2. Effect of salinity (NaCl) on secondary metabolites production in *in vitro* cultures of several species.

Culture Type	Plant Species	Changes in Secondary Metabolites Accumulation	References
Callus culture	*Carthamus tinctorius* L.	Phenolics, flavonoids ↑	[72]
	Carum copticum L.	1,8-Cineol, terpinolene, α-compheonelal, borneol, candinol, β-caryophyllene, germacrene D ↑	[77]
	Nigella sativa L.	Phenolics, flavonoids, anthocyanins ↑	[71]
	Pilocarpus microphyllus Stapf ex Wardleworth	Pilocarpine ↑	[60]
	Solanum nigrum L.	Solasodine ↑	[84]
Seed culture	*Brassica oleracea* var. *italica*	Glucoerucin, glucoalyssin, glucobrassicin, 4-hydroxy glucobrassicin, neoglucobrassicin ↑	[85]
	Carum copticum L.	Comphene, limonene, mentha-3–8- diene, terpinen-4-ol ↑	[77]
	Coelogyne ovalis Lindl.	Flavonoids, anthocyanins ↑	[83]
	Lepidium sativum L.	Phenolics ↑	[78]
	Raphanus sativus L.	Glucoraphasatin ↑	[80]
Shoot culture	*Catharanthus roseus* L. (G).	Vincristine ↑	[76]
	Lathyrus sativus L.	Phenolics ↑	[52]
	Lippia alba L.	Linalool ↑; eucalyptol ↓	[81]
	Spinacia oleracea L.	20-Hydroxyecdysone ↑	[74]
	Stevia rebaudiana Bertoni	Phenolics ↑	[82]
	Stevia rebaudiana Bertoni	Rebaudioside A, stevioside ↑	[79]
	Stevia rebaudiana Bertoni	Steviol, α-terpinolene ↑; rebaudioside A, stevioside, α and β-pinene, limonene ↓	[4]
	Swertia chirata Buch.-Ham.	Mangiferin, amaroswerin, amarogentin ↑	[75]

↑: increase, ↓: decrease.

The amounts of the main compounds of essential oils are differentially affected by salinity. For example, β-pinene occurred at a relative abundance of 63.6% in controls of *S. rebaudiana* shoots, however, this content was reduced to 40.1% in the plants grown with 100 mM NaCl. On the other hand, α-terpinolene was significantly higher in NaCl-treated cultures [4]. The highest contents of comphene, limonene, menta-3–8- diene, and terpinen-4-ol in seedlings and 1,8-cineol, terpinolene, α-compheonelal, borneol, candinol, β-caryophyllene, and germacrene D in callus of *C. copticum* were obtained also with 100 mM NaCl [77]. In shoot cultures of *Lippia alba* L., 60 mM NaCl increased linalool concentration but reduced eucalyptol levels [81].

Nutrients Deficiency

The plants' growth and development depend upon adequate amounts of nutrients. As previously mentioned, nutrient deficiency arises from the combination of other stresses, such as drought and salinity. These abiotic factors affect the availability and transport of nutrients, such as Ca^{2+}, K^+, and NO_3^-, mainly due to Na^+ and Cl^- competition [5]. The accumulation of SM in plants depends on nutrients provided to the growing cells and, usually, when plants face some stress, the production of SM enhances [3]. This increased SM accumulation occurs because growth is more inhibited than photosynthesis and, in this way, fixed carbon is mainly allocated to SM production [10]. In other words, plants allocate the extra carbon that is not utilized in the Calvin cycle to synthesize carbon-based SM [5]. In this way, macronutrients, which include nitrogen, potassium, and phosphorus, are particularly relevant for plant growth and SM biosynthesis, while micronutrients are involved in SM biosynthetic routes as enzyme activators [3]. Nitrogen is, definitely, the most studied nutrient in *in vitro* models of nutrient limitation. This macronutrient, besides being vital for plants' growth and development, is the major component of proteins, nucleic acids, and chlorophyll [86]. Its importance in plant development is evidenced in some studies, in which the limitation of nitrogen induced a decrease in growth index and biomass production [87, 88]. Moreover, this important nutrient may also influence secondary metabolism. Higher PAL activity has been found in nitrogen-stressed plants, such as *Castilleja tenuiflora* Benth [86, 87, 89] and *Ocimum basilicum* L [90]. Also, it was observed that the activity of glucose 6-phosphate dehydrogenase, another enzyme involved in the biosynthesis of phenolic compounds, is enhanced under conditions of nutritional deficiency [91].

Many reports have demonstrated that nutritional stress increased total phenolic contents in *in vitro* cultures of several species [86, 87, 89 - 91] (Table **3**). Furthermore, nitrogen limitation stimulates verbascoside, isoverbascoside, and aucubin production in *C. tenuiflora* [86, 87, 89], chlorogenic acid and isoorientin in *Cecropia obtusifolia* Bertol [88], rosmarinic and caffeic acids in *O. basilicum* [90], pilocarpine in *P. microphyllus* [60] and canophyllol in *Hippocratea excelsa* Kunth [92]. On the other hand, nitrogen deficiency decreased the biosynthesis of rosmarinic acid in *Satureja khuzistanica* Jamzad [93], canavanine in *Sutherlandia frutescens* L. R. Br [94], and hyoscyamine in *Datura stramonium* L [95].

Table 3. Effect of nutrient deficiency on secondary metabolite production in *in vitro* cultures of several species.

Nutrient Limitation	Culture Type	Plant Species	Changes in Secondary Metabolites Accumulation	References
Calcium	Callus culture	*Bellis perennis* L.	Chlorogenic, caffeic, rosmarinic, ferulic and ρ-coumaric acids, rutin hydrate ↑	[96]
	Hairy root culture	*Datura stramonium* L.	Hyoscyamine ↓	[95]
	Root culture	*Hyoscyamus niger* L.	Hyoscyamine ↑; scopolamine ↓	[97]
Iron	Root culture	*Hyoscyamus niger* L.	Hyoscyamine, scopolamine ↓	[97]
Magnesium	Callus culture	*Bellis perennis* L.	Chlorogenic, caffeic, rosmarinic, and ρ-coumaric acids, rutin hydrate ↑	[96]
	Root culture	*Hyoscyamus niger* L.	Hyoscyamine, scopolamine ↓	[97]
Nitrogen	Callus culture	*Hippocratea excelsa* Kunth	Canophyllol ↑	[92]
		Pilocarpus microphyllus Stapf ex Wardleworth	Pilocarpine ↑	[60]
	Cell suspension culture	*Cecropia obtusifolia* Bertol.	Chlorogenic acid, isoorientin ↑	[88]
		Satureja khuzistanica Jamzad	Rosmarinic acid ↓	[93]
	Hairy root culture	*Datura stramonium* L.	Hyoscyamine ↓	[95]
	Seed culture	*Ocimum basilicum* L.	Rosmarinic, caffeic acids ↑	[90]
	Shoot culture	*Castilleja tenuiflora* Benth	Verbascoside, isoverbascoside, aucubin ↑	[87]
		Castilleja tenuiflora Benth	Verbascoside, isoverbascoside ↑	[89]
		Castilleja tenuiflora Benth	Aucubin, bartsioside, tenuifloroside, 8-epiloganin, quercetin ↑	[86]
		Sutherlandia frutescens L. R. Br.	Canavanine ↓	[94]
Phosphorus	Callus culture	*Pilocarpus microphyllus* Stapf ex Wardleworth	Pilocarpine ↑	[60]
Potassium	Callus culture	*Pilocarpus microphyllus* Stapf ex Wardleworth	Pilocarpine ↓	[60]

↑: increase, ↓: decrease.

Magnesium has a crucial role in several functions in plants, such as fixation of CO_2, ATP synthesis, photosynthetic product assimilation, and chlorophyll development, and calcium is a ubiquitous signaling molecule that participates in several signal transduction routes in plant cells [3]. It has been observed that deficiencies in these nutrients may result in either increased [96] or decreased production of SM [95, 97] (Table **3**). The authors [97] studied the influence of calcium, magnesium, and iron limitation on tropane alkaloids (hyoscyamine and scopolamine) accumulation in root cultures of *Hyoscyamus niger* L. and observed that calcium deficiency improved hyoscyamine production. Also, potassium and iron deficiency reduced the concentration of the alkaloids pilocarpine [60] and hyoscyamine [97]. Phosphorus is another macronutrient involved in primary metabolism, and its deficiency could promote the production of phenolics, such as pilocarpine, in callus cultures of *P. microphyllus* [60]. Overall, there is a tendency to accumulate higher amounts of SM under nutritional limitations. This stress also causes a decrease in total chlorophyll contents [86, 87, 89], proline accumulation [91, 98], and some oxidative stress markers [89, 90, 92, 96].

Ultraviolet Radiation

Another important abiotic factor involved in metabolic production in plants is radiation. UV radiation, a form of non-ionizing radiation that is emitted by the sun or artificial sources, can redirect the carbon flux resulting in alterations in the production of several SM [6]. UV light can be divided into three ranges: UV-A (315–400 nm), UV-B (280–315 nm), and UV-C (100–280 nm). Earth's surface receives more than 70% of UV-A and about 20% of UV-B; UV-C is not received because it is completely absorbed by the stratospheric ozone. Although UV-B is in minor quantities, it has enough energy to cause photochemical damage to cellular DNA, producing serious biological damage [99]. For these reasons, the effects of UV-B are the most studied, and it has been demonstrated that this radiation could change the secondary metabolism, depending on the duration and intensity of the exposure [100]. In high doses, UV-B triggers severe problems in the photosynthetic system, nucleic acids and proteins, and, eventually, cell death [5], also decreasing the production of phenolics [100]. In contrast, several plants showed resistance against moderated UV-B radiation, being highly efficient in the biosynthesis and accumulation of phenolics [101 - 107] (Table **4**). Significant accumulation of several compounds, such as scopoletin, chlorogenic and gallic acids, rutin [106], withanolide A, withanone [105], apigenin [108, 109], camptothecin [104], scopolamine [110], isoorientin, orientin [101], isovitexin, vitexin [101, 108], artemisinin [103], ajmalicine, serpentine, lochnericine, tabersonine [111, 112], catharanthine [112, 113], ρ-coumaric, *trans*-ferulic and salicylic acids, rutin hyrate, and luteolin [109] were obtained in *in vitro* cultures of different species exposed to UV-B radiation (Table **4**).

Table 4. Effect of UV radiation on secondary metabolites production in *in vitro* cultures of several species.

UV Radiation	Culture Type	Plant Species	Changes in Secondary Metabolites Accumulation	References
UV-A	Callus culture	*Galega officinalis* L.	Apigenin, rutin hydrate, luteolin, p-coumaric, *trans*-ferulic and salicylic acids ↑; naringenin, genistein ↓	[109]
		Schisandra chinensis (Turcz.) Baill.	Angeoyl-/tigloylgomisin H and Q, benzoylgomisin P, deoxyschisandrin, gomisin A, schisandrin ↓	[125]
	Shoot culture	*Phyllanthus tenellus* Roxb.	Geraniin, ellagic acid ↑	[114]
UV-B	Callus culture	*Echium orientale* L.	Rosmarinic, chlorogenic and ferulic acids, quercetin ↑	[107]
		Galega officinalis L.	Apigenin, rutin hydrate, luteolin, p-coumaric, *trans*-ferulic and salicylic acids ↑; naringenin, genistein ↓	[109]
		Ginkgo biloba L.	Flavonoids ↑	[102]
		Jatropha curcas L.	Apigenin, vitexin, isovitexin ↑	[108]
		Passiflora quadrangularis L.	Isoorientin, orientin, isovitexin, vitexin ↑	[101]
	Cell suspension culture	*Camptotheca acuminata* Decne.	Camptothecin ↑	[104]
		Catharanthus roseus L.	Catharanthine ↑	[113]
	Hairy root culture	*Anisodus luridus* Link	Scopolamine ↑	[110]
		Catharanthus roseus L.	Ajmalicine, serpentine, catharanthine, lochnericine, tabersonine ↑; hörhammericine ↓	[111, 112]
	Shoot culture	*Artemisia annua* L.	Artemisinin ↑	[103]
		Deschampsia antarctica Desv.	Scopoletin, chlorogenic and gallic acids, rutin ↑	[106]
		Echium orientale L.	Rosmarinic acid, quercetin ↑	[107]
		Physalis peruviana L.	Withanolide A, withanone ↑	[105]
		Turnera diffusa Willd	Phenolics ↓	[100]

(Table 4) cont.....

UV Radiation	Culture Type	Plant Species	Changes in Secondary Metabolites Accumulation	References
UV-C	Callus culture	*Galega officinalis* L.	Rutin hydrate, luteolin, ρ-coumaric, *trans*-ferulic and salicylic acids ↑; naringenin, genistein ↓	[109]
		Lepidium sativum L.	Caffeic, ferulic vanillic, ρ-coumaric, sinapic, protocatechuic and chlorogenic acids, quercetin, kaempferol ↑	[115]
		Ocimum basilicum L. var *purpurascens*	Rosmarinic, chichoric and caffeic acids, cynadin, peonidin ↑	[118]
		Pyrostegia venusta (Ker Gawl.) Miers	Verbascoside, isoverbascoside leucosceptoside A ↑	[126]
	Cell suspension culture	*Morus alba* L.	Mulberroside A ↑; oxyresveratrol, resveratrol, rutin ↓	[127]
	Meristematic cell cultures	*Catharanthus roseus* (L.) G. Don	Catharanthine, vinblastine, vincristine, vindoline ↑	[117]
	Shoot culture	*Hypericum perforatum* L.	Chlorogenic acid ↑; quercetin, pseudohypericin ↓	[116]

↑: increase, ↓: decrease

High production of several phenolics, alkaloids and anthocyanins has also been obtained in plants stressed with UV-C radiation (Table **4**). Similarly, apigenin, rutin hyrate, luteolin, ρ-coumaric, *trans*-ferulic and salicylic acids [109], geraniin, and ellagic acid [114] contents were significantly improved by UV-A radiation in many species. The authors [109] tested the three types of UV radiation (UV-A, UV-B, and UV-C) for 15, 30, and 60 min and obtained the highest increase (50.63%) on total phenolics with UV-C for 30 min. Also, callus cultures of *Lepidium sativum* L. were exposed to UV-C radiation for different periods (10, 30, 60, 90, 120, and 150 min), and significant improvements in phytochemical contents were obtained, in comparison with the control, in all treatments, although the maximum phenolics accumulation occurred at 60 min, followed by 30 min [115]. These results reinforce the idea that moderated UV exposures are more beneficial for SM accumulation. Another factor that seems important to achieve higher contents of SM is the recovery of plants after UV exposure. It has been demonstrated in *Echium orientale* L. that the biosynthesis of rosmarinic, chlorogenic and ferulic acids, and quercetin increased upon UV-B exposure, however the highest contents of ferulic and rosmarinic acids raised even more after one week of recovery [107].

The mechanism behind UVs and plant SM production is still not clear, however, some studies have reported an increased PAL activity in response to UV exposure

[102, 115]. Likewise, the genes belonging to MVA/MEP and isoprenoid biosynthetic pathways showed an over-expression under 4 h of UV-B [103]. UVs activated the generation of ROS in cells of *C. roseus* [113], *A. annua* [103], *Turnera diffusa* Willd [100], and *Galega officinalis* L. [109]. To scavenge the UVs induced ROS, plants depend on their antioxidative defense machinery, in which antioxidant enzymes, such as peroxidase, superoxide dismutase, catalase, and glutathione reductase, have a key role in protecting cells from oxidative toxicity. Significant overexpression of these enzymes was observed in plants stressed with UV-B and C [103, 115]. Antioxidant [115 - 118], anticancer [117], and enzymatic and antidiabetic [115] activities were significantly enhanced in cultures exposed to UV-C.

Temperature

Elevated and low temperatures affect various molecular, biochemical, and physiological parameters of the plants [5]. Negative impacts on plant growth and productivity have been exhibited in plants grown in extreme temperatures, being 20–25 °C as the ideal temperature range to achieve the maximum biomass accumulation in many species [119 - 122]. The authors [120] obtained the highest total phenolic, flavonoid, and eleutherosides B and E1 contents in somatic embryos of *Eleutherococcus senticosus* (Rupr. & Maxim.) Maxim. at 24 °C. The highest production of ginsenoside [119], pinostrobin [121], and ascorbic acid [122] was achieved when the cultures of different species were incubated at 25 °C. Extreme temperatures caused oxidative stress in *E. senticosus* [120] and *G. officinalis* [109]. Due to these alterations, SM production is also frequently affected (Table **5**). Low-temperature treatment (4–15 °C) resulted in the highest accumulation of several pharmacologically important SM, such as genistein, apigenin, galangin [123], pinoresinol, cinnamic and caffeic acids, quercitol [122], pinocembrin [121], ρ-coumaric acid, luteolin, and rutin [109]. High (45 °C) and low (4 °C) temperatures did not significantly affect the total phenolic content and antioxidant activity of moringa callus. Nevertheless, the accumulation of chlorogenic, caffeic, and ρ-coumaric acids increased in heat-stressed callus but decreased in cultures exposed to cold for 7 days [123]. Also, a significant increase was noted in withaferin A, withanolide A and withanone [105], and naringenin [109] contents after exposure at 45 °C. The authors [124] tested the influence of 40, 45, and 50 °C in the release of betalaines from *Beta vulgaris* L. hairy roots and observed that it was directly proportional to the temperature increase. On the other hand, extreme temperatures showed to have negative impacts on the biosynthesis of some SM (*e.g.*, apigenin, genistein, myricetin, kaempferol, 3-O-β- D-glucopyranosyl, 3,3-dimethylallyl and phenyl caffeates) [109, 123]. Overall, revised studies indicate that the differences in compound production may be related to the ideal activity of enzymes at distinct temperatures [121].

Table 5. Effect of temperature on secondary metabolites production in *in vitro* cultures of several species.

Temperature	Culture Type	Plant Species	Changes in Secondary Metabolites Accumulation	References
4 °C	Callus culture	*Galega officinalis* L.	ρ-Coumaric acid, luteolin, rutin hyrate ↑; apigenin, genistein, naringenin ↓	[109]
		Moringa oleifera Lam.	Genistein, apigenin, galangin ↑; chlorogenic, caffeic and ρ-coumaric acids, rutin, myricetin, 3-O-β-D-glucopyranosyl, kaempferol ↓	[123]
15 °C	Cell suspension culture	*Boesenbergia rotunda* (L.) Mansf. Kulturpfl.	Pinocembrin ↑	[121]
	Shoot culture	*Ajuga bracteosa* Wall. ex. Benth.	Pinoresinol, cinnamic and caffeic acids, quercitol ↑	[122]
20 °C	Cell suspension culture	*Boesenbergia rotunda* (L.) Mansf. Kulturpfl.	Cardamonin ↑	[121]
24 °C	Somatic embryogenesis	*Eleutherococcus senticosus* (Rupr. & Maxim.) Maxim.	Eleutherosides B and E1; chlorogenic acid ↑	[120]
25 °C	Cell suspension culture	*Boesenbergia rotunda* (L.) Mansf. Kulturpfl.	Pinostrobin ↑	[121]
		Cynanchum wilfordii Hemsley	Gagaminine ↓	[128]
	Hairy root cultures	*Panax ginseng* C. A. Mayer	Ginsenoside ↑	[119]
	Shoot culture	*Ajuga bracteosa* Wall. ex. Benth.	Ascorbic acid ↑	[122]
30 °C	Cell suspension culture	*Boesenbergia rotunda* (L.) Mansf. Kulturpfl.	Panduratin A ↑	[121]
45 °C	Callus culture	*Galega officinalis* L.	Naringenin ↑; genistein, luteolin ↓	[109]
		Moringa oleifera Lam.	Chlorogenic, caffeic, ρ-coumaric acids, myricetin, chrysin ↑; 3,3-dimethylallyl and phenyl caffeates, rutin, galangin ↓	[123]
	Shoot culture	*Physalis peruviana* L.	Withaferin A, withanolide A and withanone ↑	[105]
50 °C	Hairy root cultures	*Beta vulgaris* L.	Betalains ↑	[124]

↑: increase, ↓: decrease

CONCLUDING REMARKS

Plants produce a high diversity of SM that have important roles in protecting plants from stress conditions. Many of these compounds have biologically active properties and, therefore, have great applicability in several industries. Abiotic stress factors, such as drought, temperature, salinity, UV radiation, and nutrient limitation, have a significant impact on the normal physiology of plants. Reviewed results indicate that although these factors usually negatively impact biomass production *in vitro*, they markedly improve the production of SM from different classes. Though abiotic factors at high intensity may have an inhibitory effect on metabolite accumulation and, thus, it is essential to know the ideal conditions for SM biosynthesis for each species in particular. PTC is a useful tool to understand plant response to abiotic stress factors, which is particularly important in the actual scenario of climate change conditions and, using these techniques, it is possible to increase the production of high-value SM as well. Besides, it allows the integration of elicitors, and it permits to optimization of other factors such as media composition, plant growth regulators, duration, and age of culture. Nevertheless, there is a need to understand the underlying mechanism of elicitors, and for that, it is crucial to a strong integration of functional genomics, namely transcriptomics, proteomics, and metabolomics.

ABBREVIATIONS

CSC   cell suspension culture

MDA   malondialdehyde

PAL   phenylalanine ammonia lyase

PEG   polyethylene glycol

PTC   plant tissue culture

ROS   reactive oxygen species

SM   secondary metabolites

ACKNOWLEDGEMENTS

This research was funded by National Funds through FCT-Foundation for Science and Technology under the Projects UIDB/05183/2020 and LA/P/0121/2020. Inês Mansinhos and Sandra Gonçalves (Grant SFRH/BD/145243/2019 and CEECINST/00052/2021) acknowledge the financial support from FCT.

REFERENCES

[1]   Lehner F, Deser C, Sanderson BM. Future risk of record-breaking summer temperatures and its mitigation. Clim Change 2018; 146(3-4): 363-75.
[http://dx.doi.org/10.1007/s10584-016-1616-2]

[2]   Arnell NW, Lowe JA, Challinor AJ, Osborn TJ. Global and regional impacts of climate change at different levels of global temperature increase. Clim Change 2019; 155(3): 377-91.
[http://dx.doi.org/10.1007/s10584-019-02464-z]

[3]   Isah T. Stress and defense responses in plant secondary metabolites production. Biol Res 2019; 52(1): 39.
[http://dx.doi.org/10.1186/s40659-019-0246-3] [PMID: 31358053]

[4]   Magangana TP, Stander MA, Masondo NA, Makunga NP. Steviol glycoside content and essential oil profiles of Stevia rebaudiana Bertoni in response to NaCl and polyethylene glycol as inducers of salinity and drought stress *in vitro*. Plant Cell Tissue Organ Cult 2021; 145(1): 1-18.
[http://dx.doi.org/10.1007/s11240-020-01972-6]

[5]   Mahajan M, Kuiry R, Pal PK. Understanding the consequence of environmental stress for accumulation of secondary metabolites in medicinal and aromatic plants. J Appl Res Med Aromat Plants 2020; 18: 100255.
[http://dx.doi.org/10.1016/j.jarmap.2020.100255]

[6]   Thoma F, Somborn-Schulz A, Schlehuber D, Keuter V, Deerberg G. Effects of light on secondary metabolites in selected leafy greens: A review. Front Plant Sci 2020; 11: 497.
[http://dx.doi.org/10.3389/fpls.2020.00497] [PMID: 32391040]

[7]   Nabi N, Singh S, Saffeullah P. Responses of *in vitro* cell cultures to elicitation: Regulatory role of jasmonic acid and methyl jasmonate: A review *In Vitro* Cell Dev Biol Plant 2021; 57: 341-55.
[http://dx.doi.org/10.1007/s11627-020-10140-6]

[8]   Chandran H, Meena M, Barupal T, Sharma K. Plant tissue culture as a perpetual source for production of industrially important bioactive compounds. Biotechnol Rep 2020; 26: e00450.
[http://dx.doi.org/10.1016/j.btre.2020.e00450] [PMID: 32373483]

[9]   Gonçalves S, Romano A. Production of plant secondary metabolites by using biotechnological tools. Secondary metabolites : Sources and applications. intechopen 2018.
[http://dx.doi.org/10.5772/intechopen.76414]

[10]   Akula R, Ravishankar GA. Influence of abiotic stress signals on secondary metabolites in plants. Plant Signal Behav 2011; 6(11): 1720-31.
[http://dx.doi.org/10.4161/psb.6.11.17613] [PMID: 22041989]

[11]   Adedeji AA, Babalola OO. Secondary metabolites as plant defensive strategy: A large role for small molecules in the near root region. Planta 2020; 252(4): 61.
[http://dx.doi.org/10.1007/s00425-020-03468-1] [PMID: 32965531]

[12]   Nascimento NC, Fett-Neto A G. Plant secondary metabolism and challenges in modifying its operation: An overview. Methods Mol Biol 2010; 643: 1-13.

[13]   Holopainen JK, Virjamo V, Ghimire RP, Blande JD, Julkunen-Tiitto R, Kivimäenpää M. Climate change effects on secondary compounds of forest trees in the northern hemisphere. Front Plant Sci 2018; 9: 1445.
[http://dx.doi.org/10.3389/fpls.2018.01445] [PMID: 30333846]

[14]   Khare S, Singh NB, Singh A, *et al.* Plant secondary metabolites synthesis and their regulations under biotic and abiotic constraints. J Plant Biol 2020; 63(3): 203-16.
[http://dx.doi.org/10.1007/s12374-020-09245-7]

[15]   Guerriero G, Berni R, Muñoz-Sanchez J, *et al.* Production of plant secondary metabolites: Examples, tips and suggestions for biotechnologists. Genes 2018; 9(6): 309.
[http://dx.doi.org/10.3390/genes9060309] [PMID: 29925808]

[16]   Ojha G, Nath Mishra K, Singh H, Kumar Mishra A. Isolation of secondary metabolites from ipomea digitata l. tuber extracts and it's effect on cardiovascular risk parameters. Orient J Chem 2020; 36(1): 76-85.
[http://dx.doi.org/10.13005/ojc/360110]

[17]   Beeby E, Magalhães M, Poças J, *et al.* Secondary metabolites (essential oils) from sand-dune plants induce cytotoxic effects in cancer cells. J Ethnopharmacol 2020; 258: 112803.
[http://dx.doi.org/10.1016/j.jep.2020.112803] [PMID: 32251759]

[18]   Silva JM, Nobre MSC, Albino SL, *et al.* Secondary metabolites with antioxidant activities for the putative treatment of amyotrophic lateral sclerosis (ALS): *Experimental Evidences*. Oxid Med Cell Longev 2020; 2020: 1-22.
[http://dx.doi.org/10.1155/2020/5642029] [PMID: 33299526]

[19]   Khani S, Barar J, Movafeghi A, Omidi Y. Production of anticancer secondary metabolites: Impacts of bioprocess engineering. Biotechnological Production of Plant Secondary Metabolites. eurekaselect 2012; pp. 215-40.

[20]   Fridlender M, Kapulnik Y, Koltai H. Plant derived substances with anti-cancer activity: From folklore to practice. Front Plant Sci 2015; 6: 799.
[http://dx.doi.org/10.3389/fpls.2015.00799] [PMID: 26483815]

[21]   Cragg GM, Newman DJ. Plants as a source of anti-cancer agents. J Ethnopharmacol 2005; 100(1-2): 72-9.
[http://dx.doi.org/10.1016/j.jep.2005.05.011] [PMID: 16009521]

[22]   Stevanato R, Bertelle M, Fabris S. Photoprotective characteristics of natural antioxidant polyphenols. Regul Toxicol Pharmacol 2014; 69(1): 71-7.
[http://dx.doi.org/10.1016/j.yrtph.2014.02.014] [PMID: 24607767]

[23]   Sarkic A, Stappen I. Essential oils and their single compounds in cosmetics :A critical review. Cosmetics 2018; 5(1): 11.
[http://dx.doi.org/10.3390/cosmetics5010011]

[24]   Gonçalves S, Romano A. Aromatic oils from forest and their application non-timber forest products : Food, healthcare and industrial applications. In: Husen A, Bachheti R K, Bachheti A, Eds. Springer 2021.

[25]   Martillanes S, Rocha-Pimienta J, Cabrera-Bañegil M, Martín-Vertedor D, Delgado-Adámez J. Application of phenolic compounds for food preservation: Food additive and active packaging. Phenolic Compounds : Biological Activity. intechopen 2017.

[26]   Ofosu FK, Daliri EBM, Elahi F, Chelliah R, Lee BH, Oh DH. New insights on the use of polyphenols as natural preservatives and their emerging safety concerns. Front Sustain Food Syst 2020; 4: 525810.
[http://dx.doi.org/10.3389/fsufs.2020.525810]

[27]   Yue W, Ming Q, Lin B, *et al.* Medicinal plant cell suspension cultures: pharmaceutical applications and high-yielding strategies for the desired secondary metabolites. Crit Rev Biotechnol 2016; 36(2): 215-32.
[http://dx.doi.org/10.3109/07388551.2014.923986] [PMID: 24963701]

[28]   Heinig U, Jennewein S. Taxol: A complex diterpenoid natural product with an evolutionarily obscure origin. African j biotech 2009; 8: 1370-85.

[29]   Ram M, Misra H. Metabolic engineering for the production of plant therapeutic compounds medicinal and aromatic plants. In: Aftab T, Hakeem KR, Eds. Academic Press 2021; pp. 169-207.

[30]   Mutanda I, Li J, Xu F, Wang Y. Recent advances in metabolic engineering, protein engineering, and transcriptome-guided insights toward synthetic production of taxol. Front Bioeng Biotechnol 2021; 9: 632269.
[http://dx.doi.org/10.3389/fbioe.2021.632269] [PMID: 33614616]

[31]   Sharifi-Rad J, Sureda A, Tenore G, *et al.* Biological activities of essential oils: From plant chemoecology to traditional healing systems. Molecules 2017; 22(1): 70.
[http://dx.doi.org/10.3390/molecules22010070] [PMID: 28045446]

[32]   Dias MI, Sousa MJ, Alves RC, Ferreira ICFR. Exploring plant tissue culture to improve the production

of phenolic compounds: A review. Ind Crops Prod 2016; 82: 9-22.
[http://dx.doi.org/10.1016/j.indcrop.2015.12.016]

[33]   Gutierrez-Valdes N, Häkkinen ST, Lemasson C, *et al.* Hairy root cultures :A versatile tool with multiple applications. Front Plant Sci 2020; 11: 33.
[http://dx.doi.org/10.3389/fpls.2020.00033] [PMID: 32194578]

[34]   Ha LT, Pawlicki-Jullian N, Pillon-Lequart M, Boitel-Conti M, Duong HX, Gontier E. Hairy root cultures of panax vietnamensis, a promising approach for the production of ocotillol-type ginsenosides. Plant Cell Tissue Organ Cult 2016; 126(1): 93-103.
[http://dx.doi.org/10.1007/s11240-016-0980-y]

[35]   Perassolo M, Cardillo AB, Mugas ML, Núñez Montoya SC, Giulietti AM, Rodríguez Talou J. Enhancement of anthraquinone production and release by combination of culture medium selection and methyl jasmonate elicitation in hairy root cultures of rubia tinctorum. Ind Crops Prod 2017; 105: 124-32.
[http://dx.doi.org/10.1016/j.indcrop.2017.05.010]

[36]   Patra N, Srivastava AK. Artemisinin production by plant hairy root cultures in gas- and liquid-phase bioreactors. Plant Cell Rep 2016; 35(1): 143-53.
[http://dx.doi.org/10.1007/s00299-015-1875-9] [PMID: 26441056]

[37]   Shajahan A, Thilip C, Faizal K, *et al.* An efficient hairy root system for withanolide production in withania somnifera (l.) dunal production of plant derived natural compounds through hairy root culture. In: Malik S, Ed. Cham: Springer International Publishing 2017; pp. 133-43.
[http://dx.doi.org/10.1007/978-3-319-69769-7_7]

[38]   Wetterauer B, Wildi E, Wink M. Production of the anticancer compound camptothecin in root and hairy root cultures of ophiorrhiza mungos l. biotechnological approaches for medicinal and aromatic plants: Conservation, genetic improvement and utilization. In: Kumar N, Ed. Singapore: Springer 2018; pp. 303-41.

[39]   Zarev Y, Popova P, Foubert K, *et al.* Biotransformation to produce the anticancer compound colchicoside using cell suspension cultures of astragalus vesicarius plant species. Natural Product Communications 2019; 14(1).
[http://dx.doi.org/10.1177/1934578X1901400108]

[40]   Zhang X, Ye M, Dong Y, *et al.* Biotransformation of bufadienolides by cell suspension cultures of Saussurea involucrata. Phytochemistry 2011; 72(14-15): 1779-85.
[http://dx.doi.org/10.1016/j.phytochem.2011.05.004] [PMID: 21636103]

[41]   Salehi M, Moieni A, Safaie N, Farhadi S. Elicitors derived from endophytic fungi chaetomium globosum and paraconiothyrium brasiliense enhance paclitaxel production in corylus avellana cell suspension culture. Plant Cell Tissue Organ Cult 2019; 136(1): 161-71.
[http://dx.doi.org/10.1007/s11240-018-1503-9]

[42]   Sharma K, Zafar R. Optimization of methyl jasmonate and β-cyclodextrin for enhanced production of taraxerol and taraxasterol in (Taraxacum officinale Weber) cultures. Plant Physiol Biochem 2016; 103: 24-30.
[http://dx.doi.org/10.1016/j.plaphy.2016.02.029] [PMID: 26950922]

[43]   Lambert C, Lemaire J, Auger H, *et al.* Optimize, modulate, and scale-up resveratrol and resveratrol dimers bioproduction in *Vitis labrusca* L. Cell Suspension from Flasks to 20 L Bioreactor. Plants 2019; 8(12): 567.
[http://dx.doi.org/10.3390/plants8120567] [PMID: 31817113]

[44]   Mounika K, Mounika K, Priya JJ, Bhuvaneswari C, Kiranmayee R, Giri A. Optimized conditions for growth kinetics and production of pharmaceutically important Kaempferol from Alpinia purpurata Cell suspensions. Res J Biotechnol 2021; 16: 1-8.

[45]   Shah M, Jan H, Drouet S, *et al.* Chitosan elicitation impacts flavonolignan biosynthesis in *Silybum marianum* (L.) Gaertn cell suspension and enhances antioxidant and anti-inflammatory activities of

cell extracts. Molecules 2021; 26(4): 791.
[http://dx.doi.org/10.3390/molecules26040791] [PMID: 33546424]

[46]   Singh B, Sharma R. Elicitation secondary metabolites of medicinal plants. John Wiley & Sons, Ltd 2020; pp. 1382-406.
[http://dx.doi.org/10.1002/9783527825578.c03-03]

[47]   Singh B, Sharma R. Immobilization secondary metabolites of medicinal plants. John Wiley & Sons, Ltd 2020; pp. 1434-8.
[http://dx.doi.org/10.1002/9783527825578.c03-07]

[48]   Kulkarni R. Metabolic engineering. Resonance 2016; 21(3): 233-7.
[http://dx.doi.org/10.1007/s12045-016-0318-4]

[49]   Mahmoud LM, Dutt M, Shalan AM, *et al.* Silicon nanoparticles mitigate oxidative stress of *in vitro*-derived banana (Musa acuminata 'Grand Nain') under simulated water deficit or salinity stress. S Afr J Bot 2020; 132: 155-63.
[http://dx.doi.org/10.1016/j.sajb.2020.04.027]

[50]   Nair DS, Manjula S. Induction of root endosymbiosis as a highly sustainable and efficient strategy for overproduction of the medicinally important diterpenoid lactone-andrographolide in Andrographis paniculata (Burm. F.) Wall. ex Nees. Ind Crops Prod 2020; 156: 112835.
[http://dx.doi.org/10.1016/j.indcrop.2020.112835]

[51]   Ahmad MA, Javed R, Adeel M, Rizwan M, Yang Y. PEG 6000-Stimulated drought stress improves the attributes of *in vitro* growth, steviol glycosides production, and antioxidant activities in *Stevia rebaudiana* Bertoni. Plants 2020; 9(11): 1552.
[http://dx.doi.org/10.3390/plants9111552] [PMID: 33198205]

[52]   Tokarz B, Wójtowicz T, Makowski W, Jędrzejczyk RJ, Tokarz KM. What is the difference between the response of grass pea (Lathyrus sativus L.) to salinity and drought stress?—a physiological study. Agronomy 2020; 10(6): 833.
[http://dx.doi.org/10.3390/agronomy10060833]

[53]   Razavizadeh R, Farahzadianpoor F, Adabavazeh F, Komatsu S. Physiological and morphological analyses of thymus vulgaris L. *in vitro* cultures under polyethylene glycol (PEG)-induced osmotic stress. *in vitro* Cell Dev Biol Plant 2019; 55(3): 342-57.
[http://dx.doi.org/10.1007/s11627-019-09979-1]

[54]   Razavizadeh R, Karami M. Antioxidant capacity and chemical composition of Carum copticum under PEG treatment. Indian J Plant Physiol 2018; 8: 2321-31.

[55]   Ghassemi-Golezani K, Farhadi N, Nikpour-Rashidabad N. Responses of *in vitro*-cultured Allium hirtifolium to exogenous sodium nitroprusside under PEG-imposed drought stress. Plant Cell Tissue Organ Cult 2018; 133(2): 237-48.
[http://dx.doi.org/10.1007/s11240-017-1377-2]

[56]   Abbaspour J, Ehsanpour AA. Sequential expression of key genes in proline, glycine betaine and artemisinin biosynthesis of artemisia aucheri boiss using salicylic acid under *in vitro* osmotic stress. Biologia 2020; 75(9): 1251-63.
[http://dx.doi.org/10.2478/s11756-020-00507-w]

[57]   Liu CZ, Cheng XY. Enhancement of phenylethanoid glycosides biosynthesis in cell cultures of Cistanche deserticola by osmotic stress. Plant Cell Rep 2008; 27(2): 357-62.
[http://dx.doi.org/10.1007/s00299-007-0443-3] [PMID: 17874242]

[58]   Kim SI, Choi HK, Kim JH, Lee HS, Hong SS. Effect of osmotic pressure on paclitaxel production in suspension cell cultures of taxus chinensis. Enzyme Microb Technol 2001; 28(2-3): 202-9.
[http://dx.doi.org/10.1016/S0141-0229(00)00292-1] [PMID: 11166813]

[59]   Gupta P, Sharma S, Saxena S. Biomass yield and steviol glycoside production in callus and suspension culture of stevia rebaudiana treated with proline and polyethylene glycol. Appl Biochem Biotechnol

2015; 176(3): 863-74.
[http://dx.doi.org/10.1007/s12010-015-1616-0] [PMID: 25940589]

[60] Abreu IN, Sawaya ACHF, Eberlin MN, Mazzafera P. Production of pilocarpine in callus of jaborandi (pilocarpus microphyllus stapf). *in vitro* Cell Dev Biol Plant 2005; 41(6): 806-11.
[http://dx.doi.org/10.1079/IVP2005711]

[61] Alzandi AA, Naguib DM. Effect of hydropriming on trigonella foenum callus growth, biochemical traits and phytochemical components under PEG treatment. Plant Cell Tissue Organ Cult 2020; 141(1): 179-90.
[http://dx.doi.org/10.1007/s11240-020-01778-6]

[62] Hosseini NS, Ghasimi Hagh Z, Khoshghalb H. Morphological, antioxidant enzyme activity and secondary metabolites accumulation in response of polyethylene glycol-induced osmotic stress in embryo-derived plantlets and callus cultures of *Salvia leriifolia* . Plant Cell Tissue Organ Cult 2020; 140(1): 143-55.
[http://dx.doi.org/10.1007/s11240-019-01718-z]

[63] Sarmadi M, Karimi N, Palazón J, Ghassempour A, Mirjalili MH. Improved effects of polyethylene glycol on the growth, antioxidative enzymes activity and taxanes production in a Taxus baccata L. callus culture. Plant Cell Tissue Organ Cult 2019; 137(2): 319-28.
[http://dx.doi.org/10.1007/s11240-019-01573-y]

[64] Yamaner O, Erdag B. Effects of sucrose and polyethylene glycol on hypericins content in Hypericum adenotrichum. EurAsian Journal of Biosciences 2013; 7: 101-10.
[http://dx.doi.org/10.5053/ejobios.2013.7.0.12]

[65] Niazian M, Howyzeh MS, Sadat-Noori SA. Integrative effects of stress- and stress tolerance-inducing elicitors on *in vitro* bioactive compounds of ajowan [Trachyspermum ammi (L.) Sprague] medicinal plant. Plant Cell Tissue Organ Cult 2021; 146(3): 589-604.
[http://dx.doi.org/10.1007/s11240-021-02096-1]

[66] Zahir A, Abbasi B H, Adil M, Anjum S, Zia M. Synergistic effects of drought stress and photoperiods on phenology and secondary metabolism of *Silybum marianum* Appl Biochem Biotechnol 2014; 174: 693-707.

[67] Wu JY, Shi M. Ultrahigh diterpenoid tanshinone production through repeated osmotic stress and elicitor stimulation in fed-batch culture of Salvia miltiorrhiza hairy roots. Appl Microbiol Biotechnol 2008; 78(3): 441-8.
[http://dx.doi.org/10.1007/s00253-007-1332-y] [PMID: 18189134]

[68] Sarmadi M, Karimi N, Palazón J, Ghassempour A, Mirjalili MH. Physiological, biochemical, and metabolic responses of a Taxus baccata L. callus culture under drought stress. *in vitro* Cell Dev Biol Plant 2020; 56(5): 703-17.
[http://dx.doi.org/10.1007/s11627-020-10128-2]

[69] Karamian R, Ghasemlou F, Amiri H. Physiological evaluation of drought stress tolerance and recovery in verbascum sinuatum plants treated with methyl jasmonate, salicylic acid and titanium dioxide nanoparticles plant biosystems. An Int J Dealing with all Aspects of Plant Biology 2020; 154: 277-87.

[70] Moharramnejad S, Sofalian O, Valizadeh M, Asgari A, Shiri M. Proline, glycine betaine, total phenolics and pigment contents in response to osmotic stress in maize seedlings undefined. 2015.

[71] Golkar P, Bakhshi G, Vahabi MR. Phytochemical, biochemical, and growth changes in response to salinity in callus cultures of Nigella sativa L. *in vitro* Cell Dev Biol Plant 2020; 56(2): 247-58.
[http://dx.doi.org/10.1007/s11627-020-10058-z]

[72] Golkar P, Taghizadeh M. *in vitro* evaluation of phenolic and osmolite compounds, ionic content, and antioxidant activity in safflower (Carthamus tinctorius L.) under salinity stress. Plant Cell Tissue Organ Cult 2018; 134(3): 357-68.
[http://dx.doi.org/10.1007/s11240-018-1427-4]

[73] Mozafari A, Ghaderi N, Havas F, Dedejani S. Comparative investigation of structural relationships among morpho-physiological and biochemical properties of strawberry (Fragaria × ananassa Duch.) under drought and salinity stresses: A study based on *in vitro* culture. Sci Hortic 2019; 256: 108601. [http://dx.doi.org/10.1016/j.scienta.2019.108601]

[74] Muchate NS, Rajurkar NS, Suprasanna P, Nikam TD. NaCl induced salt adaptive changes and enhanced accumulation of 20-hydroxyecdysone in the *in vitro* shoot cultures of Spinacia oleracea (L.). Sci Rep 2019; 9(1): 12522. [http://dx.doi.org/10.1038/s41598-019-48737-6] [PMID: 31467324]

[75] Abrol E, Vyas D, Koul S. Metabolic shift from secondary metabolite production to induction of anti-oxidative enzymes during nacl stress in swertia chirata buch.-ham. Acta Physiol Plant 2012; 34(2): 541-6. [http://dx.doi.org/10.1007/s11738-011-0851-4]

[76] Fatima S, Mujib A, Tonk D. NaCl amendment improves vinblastine and vincristine synthesis in *Catharanthus roseus*: A case of stress signalling as evidenced by antioxidant enzymes activities. Plant Cell Tissue Organ Cult 2015; 121(2): 445-58. [http://dx.doi.org/10.1007/s11240-015-0715-5]

[77] Razavizadeh R, Adabavazeh F, Komatsu S. Chitosan effects on the elevation of essential oils and antioxidant activity of Carum copticum L. seedlings and callus cultures under *in vitro* salt stress. J Plant Biochem Biotechnol 2020; 29(3): 473-83. [http://dx.doi.org/10.1007/s13562-020-00560-1]

[78] Abdelaleem KG, Khamis IM A E-W, Aldawsari OMS, Alsubaie MSA. *in vitro* Tissue culture technique as tool for micro propagation of lepidium sativum l. plant under abiotic stress conditions. >IntEnvironAgric Biotechnol 2019; 4.

[79] Javed R, Gürel E. Salt stress by NaCl alters the physiology and biochemistry of tissue culture-grownStevia rebaudiana Bertoni. Turk J Agric For 2019; 43(1): 11-20. [http://dx.doi.org/10.3906/tar-1711-71]

[80] Yuan G, Wang X, Guo R, Wang Q. Effect of salt stress on phenolic compounds, glucosinolates, myrosinase and antioxidant activity in radish sprouts. Food Chem 2010; 121(4): 1014-9. [http://dx.doi.org/10.1016/j.foodchem.2010.01.040]

[81] de Castro KM, Batista DS, Silva TD, *et al.* Salinity modulates growth, morphology, and essential oil profile in Lippia alba L. (Verbenaceae) grown *in vitro*. Plant Cell Tissue Organ Cult 2020; 140(3): 593-603. [http://dx.doi.org/10.1007/s11240-019-01755-8]

[82] Rathore S, Narender S. Influence of NaCl on biochemical parameters of two cultivars of stevia rebaudiana regenerated *in vitro*. J Stress Physiology & Biochem 2014; 10: 287-96.

[83] Singh N, Kumaria S. Molecular cloning and characterization of chalcone synthase gene from Coelogyne ovalis Lindl. and its stress-dependent expression. Gene 2020; 762: 145104. [http://dx.doi.org/10.1016/j.gene.2020.145104] [PMID: 32889060]

[84] Bhat M A, Ahmad S, Aslam J. Influence of NaCl on biochemical parameters of two cultivars of stevia rebaudiana regenerated *in vitro*. J Stress Physiology & Biochem 2008; 10: 287-96.

[85] Guo R, Yuan G, Wang Q. Effect of NaCl treatments on glucosinolate metabolism in broccoli sprouts. J Zhejiang Univ Sci B 2013; 14(2): 124-31. [http://dx.doi.org/10.1631/jzus.B1200096] [PMID: 23365011]

[86] Rubio-Rodríguez E, López-Laredo AR, Medina-Pérez V, Trejo-Tapia G, Trejo-Espino JL. Influence of spermine and nitrogen deficiency on growth and secondary metabolites accumulation in *Castilleja tenuiflora* Benth. cultured in a RITA ® temporary immersion system. Eng Life Sci 2019; 19(12): 944-54. [http://dx.doi.org/10.1002/elsc.201900040] [PMID: 32624984]

[87]   Cortes JA, López-Laredo AR, Zamilpa A, Bermúdez-Torres K, Trejo-Espino JL, Trejo-Tapia G. Morphogenesis and secondary metabolites production in the medicinal plant castilleja tenuiflora benth. under nitrogen deficiency and starvation stress in a temporary immersion system. Rev Mex Ing Quim 2018; 17(1): 229-42.
[http://dx.doi.org/10.24275/uam/izt/dcbi/revmexingquim/2018v17n1/Cortes]

[88]   Nicasio-Torres MP, Meckes-Fischer M, Aguilar-Santamaría L, Garduño-Ramírez ML, Chávez-Ávila VM, Cruz-Sosa F. Production of chlorogenic acid and isoorientin hypoglycemic compounds in Cecropia obtusifolia calli and in cell suspension cultures with nitrate deficiency. Acta Physiol Plant 2012; 34(1): 307-16.
[http://dx.doi.org/10.1007/s11738-011-0830-9]

[89]   Medina-Pérez V, López-Laredo AR, Sepúlveda-Jiménez G, Zamilpa A, Trejo-Tapia G. Nitrogen deficiency stimulates biosynthesis of bioactive phenylethanoid glycosides in the medicinal plant Castilleja tenuiflora Benth. Acta Physiol Plant 2015; 37(5): 93.
[http://dx.doi.org/10.1007/s11738-015-1841-8]

[90]   Jakovljević D, Topuzović M, Stanković M. Nutrient limitation as a tool for the induction of secondary metabolites with antioxidant activity in basil cultivars. Ind Crops Prod 2019; 138: 111462.
[http://dx.doi.org/10.1016/j.indcrop.2019.06.025]

[91]   Lattanzio V, Caretto S, Linsalata V, Colella G, Mita G. Signal transduction in artichoke [Cynara cardunculus L. subsp. scolymus (L.) Hayek] callus and cell suspension cultures under nutritional stress. Plant Physiol Biochem 2018; 127: 97-103.
[http://dx.doi.org/10.1016/j.plaphy.2018.03.017] [PMID: 29571004]

[92]   Herrera-Santoyo J, López-Delgado HA, Mora-Herrera ME. Stress in callus of hippocratea excelsa: Catalase activity hydrogen peroxide content and canophyllol accumulation. Interciencia 2007; 32: 253-6.

[93]   Sahraroo A, Mirjalili MH, Corchete P, Babalar M, Fattahi Moghadam MR. Establishment and characterization of a satureja khuzistanica jamzad (lamiaceae) cell suspension culture: A new *in vitro* source of rosmarinic acid. Cytotechnology 2016; 68(4): 1415-24.
[http://dx.doi.org/10.1007/s10616-015-9901-x] [PMID: 26264595]

[94]   Colling J, Stander MA, Makunga NP. Nitrogen supply and abiotic stress influence canavanine synthesis and the productivity of *in vitro* regenerated Sutherlandia frutescens microshoots. J Plant Physiol 2010; 167(17): 1521-4.
[http://dx.doi.org/10.1016/j.jplph.2010.05.018] [PMID: 20674074]

[95]   Amdoun R, Khelifi L, Khelifi-Slaoui M, *et al.* Influence of minerals and elicitation on Datura stramonium L. tropane alkaloid production: Modelization of the *in vitro* biochemical response. Plant Sci 2009; 177(2): 81-7.
[http://dx.doi.org/10.1016/j.plantsci.2009.03.016]

[96]   Cïngöz G, Pehlïvan Karakaş F. The effects of nutrient and macronutrient stress on certain secondary metabolite accumulations and redox regulation in callus cultures of *Bellis perennis* L. Turk J Biol 2016; 40: 1328-35.
[http://dx.doi.org/10.3906/biy-1603-73]

[97]   Matto V, Arak E, Raal A, Vardja T, Vardja R, Pudersell K. Inorganic ions in the medium modify tropane alkaloids and riboflavin output in Hyoscyamus niger root cultures. Pharmacogn Mag 2012; 8(29): 73-7.
[http://dx.doi.org/10.4103/0973-1296.93330] [PMID: 22438667]

[98]   Lattanzio V, Cardinali A, Ruta C, *et al.* Relationship of secondary metabolism to growth in oregano (Origanum vulgare L.) shoot cultures under nutritional stress. Environ Exp Bot 2009; 65(1): 54-62.
[http://dx.doi.org/10.1016/j.envexpbot.2008.09.002]

[99]   Sharma S, Chatterjee S, Kataria S, *et al.* A review on responses of plants to uv-b radiation related stress uv-b radiation. John Wiley & Sons, Ltd 2017; pp. 75-97.

[100] Soriano-Melgar L de AA, Alcaraz-Meléndez L, Méndez-Rodríguez LC, Puente ME, Rivera-Cabrera F, Zenteno-Savín T. Antioxidant responses of damiana (Turnera diffusa Willd) to exposure to artificial ultraviolet (UV) radiation in an *in vitro* model; part ii; UV-B radiation. Nutr Hosp 2014; 29(5): 1116-22.
[PMID: 24951993]

[101] Antognoni F, Zheng S, Pagnucco C, Baraldi R, Poli F, Biondi S. Induction of flavonoid production by uv-b radiation in passiflora quadrangularis callus cultures. Fitoterapia 2007; 78(5): 345-52.
[http://dx.doi.org/10.1016/j.fitote.2007.02.001] [PMID: 17512679]

[102] Hao G, Du X, Zhao F, Shi R, Wang J. Role of nitric oxide in UV-B-induced activation of PAL and stimulation of flavonoid biosynthesis in Ginkgo biloba callus. Plant Cell Tissue Organ Cult 2009; 97(2): 175-85.
[http://dx.doi.org/10.1007/s11240-009-9513-2]

[103] Pandey N, Pandey-Rai S. Short term UV-B radiation-mediated transcriptional responses and altered secondary metabolism of *in vitro* propagated plantlets of Artemisia annua L. Plant Cell Tissue Organ Cult 2014; 116(3): 371-85.
[http://dx.doi.org/10.1007/s11240-013-0413-0]

[104] Ruan J, Zhang J, Li M, *et al.* Dependence of UV-B-induced camptothecin production on nitrate reductase-mediated nitric oxide signaling in Camptotheca acuminata suspension cell cultures. Plant Cell Tissue Organ Cult 2014; 118(2): 269-78.
[http://dx.doi.org/10.1007/s11240-014-0479-3]

[105] Şahİn G, Tellİ M, ÜnlÜ E S, Pehlİvan KarakaŞ F. Effects of moderate high temperature and UV-B on accumulation of withanolides and relative expression of the squalene synthase gene in Physalis peruviana. Turk J Biol 2020; 44: 295-303.

[106] Sequeida Á, Tapia E, Ortega M, *et al.* Production of phenolic metabolites by deschampsia antarctica shoots using uv-b treatments during cultivation in a photobioreactor. Electr J Biotech 2012; 25(4).

[107] Yildirim AB. Ultraviolet-B-induced changes on phenolic compounds, antioxidant capacity and HPLC profile of *in vitro*-grown plant materials in Echium orientale L. Ind Crops Prod 2020; 153: 112584.
[http://dx.doi.org/10.1016/j.indcrop.2020.112584]

[108] Alvero-Bascos EM, Ungson LB. Ultraviolet-|B (UV-B) radiation as an elicitor of flavonoid production in callus cultures of jatropha (Jatropha curcas L.). Philippines: Philippine Agricultural Scientist 2012.

[109] Karakas FP, Bozat BG. Fluctuation in secondary metabolite production and antioxidant defense enzymes in *in vitro* callus cultures of goat's rue (Galega officinalis) under different abiotic stress treatments. Plant Cell Tissue Organ Cult 2020; 142(2): 401-14.
[http://dx.doi.org/10.1007/s11240-020-01870-x]

[110] Qin B, Ma L, Wang Y, *et al.* Effects of acetylsalicylic acid and UV-B on gene expression and tropane alkaloid biosynthesis in hairy root cultures of Anisodus luridus. Plant Cell Tissue Organ Cult 2014; 117(3): 483-90.
[http://dx.doi.org/10.1007/s11240-014-0454-z]

[111] Binder BYK, Peebles CAM, Shanks JV, San KY. The effects of UV-B stress on the production of terpenoid indole alkaloids in *Catharanthus roseus* hairy roots. Biotechnol Prog 2009; 25(3): 861-5.
[http://dx.doi.org/10.1002/btpr.97] [PMID: 19479674]

[112] Peebles CAM, Shanks JV, San KY. The role of the octadecanoid pathway in the production of terpenoid indole alkaloids in *Catharanthus roseus* hairy roots under normal and UV-B stress conditions. Biotechnol Bioeng 2009; 103(6): 1248-54.
[http://dx.doi.org/10.1002/bit.22350] [PMID: 19437555]

[113] Ramani S, Chelliah J. UV-B-induced signaling events leading to enhanced-production of catharanthine in *catharanthus roseus* cell suspension cultures. BMC Plant Biol 2007; 7(1): 61.
[http://dx.doi.org/10.1186/1471-2229-7-61] [PMID: 17988378]

[114] Victório CP, Leal-Costa MV, Schwartz Tavares E, Machado Kuster R, Salgueiro Lage CL. Effects of supplemental UV-A on the development, anatomy and metabolite production of Phyllanthus tenellus cultured *in vitro*. Photochem Photobiol 2011; 87(3): 685-9.
[http://dx.doi.org/10.1111/j.1751-1097.2011.00905.x] [PMID: 21275997]

[115] Ullah MA, Tungmunnithum D, Garros L, Drouet S, Hano C, Abbasi BH. Effect of Ultraviolet-C Radiation and melatonin stress on biosynthesis of antioxidant and antidiabetic metabolites produced in *in vitro* Callus Cultures of *Lepidium sativum* L. Int J Mol Sci 2019; 20(7): 1787.
[http://dx.doi.org/10.3390/ijms20071787] [PMID: 30978911]

[116] Eray N, Dalar A, Turker M. The effects of abiotic stressors and signal molecules on phenolic composition and antioxidant activities of *in vitro* regenerated Hypericum perforatum (St. John's Wort). S Afr J Bot 2020; 133: 253-63.
[http://dx.doi.org/10.1016/j.sajb.2020.07.037]

[117] Moon SH, Mistry B, Kim DH, Pandurangan M. Antioxidant and anticancer potential of bioactive compounds following UV-C light-induced plant cambium meristematic cell cultures. Ind Crops Prod 2017; 109: 762-72.
[http://dx.doi.org/10.1016/j.indcrop.2017.09.024]

[118] Nazir M, Asad Ullah M, Mumtaz S, *et al.* Interactive effect of melatonin and uv-c on phenylpropanoid metabolite production and antioxidant potential in callus cultures of purple basil (Ocimum basilicum L. var purpurascens). Molecules 2020; 25(5): 1072.
[http://dx.doi.org/10.3390/molecules25051072] [PMID: 32121015]

[119] Yu KW, Murthy HN, Hahn EJ, Paek KY. Ginsenoside production by hairy root cultures of Panax ginseng: influence of temperature and light quality. Biochem Eng J 2005; 23(1): 53-6.
[http://dx.doi.org/10.1016/j.bej.2004.07.001]

[120] Shohael AM, Ali MB, Yu KW, Hahn EJ, Paek KY. Effect of temperature on secondary metabolites production and antioxidant enzyme activities in Eleutherococcus senticosus somatic embryos. Plant Cell Tissue Organ Cult 2006; 85(2): 219-28.
[http://dx.doi.org/10.1007/s11240-005-9075-x]

[121] Yusuf NA, Annuar MSM, Khalid N. Physical stress for overproduction of biomass and flavonoids in cell suspension cultures of Boesenbergia rotunda. Acta Physiol Plant 2013; 35(5): 1713-9.
[http://dx.doi.org/10.1007/s11738-012-1178-5]

[122] Rani R, Khan MA, Kayani WK, Ullah S, Naeem I, Mirza B. Metabolic signatures altered by *in vitro* temperature stress in Ajuga bracteosa Wall. ex. Benth. Acta Physiol Plant 2017; 39(4): 97.
[http://dx.doi.org/10.1007/s11738-017-2394-9]

[123] Zanella L, Gismondi A, Di Marco G, *et al.* Induction of antioxidant metabolites in *Moringa oleifera* callus by abiotic stresses. J Nat Prod 2019; 82(9): 2379-86.
[http://dx.doi.org/10.1021/acs.jnatprod.8b00801] [PMID: 31430152]

[124] Thimmaraju R, Bhagyalakshmi N, Narayan MS, Ravishankar GA. Kinetics of pigment release from hairy root cultures of Beta vulgaris under the influence of pH, sonication, temperature and oxygen stress. Process Biochem 2003; 38(7): 1069-76.
[http://dx.doi.org/10.1016/S0032-9592(02)00234-0]

[125] Szopa A, Ekiert H. The importance of applied light quality on the production of lignans and phenolic acids in Schisandra chinensis (Turcz.) Baill. cultures *in vitro*. Plant Cell Tissue Organ Cult 2016; 127(1): 115-21.
[http://dx.doi.org/10.1007/s11240-016-1034-1]

[126] Reyes-Martínez A, Valle-Aguilera JR, Antunes-Ricardo M, Gutiérrez-Uribe J, Gonzalez C, Santos-Díaz MS. Callus from pyrostegia venusta (ker gawl.) miers: A source of phenylethanoid glycosides with vasorelaxant activities. Plant Cell Tissue Organ Cult 2019; 139(1): 119-29.
[http://dx.doi.org/10.1007/s11240-019-01669-5]

[127]   Pongkitwitoon B, Simpan K, Chobsri T, Sritularak B, Putalun W. Combined UV-C irradiation and precursor feeding enhances mulberroside a production in morus alba l. cell suspension cultures. Sci Asia 2020; 46(6): 679.
[http://dx.doi.org/10.2306/scienceasia1513-1874.2020.096]

[128]   Shin GH, Chio MG, Lee DW. Comparative study of the effects of various culture conditions on cell growth and gagaminine synthesis in suspension culture of cynanchum wilfordii (MAXIM.) HEMSLEY. Biol Pharm Bull 2003; 26(9): 1321-5.
[http://dx.doi.org/10.1248/bpb.26.1321] [PMID: 12951479]

Glandular Trichomes: Bio-cell Factories of Plant Secondary Metabolites

Pragya Shukla[1,2], Archana Prasad[3], Khushboo Chawda[1,4], Gauri Saxena[3], Kapil D. Pandey[2] and Debasis Chakrabarty[1,4,*]

[1] *Biotechnology and Molecular Biology Division, CSIR-National Botanical Research Institute, Lucknow, India*

[2] *Department of Botany, Institute of Science, Banaras Hindu University, Varanasi, India*

[3] *Department of Botany, University of Lucknow, Lucknow, Uttar Pradesh-226007, India*

[4] *Academy of Scientific and Innovative Research (AcSIR), Ghaziabad, India*

Abstract: Trichomes are specialised epidermal outgrowth that is present on the aerial parts of plants. On the basis of morphological and cellular variation, they are categorized into non-glandular trichomes (NGTs) and glandular trichomes (GTs). NGTs are known to be involved in the protective and defensive roles that attribute to provide structural and chemical corroboration to form specialized groups of secondary metabolites. GTs are specialized micro-organs that are considered factories for the biosynthesis of a considerable amount of different classes of bioactive metabolites. Conventionally these glandular and non-glandular trichomes are known for their protective roles against different biotic and abiotic stresses. Recently, they have attracted the interest of various researchers as a specialized organ for the production of various bioactive molecules of high pharmaceutical and commercial values. The major groups of secondary metabolites such as terpenoids, flavonoids, phenylpropanes, methyl ketones, acyl sugars and defensive proteins are reported in the trichomes of different plant species. However, the conception of the molecular regulation of their biosynthesis, storage and distribution during the development of trichomes is scattered. This review compiles structural and functional aspects of GTs and NGTs along with the molecular mechanism regulated for the production of secondary metabolite in these specialized organs. In addition, the role of several bio-physical parameters that affect the trichome biochemistry, which either directly or indirectly influence the biosynthesis of secondary metabolite, will also be focussed. The systemized knowledge of trichome biology, secondary metabolite pathway modulation and metabolic engineering at one platform will be helpful to explore recent advances in the field of trichome engineering in many medicinally important plants.

---

[*] **Corresponding author Debasis Chakrabarty:** Biotechnology and Molecular Biology Division, CSIR-National Botanical Research Institute, Lucknow, India; & Academy of Scientific and Innovative Research (AcSIR), Ghaziabad, India; E-mail: chakrabartyd@nbri.res.in

Mohammad Anis & Mehrun Nisha Khanam (Eds.)

Keywords: Glandular trichomes, Non-glandular trichomes, Secondary metabolites, Stress.

INTRODUCTION

Trichomes Greek "trichos" (hairs) are specialized epidermal outgrowth present on the aerial parts of plants. They originated by means of endo-reduplication [1 - 3]. Trichomes are the epidermal extensions, and in most of the plants, they are not connected with the vascular system of the plant, *i.e.*: they lack vasculature [4]. They exhibit great diversity in their morphological and mechanical characteristics, such as size, orientation, shape, density, and surface texture which influence the physiology and ecology of the plants [5]. Their spacial distribution also adds benefits for the identification of different plant species. More than 300 types of plant trichomes have been described by Wagner in the year 1991 [6]. These plant trichomes are specialised for performing the first line of defense mechanism against various biotic/abiotic stresses.

Trichomes can be a few micrometers to centimeters in size, unicellular or multicelluar, and exhibit enormous species-specific diversity among the plant Kingdom. Most acceptable criteria to classify these appendages is whether they are non-glandular (NGTs) or glandular (GTs). NGTs are predominantly present in angiosperms, but they are also reported in a few species of bryophytes and gymnosperms. *Arabidopsis thaliana* and cotton are two model plants that have unicellular, non-glandular structures and are used to study cell fate differentiation, cellular specification, morphogenesis and non-glandular trichome biology. However, very limited information about the synthesis of metabolites and their secretary behaviour can be obtained from NGT bearing plants.

GTs are multicellular structures containing apical, stalk and differentiated basal cells [7]. These GTs are also known for producing and reserving a significant amount of different classes of secondary metabolites. These metabolites are mainly synthesized in response to the defence mechanism and require specialized tissues/organs for their storage. Trichomes are one of specialized tissues which originate as small protrusions on the epidermis and serve as a sink for the storage of bioactive secondary metabolites in plants. The trichomes acquire these metabolites, which are not only beneficial for pharmaceutical industries but they also serve as valuable resources for the food and cosmetic industries. GTs show variability in the number of different cells as well as in their constituent of secondary metabolites and are classified into several types. The master groups of secondary metabolites that have been found to be fabricated in trichomes include terpenoids, flavonoids, phenylpropanes, methyl ketones, acyl sugars and defensive proteins. Among the two, *i.e.*; GT and NGT, GTs are special paradigms to study the biosynthesis of metabolites, storage and their secretory mechanism. Many researchers studied metabolic regulation of secondary metabolites content in different trichome bearing plants viz. Mint, Basil, *Artemisia, Nicotiana, Cannabis, etc.*, that serve as potential candidates for better understanding the biosynthetic pathway engineering in trichome biology [8 - 10].

Plants develop trichomes as a result of different defence responses against different abiotic and biotic stress responses. However, their morphology, location, metabolic constituent, ability to secrete and mode of secretion show considerable fluctuations among trichome bearing plant species. Trichome density is proportional to different environmental stimuli and their function is dependent on the trichome type and location. In the last few decades, several trichome bearing plant species have been paying attention to the accumulation of bioactive secondary metabolites and different stress related research where trichomes, either NGTs or GTs, act as active defence regulated responses to overcome different biotic/abiotic stresses. However, in several studies, NGTs are also known for their sink capacity; they act as a storage site for different toxic exudates and protect the plants from environmental and biological stresses. Although NGTs procured attention since they significantly contribute to different stress responses and the accumulation ability of metabolites [11 - 13], an update on the term 'glandular trichomes' was reported in 2020, which is based on a literature database Web of Science where a total of 2323 registered publications from 1919 to 2020 with a modest increment until 1990 were recorded. The study expeditiously plateaued at fifty publications per annum until around 2003 with the search for the very first genes involved in the biosynthesis of secondary metabolites produced in GTs of Mint. From 2005 until now, a sharp and constant speedy increase in the era of trichome research has been recorded, which reflects a large number of trichome bearing plant species such as *A. annua, C. sativa, Nicotiana, etc.*, and their functional genomics and downstream processing were investigated [14]. A key and solitary property of GT is their ability to synthesize and secrete an enormous range of specialized metabolites relative to their size. Terpenoids, flavonoids, methyl ketones, phenylpropanoids, acyl sugars, defensive proteins and alkaloids, are the constituents mainly synthesized by the GTs [15]. These qualities make GTs an excellent experimental system for biosynthesis, mechanism of regulation of natural product pathways and other molecular genetic studies. In addition, various omics-techniques have greatly contributed to unveil the experimental protocols for the enhancement and biosynthetic of metabolites in the trichomes [16]. Hence, the present chapter is an attempt to compile the systematic knowledge available for some important GTs bearing plants toward their efficacy for secondary metabolite biosynthesis and storage. The molecular cascade regulating the production of metabolites and their cross-talk with different external biotic/abiotic factors will also be focussed in the present review.

GLANDULAR TRICHOME: MORPHOLOGY, DEVELOPMENT, SECONDARY METABOLITE ACCUMULATION AND MOLECULAR REGULATION IN SOME IMPORTANT PLANTS

Insight into GT development is very limited, but due to their important and interesting specialised metabolites accumulation, most of the attention of researchers has now focused on their biosynthetic pathways regulation and production of these metabolites in the specialised microorgan-trichomes. The morphological architect of GTs varies with an abundant diversity of shape, size, and storage. It has been described in a vast number of plant species [17]. GTs are commonly multicellular structures mainly composed of three parts: base cells, a stalk and a single or group of glands on the tip [18]. The base cells connect with epidermal cells and stalk cells. Stalk cells bear the gland on the tip. Gland cells are the important structures involved in the secretion of specialized metabolites. These three cells may be unicellular or multicellular and more or less elongated. This kind of variability in cell, shape and number of trichomes accounts for high morphological diversity across GTs of different plant species. Generally, GTs are subdivided into capitate and peltate structures. Both types are frequently seen in Solanaceae, Cannabaceae and Asteraceae. The description of different types of trichomes is summarized in Fig. (**1**). Peltate types of trichomes are short structures with unicellular or bicellular stalks and a multicellular secretory cavity which contains a number of secretory cells. However, capitate trichomes consist of multicellular stalk cells, which vary with cell number and length and end up with a small unicellular head cell. Here we summarize Fig. (**1**) and Table **1** the different types of trichomes and their presence on different plant parts.

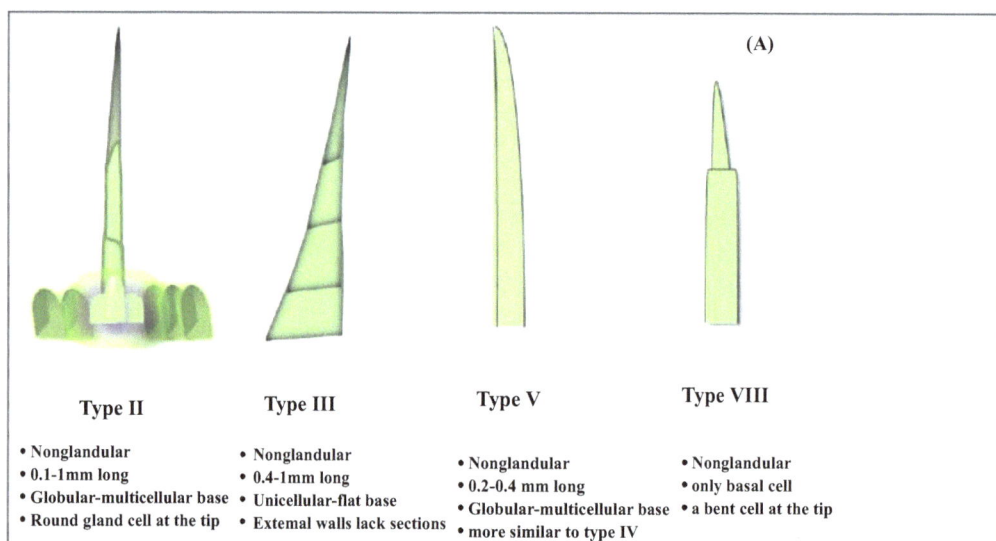

(A)

Type II	Type III	Type V	Type VIII
• Nonglandular	• Nonglandular	• Nonglandular	• Nonglandular
• 0.1-1mm long	• 0.4-1mm long	• 0.2-0.4 mm long	• only basal cell
• Globular-multicellular base	• Unicellular-flat base	• Globular-multicellular base	• a bent cell at the tip
• Round gland cell at the tip	• External walls lack sections	• more similar to type IV	

(Fig. 1) contd.....

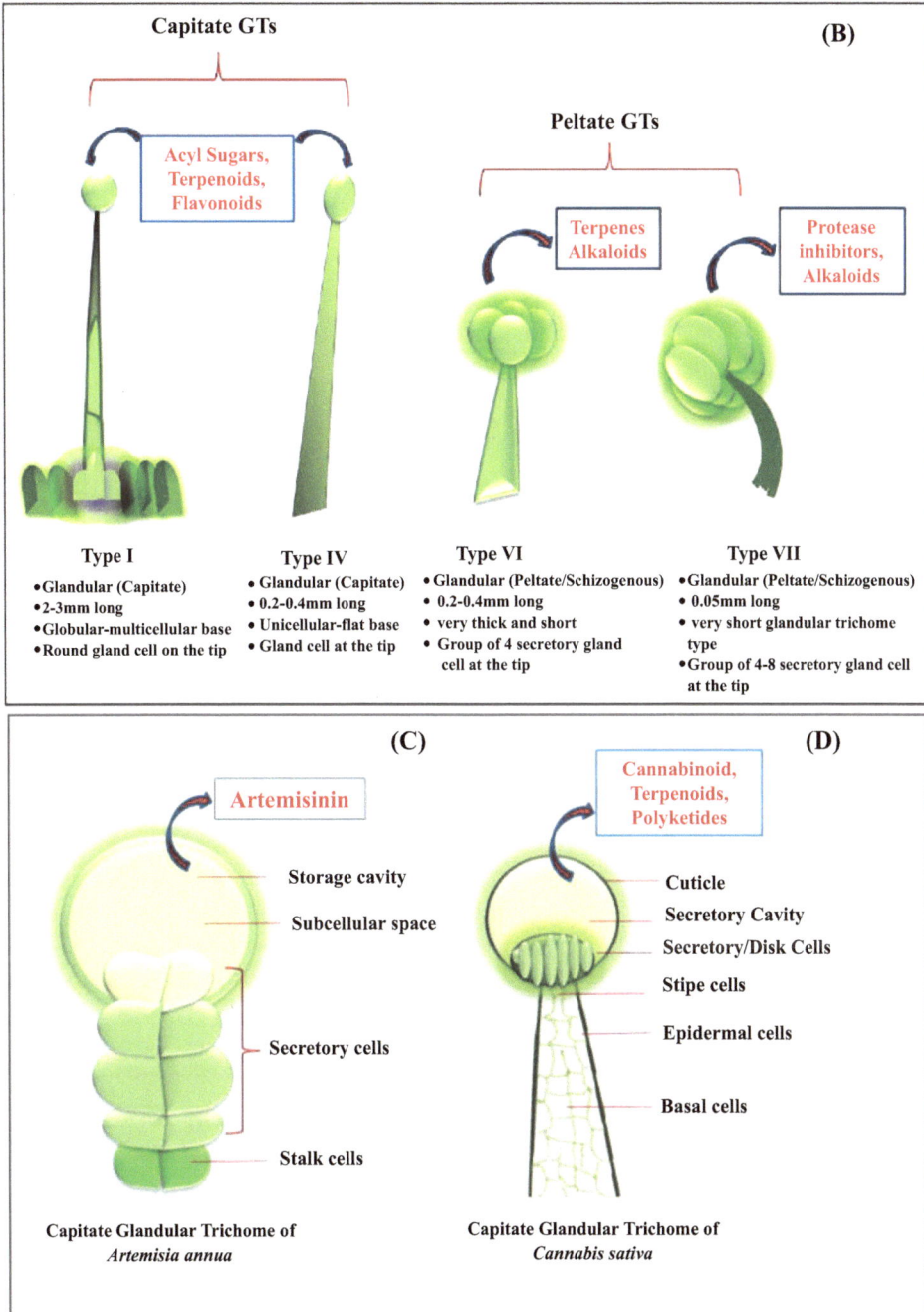

Fig. (1).   Schematic illustration of different types of trichomes. Nonglandular trichomes (NGTs), (**A**); Glandular trichomes (GTs), (**B**); Distributed across Solanums. Capitate GTs of *Artemisia annua* (**C**); *Artemisia annua* (**D**) *Cannabis sativa.*

Table 1. Trichomes present on the aerial plant parts of different families.

S. No.	Family	Plant	Trichome Type	Location/ Distribution	References
1.	Apocyanaceae	*Hibiscus esculentus.*	GTs	Seed (rare) and fruit	[22]
2.	Asteraceae	*Artemisia annua* L.	GTs	Leaves and inflorescence	[23]
		Inula britannica	NGT and biseriate GTs	Leaves	[24]
		Conyza blinii	Capitate GTs (CGTs)		[25]
		Helianthus annuus	CGTs NGTs, linear glandular trichomes (LGTs)	Leaf surfaces and the anther appendages	[26]
		Matricaria chamomilla	Canal and GTs	Stem and capitulum	[27]
3.	Cannabaceae	*Cannabis sativa*	Long-capitate stalked GTs	Floral bracts and on the margin of inflorescence leaves	[28]
			Cystolithic NGTs	Upper side of vegetative fan leaves	
			Small GTs	Omnipresent	
			Pointed non-glandular bio-mineralized	Each organ	
4.	Lamiaceae	*Schizonepeta tenuifolia* Briq.	Big peltate and small capitate GTs	Leaves	[29]
		Origanum majorana L.	NGTs and GTs		[30]
		Colquhounia vestita Wall	Peltate and capitate GTs	Leaves and stem	[31]
5.	Phrymaceae	*Mimulus guttatus*	GTs	Leaves	[32]

Plant trichome development is a complex process which is co-ordinated and regulated by different factors, such as activation/inactivation of different regulatory genes, plant growth regulators, non-coding RNA and various environmental stimuli. Among them, regulatory genes and phytohormones play a vital role in modulating trichome development [19]. Regulatory mechanisms may involve positive and negative regulation of different transcription factors (TF). Trichomes may be unicellular and multicellular, their cellular differentiation is regulated by distinguished pathways that involve different classes of regulatory proteins such as GL1, which is a crucial member of transcriptional activator ternary complex (GLABRA3/ ENHANCER of GLABRA3; GL3/EGL3)-GLABROUS1 (GL1)-TRANSPARENT TESTA GLABRA (TTG1) and regulated by C2H2-TF, which promotes the expression of GLABRA2 (GL2) to control trichome development. This complex is a central regulator of trichome initiation and maturation of NGTs in *Arabidopsis thaliana*. Mutation of GL1 produces a glabrous (*hairless*) phenotype of *A. thaliana*. However, MIXTA1 (MYB-TF) is only involved in controlling the initiation of multicellular trichomes in tobacco, *Artemisia etc*. [20, 21].

Recent advances and breakthroughs in technical and analytical technologies resulted in leading genomics and transcriptomics approaches for better understanding and investigating the mechanism of glandular trichome biology. The literature scans of the functional aspect for GTs development are mainly explored in tobacco, tomato and *Artemisia*. The present chapter is to compile the major information related to the development of trichomes and their role as a metabolite repository in several important plant species. Further, the review also gives insight into the influence of stress (biotic/abiotic) on the metabolite production/ accumulation in these micro-organs (trichomes).

Morphology, Occurrence and Biosynthetic Regulation of Metabolites in the Trichome of Some Important Plants

Solanum lycopersicum

Trichome morphology of *Solanum* species was classified based on its length, number of stalk cells, number of base cells and presence/absence of gland. Seven different types of trichomes were identified, four of them are glandular, and three are non-glandular subtypes. The work was further refined in 1992 [33, 34]. Some of the trichome types were subdivided due to the vast diversity of trichomes found on the leaf surface of *L. hirsutum*. Type VIc GTs were reported, which are capable of releasing sticky gum-like exudates, when a whitefly contacts secretory type of trichomes. The cell wall of the GTs ruptures when it interrupts with a whitefly in sticky exudates. The trichome biology of tomato achieves more insight due to their great diversity. In eight (I-VIII) types of trichomes, I, IV are capitates, type VI and VII are peltate, which are GTs, and II, III, V, and VIII are non-glandular type [35]. Schuurink and Tissier in 2020 coined the term Schizogenous for the peltate type of trichomes because trichome gland cells formed with intercellular space established by splitting or partial separation of common walls of contiguous secretory cells. These glands are used by plants as storage canals for oil, resin, acyl sugars and metabolites and are termed as schizogenous glands. GTs differ in the number of stalk, secretory cells and Type I GTs consist of six to ten cells which are 2-3 mm in length, spherical and multicellular base with round glands at the tip. Type II NGTs resemble in morphology with type I GTs except for the presence of a gland on the tip. Glands of the type I, IV, VI trichomes contain flavonoids, terpenoids and acyl sugars. Type I and IV GTs are the principal storage site of acyl sugars responsible for the viscosity of the plant surface and used by the plant during herbivory (Fig. **1**) [36, 37]. The microscopic study of type VI trichomes showed a large intercellular cavity on the trichome head of wild tomato, while a smaller cavity was observed in cultivated tomato. There are a number of studies that documented the role of type VI GTs in the biosynthesis of terpenes [38 - 40].

The varied glandular shape also defines the metabolite accumulation capacity in the case of different *Solanum* species. The study conducted on *S. habrochaites* showed 100 times more terpenoids accumulation capacity in their type VI trichomes than the cultivated variety of tomato, which lack type VI trichomes [41]. A population of Wva106 was obtained by back-cross between *S. habrochaites* LA1777 and *S. lycopersicum*, studied on the basis of their phenotyping and genotyping, where two major QTLs on chromosome number 1 and 7 governing the shape and size of the gland were identified [42]. Shotgun proteome analysis of GTs of *S. lycopersicum* revealed that proteins involved in the methylerythritol 4-phosphate (MEP) pathway are terpene and rutine [43].

The functional aspect of the development of GTs in tomato is explored by several researchers. Two main subfamilies of transcription factors (TF) viz. R2R3-MYB and HD-ZIP IV are known to involve in the development of GTs in tomato. Apart from these TFs, the role of C_2H_2 zinc-finger and bHLH proteins is also identified in GTs development [44]. Tomato *Sl* TRY and *Sl* GL3 genes are identified as orthologous to *A. thaliana* TRY and GL3 genes, respectively. *Sl* TRY and *Sl* GL3 expressions are examined in aerial parts of the plant, which suggests that the genes are involved in the trichome development of the entire tomato plant and their function is similar to CPC-like MYB-TF in *Arabidopsis*. Study concluded that trichome and root hair differentiation in *Arabidopsis* and tomato is governed by similar TF and *Sl* TRY-like R3. MYB possibly acts as a key regulator for trichome and root-hair development [45]. Another TF, *Sl* MYC1, plays a role as a positive regulator of monoterpene biosynthesis in both stem and leaf trichomes, whereas works as a negative regulator during sesquiterpene synthesis in stem trichomes. Terpenoids constitute a large family of volatile compounds, involve in the interactions between plant and abiotic/biotic stresses [46, 47]. *Sl* MYC1 also plays a vital role in GTs development and knocking down *Sl* MYC1 resulted in smaller GTs with lower densities, whereas knocking out leads to their absence which deferentially affects the accumulation of mono and sesquiterpene levels in leaf and stem trichomes. Interestingly, a new type of trichome type VII-like class was visible in the knockout lines. These may be malformed types of VI trichomes. The above results suggested the role of *Sl* MYC1 in type VI GT in the proper development and regulation of terpene biosynthesis in tomato [48, 49]. In another study, relative quantitative expression of jasmonic acid (JA) treated trichomes showed that the WRKY (*Sl* WRKY73) class and the MYC bHLH (*Sl* MYC1, MYELOCYTOMATOSIS-RELATED 1) class were involved in transient transactivation of *S. lycopersicum* terpene synthase promoters in *N. benthamiana* leaves. A recent study on another TF of tomato unveiled the role of *Sl* SCL3 (scarecrow-like subfamily) during the regulation of volatile terpene biosynthesis and the size of GTs. Downregulation of *Sl* SCL3 led to a significant decrease in terpene concentration, including the expression of terpene synthase genes. However, their overexpression leads to increased levels of volatile terpene content and the size of the GTs. The study also gives insight into the role of *Sl* SCL3 during the modulation of the terpene biosynthetic pathway genes by activation of transcriptional machinery; there was no direct protein-DNA binding, and also no interaction with studied regulators was observed. Moreover, overexpressed plants show a decreased copy of endogenously expressed *Sl* SCL3 transcript level than the heterozygous and homozygous mutants suggesting feedback repression of its own promoter [50]. MIXTA1 (MYB-TF) was involved during the control of initiation of multicellular trichomes in *Nicotiana*, *Artemisia*. *Sl* MX1 is another MIXTA like gene and belongs to the R2R3-MYB subfamily, which has been characterized as a positive regulator of GTs initiation in tomato. Down-regulation of *Sl* MX1 in tomato leads to a decrease in a number of GTs and upregulation results in an increase in their density [51]. *Sl* CD2 (CUTIN DEFEICIENT 2) belongs to the HD-ZIP IV subfamily, which is a homolog of *Artemisia Aa* HD8. Loss of function mutation in *Sl* CD2 gives rise to sticky peel mutant phenotype of tomato, which shows less number of type IV and others GTs. Their effect, particularly on type IV GTs, was eminent. WOOLLY (Wo) HD-ZIP-IV TF is one more important regulator of GT initiation. Dominant type point mutation in the C-terminus of the Wo leads to the *woolly* mutant phenotype, which is responsible for increasing the density of GTs, and reduced density is recorded in *Wo*-RNAi silencing lines. A study suggests that Wo strengthens the number of type I GTs initiation [52]. However, another recent work on *woolly* mutants suggested that the effect of dominant *woolly* point mutation showed differential trichomes on different plant parts and different developmental stages of the plant. The higher density of type IV GTs was observed in the premature leaves of *woolly* mutants [53]. In tomato, *Sl* H (HAIR) protein encodes for C_2H_2 zinc-finger protein. Deletion of the coding region of *Sl* H resulted in a hairless phenotype. Knockdown of *Sl* H and Wo suppresses the formation of type I GTs, which suggests that both the trichome regulators may function as heterodimers. Protein-protein interaction between *Sl* H and Wo was detected with the help of pull-down and yeast two-hybrid assays. Ectopic expression of *Sl* H in *Nicotiana*, and expression of their homologs from *Nicotiana* and *Capsicum,* in tomato can trigger the formation of trichomes. These results suggest that 'H' gene may functionally conserve during multicellular trichome formation in the Solanaceae family (Fig. **2**) [54].

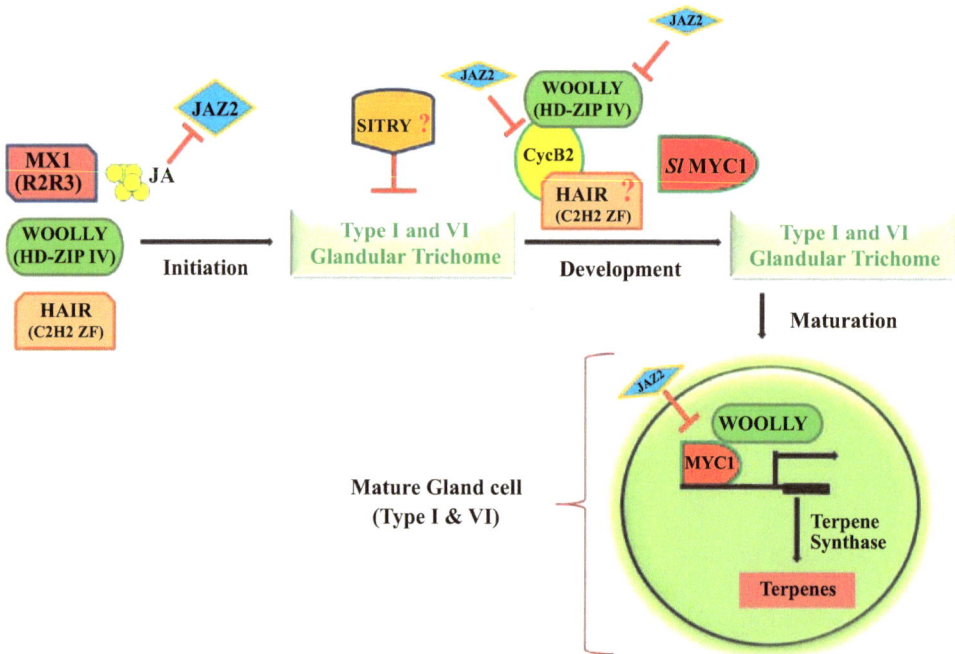

Fig. (2). Delineative representation of molecular development and metabolic regulation of tomato GT. Initiation of trichome requires WOOLLY (Wo) function. However, for the development, it interacts with HAIR (H), a C2H2 zinc finger TF. It participates in the initiation of almost all types of trichomes viz., type I, II, III, IV, and VI and is also involved during the regulation of CycB2 (*Sl* CyclinB2), which is crucial for Type I and may be for Type VI GT development. MX-1 (MIXTA-like MYB-TF) also plays a role during the initiation of GT. WOOLLY-CycB2-HAIR complex may be formed during the interaction of WOLLY with CycB2 and HAIR, and it may play a role during initiation and development. However, the existence of this complex is not studied yet. Development of GT is controlled by *Sl* MYC1 (R2R3-MYB), and it also plays an important role during terpene syntheses in a mature gland of type VI trichomes. *Sl* TRY(R3-MYB) probably plays a role in the inhibition of trichome initiation by hindering identity with adjacent epidermal cells. Jasmonic acid (JA) signalling can promote trichome initiation and terpene biosynthesis by the proteasomal degradation of JAZ2 (A repressor of WO-MYC1 expression).

Artemisia annua

In the genus *Artemisia,* biseriate and capitate GTs were prevalent. *A. annua* plant is covered with filamentous and glandular trichomes which involve in artemisinin synthesis. Comparative transcriptome analysis of both types of trichomes shows the upregulation of biosynthetic pathway genes of MVA, MEP, lipids and terpene synthase in GTs [55]. However, in self-pollinated inbreed plants of *A. annua*, NGTs also expressed artemisinin biosynthesis. However, the expression of trichome synthesis genes and artemisinin biosynthetic genes varied among the species, which resulted in differential accumulation of artemisinin. The production of artemisinin (antimalarial drug) from different plant parts was restrictedly investigated due to its limited biosynthesis. Many leaf cells such as mesophyll cells, epidermal cells and T-shaped trichomes, may lack the capacity for artemisinin biosynthesis in all ecotypes and available commercial cultivars of *A. annua*. GTs consisting of 10 cells were identified as the sole site of artemisinin biosynthesis. Researchers have cloned most transcription factors, and pathway genes of these GT cells are involved in the control of artemisinin biosynthesis [56 - 58]. Several genes involved in trichome formation, trichome branching pathways and transporters showed an efficient role in artemisinin biosynthesis. Relative expressions of three TFs genes (*Aa*-WIRKY1, *Aa*-ERF1 and *Aa*-ORA), two transporter genes (*Aa*-ABCG6 and *Aa*-ABCG7) and six terpene synthase genes (Aa-ECS, Aa-CPS, Aa-GAS, Aa-BFS, Aa-ADS, and Aa-SQS) were investigated as key genes involved in artemisinin biosynthesis in eight different *Artemisia* species. Analysis unveiled high transcript levels of *Aa* -ADS (3.33 fold), *Aa*-CPS (77.81 fold) and *Aa*-GAS (75.29 fold) in *A. deserti*. Blocking of two genes (Aa-CPS and Aa-GAS) at the branching point may be an efficient method for high artemisinin producing plants due to their large glandular size of trichomes than *A. annua,* a species found in Iran. The study on GT density and artemisinin content in different *Artemisia* species suggests that *Aa*-ABCG6 transporter plays an important role during trichome development while not involved in the transportation of artemisinin and their precursors. In contrast, some studies reported a lack of correlation between GT density and artemisinin content [58]. The biosynthesis of artemisinin takes place in 10-celled glandular trichomes in a very exclusive manner (Fig **1C**). However, some biochemicals, such as β-caryophyllene (a volatile metabolite) and β-farnesene (pheromone), are located in NGTs. Trichome morphology includes floral parts of *A. annua* plant carrying T-shaped filamentous NGTs, located on the bracts and pedicel of the capitulum and 10 celled biseriate GTs, which occur on receptacle and bracts of capitula and corolla of florets. Another type of biseriate GT is composed of 2 columns of five cells, each known as a heart-shaped GT [59].

Helianthus annuus

Helianthus annuus is known for the appearance of trichomes on leaf surfaces and anther appendages. These GTs are investigated for the production of a complex array of secondary metabolites [60]. In this family, capitate GTs are the main attraction which is common in various tribes of the family, which are known to produce thousands of sesquiterpene lactones (STLs) structures with some extent of acetophenones, flavonoids and other compounds. STL is one of the major compounds found among the diverse classes of compounds in the Compositae family. It is derived from the isoprenoid biosynthetic pathway and plays a crucial role during plant herbivory. Another class of linear glandular trichomes (LGTs) that are physiologically and metabolically active trichome was identified by Aschenbrenner *et al.*, in the year 2013. LGTs consist of 6-11 linearly arranged cells present on most of the organs of *H. annuus* connected with the plant vascular system [61, 62].

Cannabis sativa

C. sativa is one of the most important medicinal plants known for a vast range of secondary metabolites. Till now, 565 metabolites have been explored from *C. sativa*. Isoprenoids, polyketides and phenylpropanoids are the major compounds, in which around 120 correspond to cannabinoids (phytocannabinoids). Phytocannabinoids are isoprenylated polyketides that are produced in GTs [63]. Capitate stalked GTs are the most abundant type in *Cannabis sativa* L. They are abundantly present on the floral leaves and bracts of female reproductive organs. This is likely an acclimation to protect developing seeds from invaders. Cannabinoid and terpenoid biosynthesis takes place in a cluster of secretory cells situated at the base of the GTs head, named disc cells (Fig. **1D**). Stalked, pre-stalked and sessile GTs secrete and store differential proportions of monoterpenes, sesquiterpenes, and terpenophenolic cannabinoids. Sessile trichomes of *Cannabis* are more like canonical peltate GTs of the Lamiaceae family which is well known to produce many essential components such as, monoterpene-rich essential oils. Interestingly, cannabis sessile GTs contain both monoterpenes and sesquiterpenes. Monoterpene-rich cannabis GTs have a gland similar to peltate- or sessile type trichomes. However, they sit on the tip of a multicellular stalk connected with the stipe cells [64, 65]. Proteome analysis of *C. sativa* gland extracts with a mix of some epidermal tissues revealed 100 identified proteins, including zinc-finger type, F-box members and the majority of secondary metabolite synthases. However, shotgun proteomic analysis of GTs and apical buds revealed 160 proteins which include, terpene synthases, members of the cannabinoid pathway, olivetolic acid cyclase, tetrahydrocannabinolic acid synthase (THCAS), and cannabidiolic acid synthase (CBDAS) (Fig. **3**) [66]. A recent study on *C. sativa* proteomes of different parts of GTs (stalks, head cells) and late stage flower investigated with the help of quantitative time of flight mass spectrometry (QTOF-MS/MS) identified 1240 proteins in GT head, 396 proteins in GTS stalk cells and 1682 proteins in late stage flowers. On the basis of relative protein abundance data, it unveiled that GT heads are the major site for secondary metabolite biosynthesis, transport and carbon refixation. Data also suggested that floral part tissues act as sources of carbon and energy, which drive secondary metabolism synthesis into the GTs head cells that act as sinks. Apart from that, GTs stalk cells play a very lean role in secondary metabolism and perform as both source as well as sink. Chemical fingerprinting of a single GT with the help of coherent anti-Stokes Raman scattering (CARS) microscopy distinguishes the distribution and chemo-types of secondary metabolites in a non-destructive manner. $\Delta 9$ -tetrahydrocannabinolic acid was identified in the secretory cavity of drug-type of trichomes, whereas, cannabidiolic acid in the secretory cavity of fibre-type trichomes. Whereas, a unique spectral fingerprint similar to cannabigerolic acid (CBGA) was also obtained in the disk cells of drug-type trichomes, which was absent in fibre-type trichomes [67] (Fig. **3**).

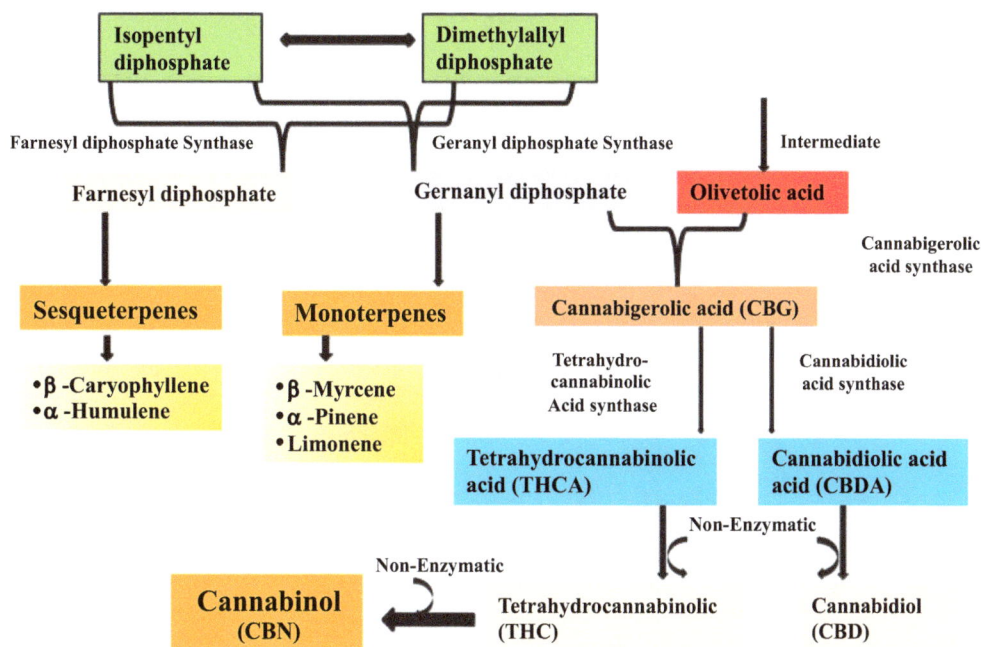

Fig. (3). Biosynthetic pathway of cannabinoids and terpenes in *Cannabis sativa*.

Withania somnifera

Micromorphology, histochemistry and ultrastructure of trichomes of *Withania somnifera* were studied [68]. Leaf of the *Withania* consists of four distinct types of trichomes including one capitate type glandular trichome and three different types of non-glandular trichomes viz. branched dendritic, bicellular and multicellular. Dendritic nonglandular trichomes of *Withania* display the 'Lotus-Effect', self-clearing property of leaf surface [68, 69]. Moreover, glandular capitate and non-glandular dendritic trichomes show aggregation on the mid-vein of young and mature leaves. Chemical constituents of glandular and non-glandular trichomes were revealed on the basis of histochemical staining which shows the presence of two major classes of phytoconstituents *i.e.*, phenolics and alkaloids.

Influence of Biotic/abiotic Stresses on Trichome Development and Metabolite Accumulation

Plants encounter a number of environmental stresses including herbivores, heavy metals, heat, cold, drought, light and wind. To overcome these stresses, plants develop a variety of defence regulatory mechanisms. Trichomes are tiny hair-like structures that cover the surface of most terrestrial plants and function as the first line of defence providing resistance to plants against various physical damages caused by biotic and abiotic stresses. These trichomes also act as a repository of some bioactive secondary metabolites. The trichomes' density and their ability to secrete secondary metabolites are resultant of plant defence mechanisms against various environmental stresses [70] (Table **2**).

Table 2. Compilation of studies on biotic and abiotic stress mediated trichome physiology, metabolite accumulation and its molecular regulators.

S. No.	Plant Species	Stress	Trichome Density	Metabolite	Molecular Regulator	References
1.	-	Arsenic	Increase	-	3-hydroxy-3-methylglutaryl coenzyme A reductase	[121, 122]
		U V –B			1-deoxy-D-xylulose-5-phosphate reducto isomerase (DXR)	[123]
2.	*Solanum lycopersicum*	Cold	Increase	Flavonoids	*CHI1*	[124]

Effect of Abiotic Stress on Trichome Physiology and Metabolic Productivity

Abiotic stresses, such as salinity, temperature, water, ultraviolet radiation, and heavy metals, are antagonistic to plant growth and development, which, in turn, affect the crop biomass and yield. A literature scan suggested that these abiotic factors significantly affect the production and accumulation of secondary metabolites in plants. Trichomes act as sinks of these metabolites and are also influenced by environmental stresses. Studies related to the variation in the occurrence of trichomes and their ability to harbour these bioactive metabolites differ according to the plants and are also highly responsive against the varied environmental influences. In this section, some abiotic factors, their effect on the trichomes and their secondary metabolite production/accumulation are summarised.

Temperature Stress

Heat and cold are the two forms of temperature stress that are known to obstruct a plant's growth, impair its plasma membranes, increase transpiration, denature proteins architect and hinder the mechanism of stomata opening. Heat stress is also reported to limit the increased membrane fluidity by changing the lipid composition of the cellular membranes [71]. GTs present on the *Wigandia urens* favour the sunlight reflection, heat dissolution and transpiration of water. Plants grown in direct sunlight have higher trichome densities than those grown in shade. Smooth leaves transpire at a slower rate than leaves with this hairy appendages. Irrigation and shade treatments also result in a decrease in trichome density, therefore, an increase in temperature is positively correlated to the increase in trichome density [72]. The plants exposed to elevated temperature stress show a special set of induced secondary metabolites, such as flavonoids, phenolics, and anthocyanins, which act as antioxidants, while osmolytes such as amino acids, sugars, and amines are produced under increased temperature, balancing the plant's osmosis [73, 74]. In *Nicotiana langsdorffii,* heat stress induced the trichomes to produce acyl sugars and glykoalkaloids. An increase in lipidic compounds, especially mono- and di- galactosyldiacylglycerols (MGDG and DGDG) and sulphoquinovosyl derivatives, was observed, which are studied to protect the photosynthetic system and to be enhanced in conditions of increased temperatures [71].

Chilling also causes injury to plants with symptoms such as cessation of protoplasmic streaming, cellular leakage, excessive water loss, diminished seedling vigour, reduced plant growth, increased impaired photosynthesis, increased susceptibility to certain diseases, and enhanced senescence [75]. The presence of the trichomes on the aerial plant parts increases the thickness of the epidermis and is involved as a physical barrier to protect from invaders [76]. Tomatoes with a lot of trichomes have been shown to be more cold tolerant in past studies [77, 78]. When the tomato plant membrane integrity is hampered by a fall in temperatures, trichome-rich plants increase their metabolic rate, resulting in reduced membrane lipids content, representing better survival. Wild tomatoes with a higher number of trichomes showed a great survival rate than common tomatoes (less number of GTs) when subjected to the same cold stress [79]. Tomatoes with a greater number of trichomes can adjust higher metabolic rates and improve tolerance against cold stress [80].

Drought and Water Stress

Water deficiency is one of the severe limiting factors that affect plant growth, development, and reproducibility. Water deficiency may lead to inhibition of photosynthesis, high rate of respiration, and deficiency of crucial mineral nutrients and may affect the lipid composition of the lipid bilayer [81]. Trichomes also play an efficient role in reducing water loss, exchange of gases and water, which reduces excessive transpiration and photoinhibition [82]. By increasing the leaf surface thickness, trichomes can reduce the absorption of temperature and radiation, which may lead to protection from drought [83]. The cooling effect of trichomes cuts water loss by 20-25% [84]. Trichomes are typically long and dense in xeromorphic plants. Many studies are being done to determine the role of trichomes in soil water deficit conditions and to examine how the trichome enhances drought resistance in plants. Leaf trichomes in *Caragana korshinskii* facilitate foliar water uptake and are reported to absorb dew that assist in partially sustaining the leaf hydraulic assimilation system and mitigating the adverse effects of drought stress [85]. Drought stress also affects the trichome density and secondary metabolism of plants. Drought affects aromatic terpenoid biosynthesis in *Nicotiana tabacum*. It altered the expression of differentially expressed genes in terpenoid backbone and diterpenoid biosynthesis, including cembratrien-ol synthase, cytochrome P450 gene *CYP71D16*, and *copalyl diphosphate synthase* (*CPS*). It also resulted in an increase in trichome density in the early stage of stress [86].

Heavy Metals Stress

The enhanced level of heavy metals in the environment is owing to increased air, water, and soil pollution. Toxic metals have a significant impact on plant growth, development, and productivity by interfering with key physiological and biochemical processes. Secretions of the trichomes are known to involve in different metal detoxification processes. As part of their elemental defence detoxification strategy, heavy metal tolerance shows plants generally accumulate heavy metals and other toxic substances in their trichomes. Trichomes aid ion and metal homeostasis by means of heavy metal sequestration, compartmentalization, accumulation, and excretion. The trichomes in Solanaceae, such as *Nicotiana*, *Solanum viarum*, are known for the detoxification of Cd, Ni, Pb, and Zn [87 - 89]. The trichomes of *A. thaliana* serve as accumulation sites for heavy metals such as Cd^{2+}, and thereby help plants to cope with both heavy metal stress and as well detoxify the soil [90]. Phenolics of the trichome cells are may involve in the metal chelating activity. The epidermis of winter cherry *W. somnifera* plants grown in the presence of different heavy metals was studied, and it was observed that the density of trichomes on the leaf apex and margin increased on both abaxial and adaxial surfaces of the plants grown in soil containing a mixture of Cd, Cr, Ni, and calcium hydroxide [91]. *Conyza blinii* also reported to show a certain tolerance against iron toxicity. On ferrous iron treatment, *C. blinii* showed a significant increase in the photosynthetic capacity and capitate glandular trichome density, providing precursors and sites for the synthesis of blinin which actively participates in the process of resistance to stress and other damage. The distribution and density of trichomes increased significantly in *Matricaria chamomilla* L. on cadmium treatment. Under Cd stress, the MDA content enhanced in chamomile flowers increasing the ROS levels, which enhanced the production of apigenin showing defence response due to its antioxidant and sequestering properties. The Pb enters the cellular space of trichomes in *Brassica rapa* ssp. *pekinensis* and accumulates in the basal compartment, enhancing foliar Pb uptake in the edible leaves of cabbage [92].

Salinity Stress

High salinity-induced Na^+ toxicity and osmotic stress in the rhizosphere environment jeopardize and limit plant growth, development and hence, crop productivity. Salinity is well known for causing oxidative damage, primarily through the production of excessive ROS, which alters proteins, carbohydrates, DNA, and lipids. Secondary metabolites such as phenolic and flavonoid compounds are produced by plants as a result of defence mechanisms operated in response to ROS detoxification in salinity exposed plants [93, 94]. Salinity is reported to induce the accumulation of terpenoid secondary metabolites such as artemisinin (having antioxidant activity) in the GTs in *A. annua* [95]. Changes in cellular redox homeostasis are thought to stir up MYB transcription factors, which are involved in the biosynthesis of flavonoids, particularly flavonols [96]. Salinity stress increases the trichome density in borage (*Borago officinalis* L.), which helps the plants to deal with salt stress by reducing the evapo-transpiration rate under conditions of salinity stress [97].

Ozone Stress

Ozone (O_3) is a toxic, strong polar oxidant that primarily enters the plant through the stomata. Trichomes provide protection against O_3 damage on the leaf surface. Glandular trichomes play a protective role against O_3 stress which is associated with the type and density of glandular trichomes across a highly diverse set of species [98]. Trichomes promote the formation of a thick, moist boundary layer that can act as an ozone sink [99]. *Nicotiana tabacum* GTs secrete semi-volatile organic compounds (such as the diterpenoidcis-abienol) that act as an efficient O_3 sink [100]. GTs are said to act as a chemical barrier, reducing ozone uptake and toxicity in the leaves. Their density is linked to the plant's ozone sensitivity, as indicated by visible leaf injuries and lipoxygenase (LOX) product emissions. Thus, ozone stress is found to be more vulnerable in species with fewer glandular trichomes on their leaf surface than those with a higher density.

Light and Wind Stress

Plant growth and development are strongly influenced by the photosynthetically active radiation (PAR; 400–700 nm). Increased PAR may influence the synthesis of carbon-based metabolites like phenolics and terpenes. In particular, trichomes can diminish the absorbance of overabundance solar radiation by the mesophyll cells. They may facilitate the condensation of moisture present in the air [101]. Positive correlation of leaf trichomes and reflectance of PAR have been documented in several metabolite rich plants. Trichome density is enhanced when the water potential is reduced in the plant, resulting in increased leaf reflectance of PAR. A higher density of trichomes reflects more light which may facilitate the temperature regulation of plants. Researchers also revealed the role of near-infrared light during improved reflectance by trichomes [102]. Type VI structures are the most prominent GTs present on the leaf surface of *S. lycopersicum* (cultivated tomatoes), which mainly contribute during physical defences. An increase in PAR induces the type VI GTs in the leaves of cultivated tomatoes. Shift in light intensity is responsible for the induction of type VI GTs density and stored metabolites. Elevated light intensity is responsible for induced expression of jasmonic acid responsive defence genes. An increase in trichome density is proportional to higher production of trichome associated phytoconstituents such as terpenes and phenolics. These trichome associated chemicals provide defence against thrips (*Frankliniella occidentalis*). Cannabinoids are unique bio-active compounds that are known to be affected by the influence of light. The ratio of different wavelengths of light affects the metabolism of cannabinoids. Increased yields were procured when the Blue:Red light ranges at 1:1. However, white light along with Blue:Red light gives an adverse effect on trichome density and yield. Blue rich light gives a stimulatory effect on CBGA accumulation as compared to Red light. Along with CBGA, other major cannabinoids, *i.e.*, CBDA, CBCA and THCA, were also influenced by light quality [103].

Increased density of trichomes provides high resistance to mechanical damage which influenced by wind and sand particles. More than 85% of particulate matters (PM) dispersal takes place by wind at the plants which lack trichomes at their leaf surface. However, trichome bearing plants show lesser extent of PM adsorption and resuspension [104].

EFFECT OF BIOTIC STRESS ON TRICHOME PHYSIOLOGY AND METABOLITE PRODUCTIVITY

Plants are damaged by more than ten thousand insects and one million pathogens. The structural anatomy of plants plays a very important role in mechanical defence or delivery of the chemicals through pores or glands. Several leaf anatomical traits, such as the presence and density of trichomes, and leaf cuticular thickness, impact the interaction with various pests and insects; thereby influencing their plant-insects' interaction [105].

Pathogens

Pathogens are a major threat to plant growth, development, and yield among the various biotic stresses. Trichome density is connected with resistance to different pathogens in various crops. Trichomes provide host resistance because of their habit to entrap spores, thereby preventing the attraction of spores to the epidermis. In wheat, trichomes entrap fungal spores (*Parastagonospora nodorum*) and, thus, prevent germ tubes from reaching the epidermis, providing resistance to the host from *Septoria nodorum* blotch [106]. High trichome density reduces surface wettability required for spore germination of many pathogens. In wheat, the high density of trichomes on the adaxial surface of flag leaves entraps *Bipolaris sorokiniana* spores. It also restricts the dew droplet size on the flag leaves and thus prevents direct connection between the pathogenic spores and the plant epidermis [107]. *Nicotana tabacum*'s GTs secretes phylloplanins, a protein inhibitor that prevents spore germination and infection by the pathogen *Peronospora tabacina* [108]. In *Artemisia annua*, enhancing artemisinin content in trichomes by the overexpression of transcription factors, *AaWRKY17* and *AaORA* provide tolerance towards *Pseudomonas syringae* and *Botrytis cinerea* infections, respectively [109, 110].

Insects

Trichomes act as a physical barrier against insects either by attacking or killing the insects directly or by retarding their growth and population. Trichomes can act as an additional line of defence against foliar secondary metabolites, and they are even effective against specialist herbivores. Plant trichomes create hindrances to the free movement of insects and may secrete volatile or non-volatile toxic chemicals, making it very tough for pests to feed on the plant surface and thus affecting insect feeding positions. Flavonoids and terpenes are secreted by anemones with long glandular trichomes to keep leafhoppers away from the plants [111]. Recent studies provide relevant evidence that trichomes may perform functions as sensors for detecting movements of insect on the leaf surface [112]. Sucking pest resistance is aided by the presence of trichomes on the lower surface of cotton leaves. In sunflowers, the presence of trichome density confers insect resistance. Trichomes have been found to play a role in the defence of chilli plants, both directly and indirectly. Thrips (*Scirtothrips dorsalis*), for example, avoided a large number of trichomes that restricted their movement on chilli. *Capsicum annuum* also produces terpene volatiles that keep whiteflies (*Bemisia tabaci*) away from the plant [113]. Tomato glandular trichomes have been reported to emit terpene volatiles, which reduce thrips infestation on plants [114, 115]. Tarweed (*Madia elegans*) GTs trap insects by releasing sticky chemicals and provide carrion as a food source for predators. Under natural field conditions, this indirect defence effectively reduces herbivore activity while increasing plant fitness [116]. Stellate trichomes and internodal spines may be a key towards mitigating interactions between *Manduca sexta* and *Solanum carolinense*. These structural defences damaged the peritrophic membrane of *M. sexta*, along with deterring their feeding as well as negatively affecting their growth [117]. *Tetranychus urticae* encounters difficulties on *Solanum pennellii* plant leaf's surface due to the presence of a high density of type IV GTs, positively related to acyl sugar production. On *S. pennellii*, nymphs and adult females showed high mortality rate, adult females had a low rate for oviposition, the duration of the egg incubation period increased, and viability of the egg and mite declined [118]. Spider mites travelled shorter distances in tomato plants with high type IV and VI densities corresponding to high zingiberene content. Also, the number of whitefly eggs and nymphs was lower in these plants. Higher zingiberene contents affected negatively both the spider mite and the whitefly behaviour [119, 120].

CONCLUDING REMARKS AND FUTURE PROSPECTIVE

Glandular trichomes (GTs) are valuable bio-repertoires as they synthesize and store different plant secondary metabolites. Over the years, studies on GTs and NGTs are emerging with the advancement of transcriptome, metabolome, and proteomic techniques. Different studies suggested that the demand for plant based secondary metabolites in drug industry was rising over synthetic drugs. Hence, the present chapter focuses on comprehending the knowledge of GT development and secondary metabolite biosynthesis and its regulation.

Trichome initiation is a controlled developmental process mediated by different transcription factors (TF), cyclins or their complexes. Further research is required to investigate other similar TF and their complexes' involvement in trichome biology across the medicinally important plant species. MYC1, a bHLH TF, MX1, a R2R3-MYB TF, and CD2, a HD-ZIP IV TF participate in the tomato glandular trichome initiation. MYC1 is the only identified gene involved in the GT development of tomato. The study should also be conducted to know that, are molecular regulators involved in the GT initiation and development process conserved in similar plant lineages? On the basis of compiled literature, we can interpret the conserved function of H, CycB2 and Wo genes among the Solanaceae family. To further explore the functions of identified genes and characterization of novel regulators in trichome development, recent advances, such as targeted based mutagenesis approaches, such as, CRISPR-Cas9 (Clustered Regularly Interspaced Short Palindromic Repeats-CRISPR-associated protein 9) and TILLING (Targeting Induced Local Lesions In Genomes), can be focused. On the other hand, comparative analysis of type-V glandular trichomes with type IV may also provide information related to glandular cell differentiation due to their morphological similarity except the gland cell. In addition, environmental factors both biotic as well as abiotic significantly influence the biosynthesis and accumulation of bioactive metabolites in the glandular trichomes. They can be further explored by investigators using different elicitors and precursor feeding strategies to not only design a high yielding crop but also provide two contrasting types that insight into the biosynthetic regulatory mechanism operating in these GTs.

ACKNOWLEDGEMENTS

"The authors are thankful to the Director, CSIR-National Botanical Research Institute, Lucknow. PS is indebted to Banaras Hindu University, Varanasi, India for the registration (Sept.-2017/358). AP is thankful to UGC No. (F.4-2/2006 (BSR)/BL/18-19/0078) New Delhi, India for the financial support provided during the present work." This MS bears NBRI communication number CSIR-NBRI_MS/2022/03/09.

REFERENCES

[1]   Yang C, Ye Z. Trichomes as models for studying plant cell differentiation. Cell Mol Life Sci 2013; 70(11): 1937-48.
[http://dx.doi.org/10.1007/s00018-012-1147-6] [PMID: 22996257]

[2]   Ma ZY, Wen J, Ickert-Bond SM, Chen LQ, Liu XQ. Morphology, structure, and ontogeny of trichomes of the grape genus (*Vitis,* Vitaceae). Front Plant Sci 2016; 7: 704.
[http://dx.doi.org/10.3389/fpls.2016.00704] [PMID: 27252720]

[3]   Schuurink R, Tissier A. Glandular trichomes: Micro-organs with model status? New Phytol 2020; 225(6): 2251-66.
[http://dx.doi.org/10.1111/nph.16283] [PMID: 31651036]

[4]   Pandey S, Goel R, Bhardwaj A, Asif MH, Sawant SV, Misra P. Transcriptome analysis provides insight into prickle development and its link to defense and secondary metabolism in *Solanum viarum* Dunal. Sci Rep 2018; 8(1): 17092.
[http://dx.doi.org/10.1038/s41598-018-35304-8] [PMID: 30459319]

[5]   Doolabh K, Naidoo Y, Dewir YH, Al-Suhaibani N. Micromorphology, ultrastructure and histochemistry of *Commelina benghalensis* L. leaves and stems. Plants 2021; 10(3): 512.
[http://dx.doi.org/10.3390/plants10030512] [PMID: 33803463]

[6]   Wagner GJ. Secreting glandular trichomes: More than just hairs. Plant Physiol 1991; 96(3): 675-9.
[http://dx.doi.org/10.1104/pp.96.3.675] [PMID: 16668241]

[7]   Glas J, Schimmel B, Alba J, Escobar-Bravo R, Schuurink R, Kant M. Plant glandular trichomes as targets for breeding or engineering of resistance to herbivores. Int J Mol Sci 2012; 13(12): 17077-103.
[http://dx.doi.org/10.3390/ijms131217077] [PMID: 23235331]

[8]   Cui H, Zhang ST, Yang HJ, Ji H, Wang XJ. Gene expression profile analysis of tobacco leaf trichomes. BMC Plant Biol 2011; 11(1): 76.
[http://dx.doi.org/10.1186/1471-2229-11-76] [PMID: 21548994]

[9]   Huchelmann A, Boutry M, Hachez C. Plant glandular trichomes: Natural cell factories of high biotechnological interest. Plant Physiol 2017; 175(1): 6-22.
[http://dx.doi.org/10.1104/pp.17.00727] [PMID: 28724619]

[10] Tissier A. Glandular trichomes: What comes after expressed sequence tags? Plant J 2012; 70(1): 51-68.
[http://dx.doi.org/10.1111/j.1365-313X.2012.04913.x] [PMID: 22449043]

[11] Tripathi DK, Singh VP, Chauhan DK, Eds., *et al.* Plant Life Under Changing Environment: Responses and Management. Academic Press 2020.

[12] Mishra A, Lal RK, Chanotiya CS, Dhawan SS. Genetic elaborations of glandular and non-glandular trichomes in *Mentha arvensis* genotypes: Assessing genotypic and phenotypic correlations along with gene expressions. Protoplasma 2017; 254(2): 1045-61.
[http://dx.doi.org/10.1007/s00709-016-1011-x] [PMID: 27515313]

[13] Koudounas K, Manioudaki ME, Kourti A, Banilas G, Hatzopoulos P. Transcriptional profiling unravels potential metabolic activities of the olive leaf non-glandular trichome. Front Plant Sci 2015; 6: 633.
[http://dx.doi.org/10.3389/fpls.2015.00633] [PMID: 26322070]

[14] Feng Z, Bartholomew ES, Liu Z, *et al.* Glandular trichomes: New focus on horticultural crops. Hortic Res 2021; 8(1): 158.
[http://dx.doi.org/10.1038/s41438-021-00592-1] [PMID: 34193839]

[15] Jing H, Liu J, Liu H, Xin H. Histochemical investigation and kinds of alkaloids in leaves of different developmental stages in *Thymus quinquecostatus*. ScientWorldJ 2014; 2014: 1-6.
[http://dx.doi.org/10.1155/2014/839548] [PMID: 25101324]

[16] Wang G. Recent progress in secondary metabolism of plant glandular trichomes. Plant Biotechnol 2014; 31(5): 353-61.
[http://dx.doi.org/10.5511/plantbiotechnology.14.0701a]

[17] Tissier A. Glandular trichomes: What comes after expressed sequence tags? Plant J 2012; 70(1): 51-68.
[http://dx.doi.org/10.1111/j.1365-313X.2012.04913.x] [PMID: 22449043]

[18] Lange BM. The evolution of plant secretory structures and emergence of terpenoid chemical diversity. Annu Rev Plant Biol 2015; 66(1): 139-59.
[http://dx.doi.org/10.1146/annurev-arplant-043014-114639] [PMID: 25621517]

[19] Wang X, Shen C, Meng P, Tan G, Lv L. Analysis and review of trichomes in plants. BMC Plant Biol 2021; 21(1): 70.
[http://dx.doi.org/10.1186/s12870-021-02840-x] [PMID: 33526015]

[20] Li R, Wang X, Zhang S, *et al.* Two zinc-finger proteins control the initiation and elongation of long stalk trichomes in tomato. J Genet Genomics 2021; 48(12): 1057-69.
[http://dx.doi.org/10.1016/j.jgg.2021.09.001] [PMID: 34555548]

[21] An L, Zhou Z, Yan A, Gan Y. Progress on trichome development regulated by phytohormone signaling. Plant Signal Behav 2011; 6(12): 1959-62.
[http://dx.doi.org/10.4161/psb.6.12.18120] [PMID: 22105030]

[22] Werker E. Trichome diversity and development. Adv Botan Res 2000; 31: 1-35.

[23] Yadav RK, Sangwan RS, Sabir F, Srivastava AK, Sangwan NS. Effect of prolonged water stress on specialized secondary metabolites, peltate glandular trichomes, and pathway gene expression in *Artemisia annua* L. Plant Physiol Biochem 2014; 74: 70-83.
[http://dx.doi.org/10.1016/j.plaphy.2013.10.023] [PMID: 24269871]

[24] Stanojković J, Todorović S, Pećinar I, Lević S, Ćalić S, Janošević D. Leaf glandular trichomes of micropropagated *Inula britannica* – Effect of sucrose on trichome density, distribution and chemical profile. Ind Crops Prod 2021; 160: 113101.
[http://dx.doi.org/10.1016/j.indcrop.2020.113101]

[25] Zheng T, Wang M, Zhan J, *et al.* Ferrous iron-induced increases in capitate glandular trichome density

and upregulation of CbHO-1 contributes to increases in blinin content in *Conyza blinii*. Planta 2020; 252(5): 81.
[http://dx.doi.org/10.1007/s00425-020-03492-1] [PMID: 33037484]

[26]   Gao QM, Kane NC, Hulke BS, *et al*. Genetic architecture of capitate glandular trichome density in florets of domesticated sunflower (*Helianthus annuus* L.). Front Plant Sci 2018; 8: 2227.
[http://dx.doi.org/10.3389/fpls.2017.02227] [PMID: 29375602]

[27]   Zarinkamar F, Moradi A, Davoodpour M. Ecophysiological, anatomical, and apigenin changes due to uptake and accumulation of cadmium in *Matricaria chamomilla* L. flowers in hydroponics. Environ Sci Pollut Res Int 2021; 28(39): 55154-65.
[http://dx.doi.org/10.1007/s11356-021-14000-7] [PMID: 34128167]

[28]   Bar M, Shtein I. Plant trichomes and the biomechanics of defense in various systems, with Solanaceae as a model. Botany 2019; 97(12): 651-60.
[http://dx.doi.org/10.1139/cjb-2019-0144]

[29]   Zhou Y, Tang N, Huang L, Zhao Y, Tang X, Wang K. Effects of salt stress on plant growth, antioxidant capacity, glandular trichome density, and volatile exudates of *Schizonepeta tenuifolia* Briq. Int J Mol Sci 2018; 19(1): 252.
[http://dx.doi.org/10.3390/ijms19010252] [PMID: 29342961]

[30]   Olfa B, Imen T, Mohamed C, Nasri-Ayachi M B. Essential oil and trichome density from *Origanum majorana* L. shoots affected by leaf age and salinity. Biosci J 2016; 32(1): 238-45.
[http://dx.doi.org/10.14393/BJ-v32n1a2016-30323]

[31]   Tang T, Li CH, Li DS, *et al*. Peltate glandular trichomes of Colquhounia vestita harbor diterpenoid acids that contribute to plant adaptation to UV radiation and cold stresses. Phytochemistry 2020; 172: 112285.
[http://dx.doi.org/10.1016/j.phytochem.2020.112285] [PMID: 32035325]

[32]   Haber AI, Rivera Sustache J, Carr DE. A generalist and a specialist herbivore are differentially affected by inbreeding and trichomes in *Mimulus guttatus*. Ecosphere 2018; 9(2): e02130.
[http://dx.doi.org/10.1002/ecs2.2130]

[33]   Luckwill LC. The genus Lycopersicon: an historical, biological, and taxonomic survery of the wild and cultivated tomatoes (No BOOK). Aberdeen University Press 1943.

[34]   Channarayappa C, Shivashankar G, Muniyappa V, Frist RH. Resistance of *Lycopersicon* species to *Bemisia tabaci*, a tomato leaf curl virus vector. Can J Bot 1992; 70(11): 2184-92.
[http://dx.doi.org/10.1139/b92-270]

[35]   McDowell ET, Kapteyn J, Schmidt A, *et al*. Comparative functional genomic analysis of Solanum glandular trichome types. Plant Physiol 2011; 155(1): 524-39.
[http://dx.doi.org/10.1104/pp.110.167114] [PMID: 21098679]

[36]   Calo L, García I, Gotor C, Romero LC. Leaf hairs influence phytopathogenic fungus infection and confer an increased resistance when expressing a Trichoderma -1,3-glucanase. J Exp Bot 2006; 57(14): 3911-20.
[http://dx.doi.org/10.1093/jxb/erl155] [PMID: 17043085]

[37]   Li C, Wang Z, Jones AD. Chemical imaging of trichome specialized metabolites using contact printing and laser desorption/ionization mass spectrometry. Anal Bioanal Chem 2014; 406(1): 171-82.
[http://dx.doi.org/10.1007/s00216-013-7444-6] [PMID: 24220760]

[38]   Bennewitz S, Bergau N, Tissier A. QTL mapping of the shape of type VI glandular trichomes in tomato. Front Plant Sci 2018; 9: 1421.
[http://dx.doi.org/10.3389/fpls.2018.01421] [PMID: 30319679]

[39]   Xu J, Van Herwijnen ZO, Dräger DB, Sui C, Haring MA, Schuurink RC. SlMYC1 regulates type VI glandular trichome formation and terpene biosynthesis in tomato glandular cells. Plant Cell 2018; 30(12): 2988-3005.

[http://dx.doi.org/10.1105/tpc.18.00571] [PMID: 30518626]

[40]   Bergau N, Bennewitz S, Syrowatka F, Hause G, Tissier A. The development of type VI glandular trichomes in the cultivated tomato *Solanum lycopersicum* and a related wild species *S. habrochaites*. BMC Plant Biol 2015; 15(1): 289.
[http://dx.doi.org/10.1186/s12870-015-0678-z] [PMID: 26654876]

[41]   Balcke GU, Bennewitz S, Bergau N, *et al*. Multi-omics of tomato glandular trichomes reveals distinct features of central carbon metabolism supporting high productivity of specialized metabolites. Plant Cell 2017; 29(5): 960-83.
[http://dx.doi.org/10.1105/tpc.17.00060] [PMID: 28408661]

[42]   Bennewitz S, Bergau N, Tissier A. QTL mapping of the shape of type VI glandular trichomes in tomato. Front Plant Sci 2018; 9: 1421.
[http://dx.doi.org/10.3389/fpls.2018.01421] [PMID: 30319679]

[43]   Conneely LJ, Mauleon R, Mieog J, Barkla BJ, Kretzschmar T. Characterization of the *Cannabis sativa* glandular trichome proteome. PLoS One 2021; 16(4): e0242633.
[http://dx.doi.org/10.1371/journal.pone.0242633] [PMID: 33793557]

[44]   Chalvin C, Drevensek S, Dron M, Bendahmane A, Boualem A. Genetic control of glandular trichome development. Trends Plant Sci 2020; 25(5): 477-87.
[http://dx.doi.org/10.1016/j.tplants.2019.12.025] [PMID: 31983619]

[45]   Tominaga-Wada R, Nukumizu Y, Sato S, Wada T. Control of plant trichome and root-hair development by a tomato (*Solanum lycopersicum*) R3 MYB transcription factor. PLoS One 2013; 8(1): e54019.
[http://dx.doi.org/10.1371/journal.pone.0054019] [PMID: 23326563]

[46]   Zhou F, Pichersky E. The complete functional characterisation of the terpene synthase family in tomato. New Phytol 2020; 226(5): 1341-60.
[http://dx.doi.org/10.1111/nph.16431] [PMID: 31943222]

[47]   Tissier A, Morgan JA, Dudareva N. Plant volatiles: Going 'in' but not 'out'of trichome cavities. Trends Plant Sci 2017; 22(11): 930-8.
[http://dx.doi.org/10.1016/j.tplants.2017.09.001] [PMID: 28958712]

[48]   Spyropoulou EA, Haring MA, Schuurink RC. RNA sequencing on *Solanum lycopersicum* trichomes identifies transcription factors that activate terpene synthase promoters. BMC Genomics 2014; 15(1): 402.
[http://dx.doi.org/10.1186/1471-2164-15-402] [PMID: 24884371]

[49]   Flood P J. The smell of transcription: The SlMYC1 transcription factor makes tomato plants smelly. Plant Cell 2019; 31(1): 2.

[50]   Yang C, Marillonnet S, Tissier A. The scarecrow-like transcription factor SlSCL3 regulates volatile terpene biosynthesis and glandular trichome size in tomato (*Solanum lycopersicum*). Plant J 2021; 107(4): 1102-18.
[http://dx.doi.org/10.1111/tpj.15371] [PMID: 34143914]

[51]   Ewas M, Gao Y, Wang S, *et al*. Manipulation of *Sl*MX1 for enhanced carotenoids accumulation and drought resistance in tomato. Sci Bull 2016; 61(18): 1413-8.
[http://dx.doi.org/10.1007/s11434-016-1108-9]

[52]   Yang C, Li H, Zhang J, *et al*. A regulatory gene induces trichome formation and embryo lethality in tomato. Proc Natl Acad Sci 2011; 108(29): 11836-41.
[http://dx.doi.org/10.1073/pnas.1100532108] [PMID: 21730153]

[53]   Vendemiatti E, Zsögön A, Silva GFF, *et al*. Loss of type-IV glandular trichomes is a heterochronic trait in tomato and can be reverted by promoting juvenility. Plant Sci 2017; 259: 35-47.
[http://dx.doi.org/10.1016/j.plantsci.2017.03.006] [PMID: 28483052]

[54]   Chang J, Yu T, Yang Q, *et al*. *Hair*, encoding a single C2H2 zinc-finger protein, regulates

multicellular trichome formation in tomato. Plant J 2018; 96(1): 90-102.
[http://dx.doi.org/10.1111/tpj.14018] [PMID: 29981215]

[55] Soetaert SSA, Van Neste CMF, Vandewoestyne ML, *et al.* Differential transcriptome analysis of glandular and filamentous trichomes in *Artemisia annua.* BMC Plant Biol 2013; 13(1): 220.
[http://dx.doi.org/10.1186/1471-2229-13-220] [PMID: 24359620]

[56] Pandey N, Tiwari A, Rai S K, Pandey-Rai S. Accumulation of secondary metabolites and improved size of glandular trichomes in artemisia annua. Plant Cell and Tissue Differentiation and Secondary Metabolites: Fundamentals and Applications 2021; 99-116.

[57] Judd R, Bagley MC, Li M, *et al.* Artemisinin biosynthesis in non-glandular trichome cells of *Artemisia annua.* Mol Plant 2019; 12(5): 704-14.
[http://dx.doi.org/10.1016/j.molp.2019.02.011] [PMID: 30851440]

[58] Salehi M, Karimzadeh G, Naghavi MR, Naghdi Badi H, Rashidi Monfared S. Expression of key genes affecting artemisinin content in five *Artemisia* species. Sci Rep 2018; 8(1): 12659.
[http://dx.doi.org/10.1038/s41598-018-31079-0]

[59] Janick J, Janick J. Floral morphology of *Artemisia annua* with special reference to trichomes. Int J Plant Sci 1995; 156(6): 807-15.
[http://dx.doi.org/10.1086/297304]

[60] Rowe HC, Ro D, Rieseberg LH. Response of sunflower (*Helianthus annuus* L.) leaf surface defenses to exogenous methyl jasmonate. PLoS One 2012; 7(5): e37191.
[http://dx.doi.org/10.1371/journal.pone.0037191] [PMID: 22623991]

[61] Aschenbrenner AK, Horakh S, Spring O. Linear glandular trichomes of *Helianthus* (Asteraceae): Morphology, localization, metabolite activity and occurrence. AoB Plants 2013; 5(0): plt028.
[http://dx.doi.org/10.1093/aobpla/plt028]

[62] Amrehn E, Spring O. Ultrastructural alterations in cells of sunflower linear glandular trichomes during maturation. Plants 2021; 10(8): 1515.
[http://dx.doi.org/10.3390/plants10081515] [PMID: 34451559]

[63] Romero P, Peris A, Vergara K, Matus JT. Comprehending and improving cannabis specialized metabolism in the systems biology era. Plant Sci 2020; 298: 110571.
[http://dx.doi.org/10.1016/j.plantsci.2020.110571] [PMID: 32771172]

[64] Tanney CAS, Backer R, Geitmann A, Smith DL. Cannabis glandular trichomes: A cellular metabolite factory. Front Plant Sci 2021; 12: 721986.
[http://dx.doi.org/10.3389/fpls.2021.721986] [PMID: 34616415]

[65] Livingston SJ, Quilichini TD, Booth JK, *et al.* Cannabis glandular trichomes alter morphology and metabolite content during flower maturation. Plant J 2020; 101(1): 37-56.
[http://dx.doi.org/10.1111/tpj.14516] [PMID: 31469934]

[66] Vincent D, Rochfort S, Spangenberg G. Optimisation of protein extraction from medicinal cannabis mature buds for bottom-up proteomics. Molecules 2019; 24(4): 659.
[http://dx.doi.org/10.3390/molecules24040659] [PMID: 30781766]

[67] Ebersbach P, Stehle F, Kayser O, Freier E. Chemical fingerprinting of single glandular trichomes of *Cannabis sativa* by coherent anti-stokes raman scattering (CARS) microscopy. BMC Plant Biol 2018; 18(1): 275.
[http://dx.doi.org/10.1186/s12870-018-1481-4] [PMID: 30419820]

[68] Munien P, Naidoo Y, Naidoo G. Micromorphology, histochemistry and ultrastructure of the foliar trichomes of Withania somnifera (L.) Dunal (Solanaceae). Planta 2015; 242(5): 1107-22.
[http://dx.doi.org/10.1007/s00425-015-2341-1] [PMID: 26063189]

[69] Bhatt A, Naidoo Y, Nicholas A. The foliar trichomes of *Hypoestes aristata* (Vahl) Sol. ex Roem. & Schult var aristata (Acanthaceae) a widespread medicinal plant species in tropical sub-Saharan Africa: with comments on its possible phylogenetic significance. Biol Res 2010; 43(4): 403-9.

[http://dx.doi.org/10.4067/S0716-97602010000400004] [PMID: 21526266]

[70] Zhang H, Liu P, Wang B, Yuan F. The roles of trichome development genes in stress resistance. Plant Growth Regul 2021; 95(2): 137-48.
[http://dx.doi.org/10.1007/s10725-021-00733-5]

[71] Scalabrin E, Radaelli M, Rizzato G, *et al.* Metabolomic analysis of wild and transgenic *Nicotiana langsdorffii* plants exposed to abiotic stresses: Unraveling metabolic responses. Anal Bioanal Chem 2015; 407(21): 6357-68.
[http://dx.doi.org/10.1007/s00216-015-8770-7] [PMID: 26014284]

[72] Pérez-Estrada LB, Cano-Santana Z, Oyama K. Variation in leaf trichomes of *Wigandia urens*: environmental factors and physiological consequences. Tree Physiol 2000; 20(9): 629-32.
[http://dx.doi.org/10.1093/treephys/20.9.629] [PMID: 12651428]

[73] Lipiec J, Doussan C, Nosalewicz A, Kondracka K. Effect of drought and heat stresses on plant growth and yield: A review. Int Agrophys 2013; 27(4): 463-77.
[http://dx.doi.org/10.2478/intag-2013-0017]

[74] Bartwal A, Mall R, Lohani P, Guru SK, Arora S. Role of secondary metabolites and brassinosteroids in plant defense against environmental stresses. J Plant Growth Regul 2013; 32(1): 216-32.
[http://dx.doi.org/10.1007/s00344-012-9272-x]

[75] Saltveit ME, Hepler PK. Effect of heat shock on the chilling sensitivity of trichomes and petioles of African violet (Saintpaulia ionantha). Physiol Plant 2004; 121(1): 35-43.
[http://dx.doi.org/10.1111/j.0031-9317.2004.00288.x] [PMID: 15086815]

[76] Kang JH, Liu G, Shi F, Jones AD, Beaudry RM, Howe GA. The tomato *odorless-2* mutant is defective in trichome-based production of diverse specialized metabolites and broad-spectrum resistance to insect herbivores. Plant Physiol 2010; 154(1): 262-72.
[http://dx.doi.org/10.1104/pp.110.160192] [PMID: 20668059]

[77] Agrawal AA, Fishbein M. Plant defense syndromes. Ecology 2006; 87(sp7) (Suppl.): S132-49.
[http://dx.doi.org/10.1890/0012-9658(2006)87[132:PDS]2.0.CO;2] [PMID: 16922309]

[78] Traw MB, Bergelson J. Interactive effects of jasmonic acid, salicylic acid, and gibberellin on induction of trichomes in *Arabidopsis*. Plant Physiol 2003; 133(3): 1367-75.
[http://dx.doi.org/10.1104/pp.103.027086] [PMID: 14551332]

[79] Zhu W, Li J, Wang A. Effect of low temperature stress on physiological and biochemical characteristics of *Lycopersicon hirsutum* seedlings. Dongbei Nongye Daxue Xuebao 2011; 42: 57-61.

[80] Zhang Y, Song H, Wang X, *et al.* The roles of different types of trichomes in tomato resistance to cold, drought, whiteflies, and botrytis. Agronomy 2020; 10(3): 411.
[http://dx.doi.org/10.3390/agronomy10030411]

[81] Yordanov I, Velikova V, Tsonev T. Plant responses to drought, acclimation, and stress tolerance. Photosynthetica 2000; 38(2): 171-86.
[http://dx.doi.org/10.1023/A:1007201411474]

[82] Ning P, Wang J, Zhou Y, Gao L, Wang J, Gong C. Adaptional evolution of trichome in *Caragana korshinskii* to natural drought stress on the Loess Plateau, China. Ecol Evol 2016; 6(11): 3786-95.
[http://dx.doi.org/10.1002/ece3.2157] [PMID: 28725356]

[83] Schreuder MDJ, Brewer CA, Heine C. Modelled influences of non-exchanging trichomes on leaf boundary layers and gas exchange. J Theor Biol 2001; 210(1): 23-32.
[http://dx.doi.org/10.1006/jtbi.2001.2285] [PMID: 11343428]

[84] Shahzad M, Khan Z, Hussain SI, *et al.* A review on role of trichomes in plant physiology and genetic mechanism involved in trichome regulation in cotton. Pure Appl Biol 2021; 10(2): 458-64.
[http://dx.doi.org/10.19045/bspab.2021.100049]

[85] Waseem M, Nie ZF, Yao GQ, Hasan M, Xiang Y, Fang XW. Dew absorption by leaf trichomes in

Caragana korshinskii : An alternative water acquisition strategy for withstanding drought in arid environments. Physiol Plant 2021; 172(2): 528-39.
[http://dx.doi.org/10.1111/ppl.13334] [PMID: 33452683]

[86]   Wang J, Wang H, Fu Y, Huang T, Liu Y, Wang X. Genetic variance and transcriptional regulation modulate terpenoid biosynthesis in trichomes of *Nicotiana tabacum* under drought. Ind Crops Prod 2021; 167: 113501.
[http://dx.doi.org/10.1016/j.indcrop.2021.113501]

[87]   Koul M, Thomas L, Karmakar K. Functional aspects of solanaceae trichomes in heavy metal detoxification. Nord J Bot 2021; 39(5): njb.03171.
[http://dx.doi.org/10.1111/njb.03171]

[88]   Pandey S, Shukla P, Misra P. Physical state of the culture medium triggers shift in morphogenetic pattern from shoot bud formation to somatic embryo in *Solanum khasianum*. Physiology and molecular biology of plants: an international journal of functional plant biology 2018; 24: 1295-305.

[89]   Shukla P, Kidwai M, Narayan S, *et al.* Phytoremediation potential of *Solanum viarum* Dunal and functional aspects of their capitate glandular trichomes in lead, cadmium, and zinc detoxification. Environ Sci Pollut Res Int 2023; 30(14): 41878-99.
[http://dx.doi.org/10.1007/s11356-023-25174-7] [PMID: 36640234]

[90]   Guo C, Hu J, Gao W, *et al.* Mechanosensation triggers enhanced heavy metal ion uptake by non-glandular trichomes. J Hazard Mater 2022; 426: 127983.
[http://dx.doi.org/10.1016/j.jhazmat.2021.127983] [PMID: 34923380]

[91]   Saidulu CH, Venkateshwar C, Gangadhar Rao S. Foliar epidermal study of *Withania somnifera* grown in heavy metal treated soil. Res Rev BioSci 2016; 11: 107.

[92]   Gao PP, Zhang XM, Xue PY, *et al.* Mechanism of Pb accumulation in Chinese cabbage leaves: Stomata and trichomes regulate foliar uptake of Pb in atmospheric $PM_{2.5}$. Environ Pollut 2022; 293: 118585.
[http://dx.doi.org/10.1016/j.envpol.2021.118585] [PMID: 34848290]

[93]   Ahmad F, Kamal A, Singh A, *et al.* Seed priming with gibberellic acid induces high salinity tolerance in *Pisum sativum* through antioxidants, secondary metabolites and up-regulation of antiporter genes. Plant Biol 2021; 23(S1) (1): 113-21.
[http://dx.doi.org/10.1111/plb.13187] [PMID: 32989871]

[94]   Salem N, Msaada K, Dhifi W, Limam F, Marzouk B. Effect of salinity on plant growth and biological activities of *Carthamus tinctorius* L. extracts at two flowering stages. Acta Physiol Plant 2014; 36(2): 433-45.
[http://dx.doi.org/10.1007/s11738-013-1424-5]

[95]   Yadav RK, Sangwan RS, Srivastava AK, Sangwan NS. Prolonged exposure to salt stress affects specialized metabolites-artemisinin and essential oil accumulation in *Artemisia annua* L.: metabolic acclimation in preferential favour of enhanced terpenoid accumulation accompanying vegetative to reproductive phase transition. Protoplasma 2017; 254(1): 505-22.
[http://dx.doi.org/10.1007/s00709-016-0971-1] [PMID: 27263081]

[96]   Taylor LP, Grotewold E. Flavonoids as developmental regulators. Curr Opin Plant Biol 2005; 8(3): 317-23.
[http://dx.doi.org/10.1016/j.pbi.2005.03.005] [PMID: 15860429]

[97]   Torabi F, Majd A, Enteshari S. The effect of silicon on alleviation of salt stress in borage (*Borago officinalis* L.). Soil Sci Plant Nutr 2015; 61(5): 788-98.
[http://dx.doi.org/10.1080/00380768.2015.1005540]

[98]   Li S, Tosens T, Harley PC, *et al.* Glandular trichomes as a barrier against atmospheric oxidative stress: Relationships with ozone uptake, leaf damage, and emission of LOX products across a diverse set of species. Plant Cell Environ 2018; 41(6): 1263-77.
[http://dx.doi.org/10.1111/pce.13128] [PMID: 29292838]

[99] Gasche R, Papen H, Rennenberg H, Eds. Trace gas exchange in forest ecosystems. Kluwer Academic Publishers 2002.
[http://dx.doi.org/10.1007/978-94-015-9856-9]

[100] Jud W, Fischer L, Canaval E, Wohlfahrt G, Tissier A, Hansel A. Plant surface reactions: An ozone defence mechanism impacting atmospheric chemistry. Atmos Chem Phys Discuss 2015; 15: 19873-902.
[http://dx.doi.org/10.5194/acpd-15-19873-2015]

[101] Leiss KA, Choi YH, Abdel-Farid IB, Verpoorte R, Klinkhamer PGL. NMR metabolomics of thrips (*Frankliniella occidentalis*) resistance in Senecio hybrids. J Chem Ecol 2009; 35(2): 219-29.
[http://dx.doi.org/10.1007/s10886-008-9586-0] [PMID: 19169751]

[102] Escobar-Bravo R, Ruijgrok J, Kim HK, *et al.* Light intensity-mediated induction of Trichome-associated allelochchemicals increases resistance against thrips in tomato. Plant Cell Physiol 2018; 59(12): 2462-75.
[PMID: 30124946]

[103] Danziger N, Bernstein N. Light matters: Effect of light spectra on cannabinoid profile and plant development of medical cannabis (Cannabis sativa L.). Ind Crops Prod 2021; 164: 113351.
[http://dx.doi.org/10.1016/j.indcrop.2021.113351]

[104] Zhang R, Zheng G, Li P. Effects of foliar trichomes on the accumulation of atmospheric particulates in *Tillandsia brachycaulos*. Open Life Sci 2019; 14(1): 580-7.
[http://dx.doi.org/10.1515/biol-2019-0065] [PMID: 33817195]

[105] Maiti R K. Potential morpho-physiological trait selection criteria for biotic and abiotic stress resistance in crops. Int J Bio-res and Stress Manag 2012.

[106] Zelinger E, Hawes CR, Gurr SJ, Dewey FM. Attachment and adhesion of conidia of *Stagonospora nodorum* to natural and artificial surfaces. Physiol Mol Plant Pathol 2006; 68(4-6): 209-15.
[http://dx.doi.org/10.1016/j.pmpp.2006.11.002]

[107] Gupt SK, Chand R, Mishra VK, Ahirwar RN, Bhatta M, Joshi AK. Spot blotch disease of wheat as influenced by foliar trichome and stomata density. J Agricul Food Res 2021; 6: 100227.
[http://dx.doi.org/10.1016/j.jafr.2021.100227]

[108] Shepherd RW, Bass WT, Houtz RL, Wagner GJ. Phylloplanins of tobacco are defensive proteins deployed on aerial surfaces by short glandular trichomes. Plant Cell 2005; 17(6): 1851-61.
[http://dx.doi.org/10.1105/tpc.105.031559] [PMID: 15894716]

[109] Chen T, Li Y, Xie L, *et al. Aa*WRKY17, a positive regulator of artemisinin biosynthesis, is involved in resistance to *Pseudomonas syringae* in *Artemisia annua*. Hortic Res 2021; 8(1): 217.
[http://dx.doi.org/10.1038/s41438-021-00652-6] [PMID: 34593786]

[110] Lu X, Zhang L, Zhang F, *et al. AaORA*, a trichome-specific AP 2/ ERF transcription factor of *Artemisia annua*, is a positive regulator in the artemisinin biosynthetic pathway and in disease resistance to *Botrytis cinerea*. New Phytol 2013; 198(4): 1191-202.
[http://dx.doi.org/10.1111/nph.12207] [PMID: 23448426]

[111] Williamson B, Tudzynski B, Tudzynski P, Van Kan JAL. *Botrytis cinerea*: The cause of grey mould disease. Mol Plant Pathol 2007; 8(5): 561-80.
[http://dx.doi.org/10.1111/j.1364-3703.2007.00417.x] [PMID: 20507522]

[112] Peiffer M, Tooker JF, Luthe DS, Felton GW. Plants on early alert: Glandular trichomes as sensors for insect herbivores. New Phytol 2009; 184(3): 644-56.
[http://dx.doi.org/10.1111/j.1469-8137.2009.03002.x] [PMID: 19703113]

[113] Saad KA, Mohamad Roff MN, Hallett RH, Abd-Ghani IB. Effects of cucumber mosaic virus-infected chilli plants on non-vector *Bemisia tabaci* (Hemiptera: Aleyrodidae). Insect Sci 2019; 26(1): 76-85.
[http://dx.doi.org/10.1111/1744-7917.12488] [PMID: 28594105]

[114] Escobar-Bravo R, Klinkhamer PGL, Leiss KA. Induction of jasmonic acid-associated defenses by thrips alters host suitability for conspecifics and correlates with increased trichome densities in tomato. Plant Cell Physiol 2017; 58(3): 622-34.
[http://dx.doi.org/10.1093/pcp/pcx014] [PMID: 28158865]

[115] Chen G, Klinkhamer PGL, Escobar-Bravo R, Leiss KA. Type VI glandular trichome density and their derived volatiles are differently induced by jasmonic acid in developing and fully developed tomato leaves: Implications for thrips resistance. Plant Sci 2018; 276: 87-98.
[http://dx.doi.org/10.1016/j.plantsci.2018.08.007] [PMID: 30348331]

[116] Krimmel BA, Pearse IS. Sticky plant traps insects to enhance indirect defence. Ecol Lett 2013; 16(2): 219-24.
[http://dx.doi.org/10.1111/ele.12032] [PMID: 23205839]

[117] Kariyat RR, Smith JD, Stephenson AG, De Moraes CM, Mescher MC. Non-glandular trichomes of *Solanum carolinense* deter feeding by *Manduca sexta* caterpillars and cause damage to the gut peritrophic matrix. Proc Biol Sci 2017; 284(1849): 20162323.
[http://dx.doi.org/10.1098/rspb.2016.2323] [PMID: 28228510]

[118] Lucini T, Faria MV, Rohde C, Resende JTV, de Oliveira JRF. Acylsugar and the role of trichomes in tomato genotypes resistance to *Tetranychus urticae*. Arthropod-Plant Interact 2015; 9(1): 45-53.
[http://dx.doi.org/10.1007/s11829-014-9347-7]

[119] Lima IP, Resende JTV, Oliveira JRF, Faria MV, Dias DM, Resende NCV. Selection of tomato genotypes for processing with high zingiberene content, resistant to pests. Hortic Bras 2016; 34(3): 387-91.
[http://dx.doi.org/10.1590/S0102-05362016003013]

[120] De Oliveira JRF, de Resende JTV, Maluf WR, *et al.* Trichomes and allelochemicals in tomato genotypes have antagonistic effects upon behavior and biology of *Tetranychus urticae*. Front Plant Sci 2018; 9: 1132.
[http://dx.doi.org/10.3389/fpls.2018.01132] [PMID: 30154808]

[121] Rai R, Meena RP, Smita SS, Shukla A, Rai SK, Pandey-Rai S. UV-B and UV-C pre-treatments induce physiological changes and artemisinin biosynthesis in *Artemisia annua* L. : An antimalarial plant. J Photochem Photobiol B 2011; 105(3): 216-25.
[http://dx.doi.org/10.1016/j.jphotobiol.2011.09.004] [PMID: 22019553]

[122] Rai R, Pandey S, Rai SP. Arsenic-induced changes in morphological, physiological, and biochemical attributes and artemisinin biosynthesis in *Artemisia annua*, an antimalarial plant. Ecotoxicology 2011; 20(8): 1900-13.
[http://dx.doi.org/10.1007/s10646-011-0728-8] [PMID: 21710305]

[123] Pandey N, Pandey-Rai S. Short term UV-B radiation-mediated transcriptional responses and altered secondary metabolism of *in vitro* propagated plantlets of *Artemisia annua* L. Plant Cell Tissue Organ Cult 2014; 116(3): 371-85.
[http://dx.doi.org/10.1007/s11240-013-0413-0]

[124] Kang JH, McRoberts J, Shi F, Moreno JE, Jones AD, Howe GA. The flavonoid biosynthetic enzyme chalcone isomerase modulates terpenoid production in glandular trichomes of tomato. Plant Physiol 2014; 164(3): 1161-74.
[http://dx.doi.org/10.1104/pp.113.233395] [PMID: 24424324]

CHAPTER 6

Role of Plant Growth Regulators for Augmenting Secondary Metabolites Production in Medicinal Plants

Harsh Kumar Chauhan[1], **Anil Kumar Bisht**[1] and **Indra Dutt Bhatt**[2,*]

[1] *Department of Botany, Kumaun University, Nainital, India*

[2] *G.B. Pant National Institute of Himalayan Environment, Kosi-Katarmal, Almora-263643, Uttarakhand, India*

Abstract: Plants are an important source of natural products for health care throughout the globe. Recent trends show an abrupt increase in the demand for medicinal plants due to their cost-efficiency, safety, and potency. The medicinal properties of the plants are attributable to the presence of secondary metabolites, which accumulate as the natural defense against herbivory and other interspecies defenses. Along with their medicinal uses, secondary metabolites are also used in flavorings, agrochemicals, fragrances, bio-pesticides, and food additives. The demand for secondary metabolites is mainly expedited through the collection of medicinal plants from the wild. This has provided an impetus for overharvesting medicinal plants from the wild, and many of them are threatened. The accumulation of secondary metabolites in medicinal plants is limited, and therefore diverse strategies for improving the production of secondary metabolites are a priority. Biotechnological applications, especially plant tissue culture techniques, offer a viable alternative for obtaining secondary metabolites. Along with the optimization of growth media and culture conditions, the role of plant growth regulators is vital in enhancing biomass and secondary metabolite accumulation in the culture medium. The present chapter demonstrates the types and uses of plant growth regulators with a focus on the application of plant growth regulators for the production of secondary metabolites from medicinal plants.

Keywords: *In-vitro* propagation, Medicinal plants, Natural products, Plant growth regulators, Plant tissue culture, Secondary metabolites.

INTRODUCTION

Natural products obtained from plants are valued for health care throughout the globe. About 60,000 plant species are used as medicine, nutritional supplement, and aromatic in the world [1]. Recent trends show an abrupt increase in the

* Corresponding author Indra Dutt Bhatt: G.B. Pant National Institute of Himalayan Environment, Kosi-Katarmal, Almora-263643, Uttarakhand, India; E-mail: id_bhatt@yahoo.com

demand for medicinal plants [2] which is more likely attributable to cost-efficiency, safety, and potency. At present, there are about 90 plant species used to develop 121 clinically prescribed drugs in the market [3]. Several new plants are being screened for their pharmacological activities for developing new drugs. The global herbal market has increased from $1.2 billion in 1990 to $ 25.6 billion in 2015 [4, 5] with an expectation to reach $ 5 trillion by the year 2050 [6]. High demand has provided an impetus for overharvesting from the wild and about 21% of medicinal plant species used in herbal preparation are endangered [7].

Plants produce compounds with toxic and hallucinogenic properties as the natural defense against herbivory and other interspecies defenses. These plants often contain secondary metabolites which modulate a corresponding molecular target (neuroreceptor, enzymes that degrade neurotransmitters, ion channels, ion pumps, or the elements of the cytoskeleton) in animals and humans [8]. Large numbers of secondary metabolites are extracted and used in the synthesis of modern medicines. Along with their utility as medicine, secondary metabolites are also used as flavorings, pharmaceuticals, agrochemicals, fragrances, bio-pesticides, and food additives. As such, plants produce more than 100,000 secondary metabolites, this number may exceed over 500,000 once we know the structural characterization [9]. Plants continue to be the principal source of many important bioactive molecules/pharmacophores [10]. Interestingly, one-fourth of the prescribed drugs across the globe contain chemical compounds (secondary metabolites) directly, indirectly, or semi-synthetically obtained from plants [11].

Medicinal plants from the wild are the major source of raw material for obtaining secondary metabolites. The accumulation of secondary metabolites is limited, and alternative methods for the production of secondary metabolites are being focused by the pharmaceutical firms under controlled conditions. Plant tissue culture provides a promising outlet for the mass propagation of medicinal plants as well as the production of bioactive compounds (secondary metabolites) under *in vitro* conditions. Cell suspension cultures often accumulate desired natural target compounds. Advancements in molecular biology and fermentation technology of plant cells suggest that these techniques will be a viable source of obtaining secondary metabolites [12]. Along with the optimization of growth media and culture conditions, the role of plant growth regulators (PGRs) is vital for stimulating diverse secondary metabolites from medicinal plants [13, 14]. The mechanism of PGRs varies considerably and hence the production of secondary metabolites is unpredictable in terms of quality, quantity, and diversity [15]. Enhancement of secondary metabolites by optimizing PGRs has provoked their commercial application. Hence, it becomes imperative to review the application of PGRs for the production of secondary metabolites from medicinal plants.

PLANT GROWTH REGULATORS (PGRs)

PGRs can be defined as natural or synthetic compounds that regulate the development or metabolic activities of plants (mostly at low concentrations). These compounds can be associated primarily with an increase or reduction of plant growth along with effects on other physiological processes like flowering, fruit formation, fruit ripening, fruit drop, and defoliation or quality traits. PGRs may act at the site of synthesis or are translocated to the target sites. Meristems tissues and growing fruits are the major sites for their production in plants. Various groups of hormones often interact synergistically or antagonistically to control physiological activities in plants. This provokes the need for understanding their structure, function, and production complexities to get the desired performance of the plant. Unlike animals, plants produce hormones in many cells, playing multiple regulatory roles thereby affecting several aspects of plant development.

The credit for the discovery of plant hormones goes to Neljubow [16], who demonstrated the triple response (horizontal growth, inhibition of elongation, and radial swelling) of pea seedlings to ethylene. The systematic use of PGRs began in the 1930s with the use of ethylene for flower induction and fruit formation in pineapple [17]. Since then, PGRs have been used in agriculture, horticulture, and viticulture to improve the qualitative and quantitative traits of the plants.

Types of PGRs

Auxins, cytokinins, gibberellins, abscisic acid, and ethylene are the main PGRs (Fig. **1**) involved in the vital physiological processes of the plants, and hence this group is termed as the "classic group" of plant hormones. Brassinosteroids and jasmonates are also known for phytohormonal activities, but the classification of polyamines and other compounds is still controversial [18].

Auxins

Auxins are plant-growth regulators with some morphogen-like characteristics. Auxins are organic acids that play a cardinal role in the coordination of cell expansion, division, elongation, and differentiation, thereby affecting the shape and function of cells and tissues in plants [19]. The work of Charles Darwin and his son Francis in the 1880s, followed by Frits W. Went in the 1920s on photoperiodism, led to the discovery of auxin. The first chemical structure of plant auxin, indole-3-acetic acid (IAA) was deduced in the 1930s. Five auxins (indole-3-acetic acid, 4-chloroindole-3-acetic acid, phenylacetic acid, indole-3-butyric acid, and indole-3-propionic acid) are known to occur naturally in plants [20]; several others are synthetic auxin analogs (Fig. **1**). Auxins are known for stimulating cell elongation and division. They are also involved in phototropic and gravitropic reactions. The major function of auxins and their role in plant tissue culture are briefly summarized in Table **1**.

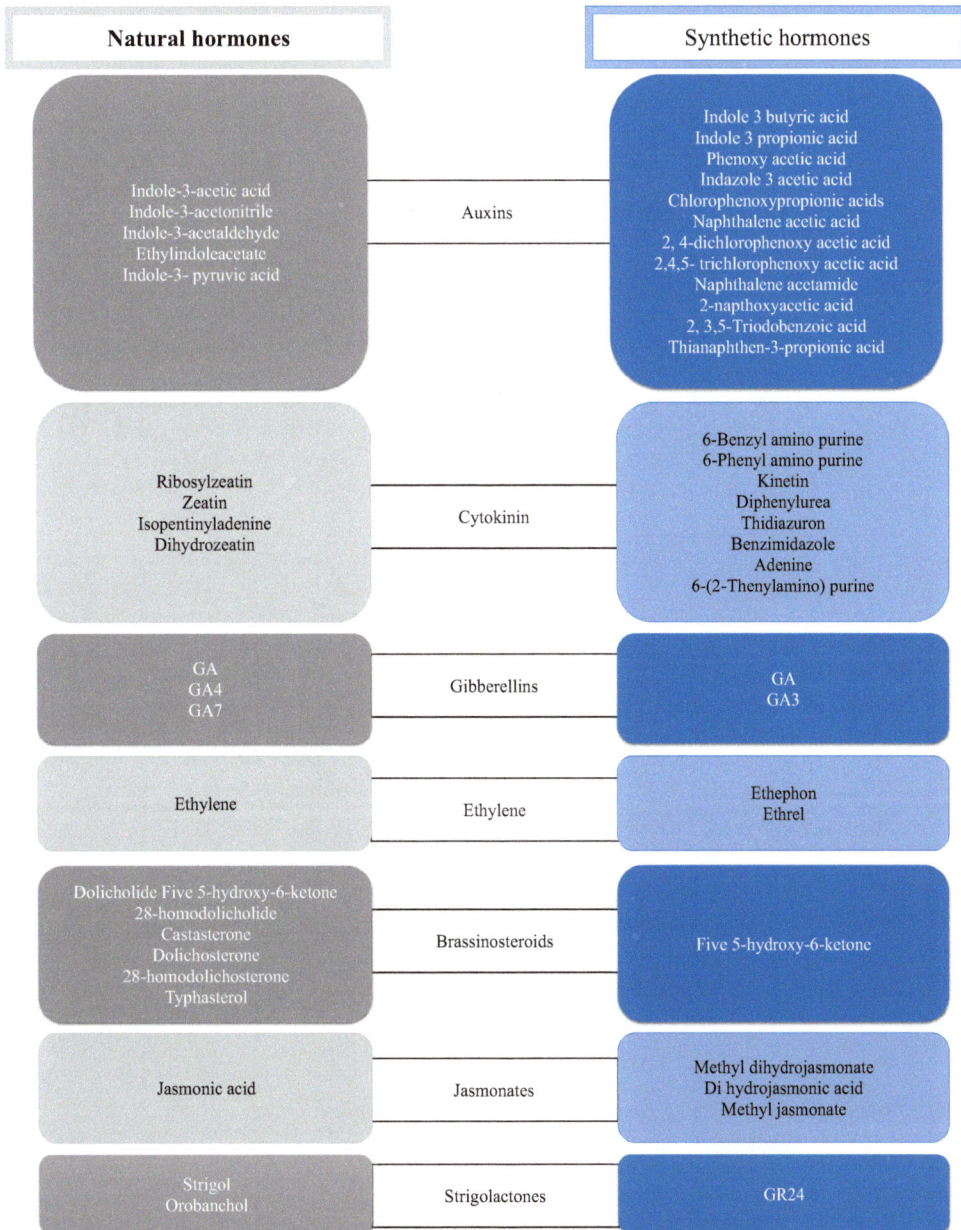

Natural hormones		Synthetic hormones
Indole-3-acetic acid Indole-3-acetonitrile Indole-3-acetaldehyde Ethylindoleacetate Indole-3- pyruvic acid	Auxins	Indole 3 butyric acid Indole 3 propionic acid Phenoxy acetic acid Indazole 3 acetic acid Chlorophenoxypropionic acids Naphthalene acetic acid 2, 4-dichlorophenoxy acetic acid 2,4,5- trichlorophenoxy acetic acid Naphthalene acetamide 2-napthoxyacetic acid 2, 3,5-Triodobenzoic acid Thianaphthen-3-propionic acid
Ribosylzeatin Zeatin Isopentinyladenine Dihydrozeatin	Cytokinin	6-Benzyl amino purine 6-Phenyl amino purine Kinetin Diphenylurea Thidiazuron Benzimidazole Adenine 6-(2-Thenylamino) purine
GA GA4 GA7	Gibberellins	GA GA3
Ethylene	Ethylene	Ethephon Ethrel
Dolicholide Five 5-hydroxy-6-ketone 28-homodolicholide Castasterone Dolichosterone 28-homodolichosterone Typhasterol	Brassinosteroids	Five 5-hydroxy-6-ketone
Jasmonic acid	Jasmonates	Methyl dihydrojasmonate Di hydrojasmonic acid Methyl jasmonate
Strigol Orobanchol	Strigolactones	GR24

Fig. (1). Types of Plant Growth Regulators (PGRs) and their natural and synthetic representatives.

Table 1. Plant growth regulators and their role in plant tissue culture.

S. No.	Plant Growth Regulator	Major Production Sites	Major Role in Plant Tissue Culture (PTC)
1.	Auxins	Stem, buds, root tips, shoot apical meristems, young leaves, developing fruits and seeds	Promote stem elongation, inhibit the growth of lateral buds and leaf abscission, and promote adventitious root initiation and fruit growth. **Specific to PTC** Adventitious root formation (at higher concentration) Adventitious shoot formation (at low concentration) Callus formation and growth Somatic embryo induction Inhibition of root growth
2.	Cytokinins	Meristematic region and growing tissues; Believed to be synthesized in roots and translocated *via* xylem to shoots	Promote cell growth, development and differentiation, inhibit leaf senescence, promote cell division and lateral bud outgrowth, and affect root growth. **Specific to PTC** Adventitious shoot formation (at high concentration) Inhibition of root formation Callus formation and growth Axillary buds outgrowth stimulation Inhibition of leaf senescence
3.	Gibberellins	Young tissues and developing seed	Promote cell division and elongation, seed germination, stem and hypocotyl elongation and flower induction. It also regulates plant adaptation to biotic and abiotic stress. **Specific to PTC** Shoot elongation Breaking the dormancy of seeds, embryos, apical buds, and bulbs. Inhibit adventitious root formation
4.	Ethylene	In tissues undergoing senescence or ripening	Ethylene has profound effects on plant adaptation. Control growth, development, reproduction (germination), cell elongation, fruit ripening and senescence. **Specific to PTC** Senescence of leaves Ripening of fruits
5.	Abscisic Acid	Almost all cells that contain chloroplast and plastid	Promote embryo development, seed maturation, seed dormancy, stomatal movement, flowering, pathogen response and senescence. The hormone is also known as stress hormone. **Specific to PTC** Somatic embryo maturation Acclimatization Bulbs and tuber formation Dormancy development

Cytokinins

Cytokinins are adenine derivates that stimulate cell division in meristematic tissues, counteract auxins in apical dominance, delay leaf senescence and attract assimilates into sinks [18]. The first cytokinin was isolated by Miller and his coworkers from the University of Wisconsin-Madison from herring sperm in 1955. Since then, several natural cytokinins have been isolated and synthetic cytokinins have been formulated in the laboratory (Fig. **1**). Kinetin [N-(2furylmethyl)-3H-purin-6-amine] and 6-benzyleadenine have practical relevance in plant tissue culture. Cytokinin is an N-adenine derivative, a phenyl urea compound involved in almost all aspects of plant growth and development (Table **1**).

Gibberellins

Gibberellins (GAs) are a class of tetracyclic diterpenoid phytohormones produced by plants and some fungi. Gibberellins were first discovered by Kurosawa in Japan while studying the fungal disease of rice ('bakanae') caused by *Gibberella fujikuroi* (imperfect stage of *Fusarium moniliforme* later corrected to *F. fujikuroi*). The diseased plant showed abnormal growth promoted by the fungi due to the compounds (Gibberellins) produced by *G. fujikuroi*. Since then, about 136 gibberellins molecules have been discovered, however only a few, such as GA1, GA3, GA4, and GA7, are bioactive [21]. GA functions are diverse, influencing stem elongation, seed germination, dormancy, flowering, sex expression, *etc.* (Table **1**).

Ethylene

Ethylene, unlike other plant hormones, is a gaseous hormone that regulates numerous processes in plant growth, development, and response to biotic and abiotic stresses. It is known for its effect on fruit ripening and has commercial importance in agriculture [22]. Ethylene is also famous for its triple response (treatment of pea seedlings with ethylene inhibited internodal elongation, and increased stem thickness and horizontal growth).

Abscisic Acid (ABA)

Often known as the 'stress hormone', abscisic acid plays a major role in protecting plants against biotic stress. The hormone was discovered by F.T. Addicott and co-workers while studying abscission in cotton fruits. ABA is a single compound. ABA leads to stomatal closure under drought stress. It inhibits stem elongation and germination and maintains dormancy. The synthesis of ABA is complicated and not suited for commercial purposes [18].

SECONDARY METABOLITES

Plants produce several economically useful chemical compounds. Secondary metabolites are organic molecules produced by plants that are not essential for their growth, development, and performing vital functions. The function of secondary metabolites is mainly associated with the defense against pests and pathogens. Some of them, such as alkaloids, have immense value in medicine. Based on the biosynthetic pathway, secondary metabolites can be classified into three groups, *i.e.*, terpenes, phenolics and nitrogen, and sulphur comprising compounds (Fig. **2**). Terpenes are composed of a 5-C isopentanoid unit. Phenolics are synthesized from products of the shikimic pathway, while Nitrogen and Sulphur containing compounds are synthesized from common amino acids [23].

Terpenes

Terpenes are the most largest and diverse class of secondary metabolites. They are synthesized from acetyl-CoA or glycolytic intermediates. They are hydrocarbons with five-carbon isoprene as the building having a molecular formula of $(C_5H_8)n$; n indicates the number of units involved. Terpenes are classified according to isoprene units (Fig. **2**): Monoterpenes (2 isoprene and 10 carbon atom) Sesquiterpenes (3 isoprene and 15 carbon atom), Diterpenes (4 isoprene and 20 carbon atom), Triterpenes (6 isoprene and 30 carbon atom), Tetraterpenes (8 isoprene and 40 carbon atom), Polyterpenes (more than 8 isoprene and 40 carbon atom). Most of the terpenes are produced by plants are believed to provide defense as toxins to prevent themselves from consumption by insects and mammals [24]. They are the primary constituents of essential oils in many plants and flowers. Some other functions include cell growth modulation and plant elongation, light harvest action, photoprotection, and membrane permeability and fluidity control [25]. Consumption of terpenes in diet can protect against many diseases, such as cancer [26]. Several plant species are known to produce terpenes, however, the most common plant families producing terpenes are Lamiaceae (*Melissa officinalis, Agastache rugosa, Rosmarinus officinalis, Lavandula officinalis, Mentha* spp.), Coniferae (*Thuja occidentalis, Pinus* spp.), Compositae (*Artemisia* spp.), Leguminosae (*Glycyrrhizae* spp.), Taxaceae (*Taxus* spp.) [27].

Some plant species (about 17) have genes that encode for the enzyme terpenoid synthase and cytochrome P450s, which help in the conversion of terpenes to terpenoids [28, 29]. Terpenoids are used in several traditional medicines. They contribute to the scent of Eucalyptus, the flavor of cinnamon, cloves, and ginger, the red color of tomatoes, and the yellow color of sunflowers [30]. Steroids and sterols are biologically produced from terpenoid precursors. Terpenes have several medicinal properties, such as anticancer, antimicrobial, anti-fungal antiviral, anti-hyperglycemic, analgesic, anti-inflammatory, and anti-parasitic [31]. Terpenes enhance skin penetration and are nowadays being used for the production of several drugs [32].

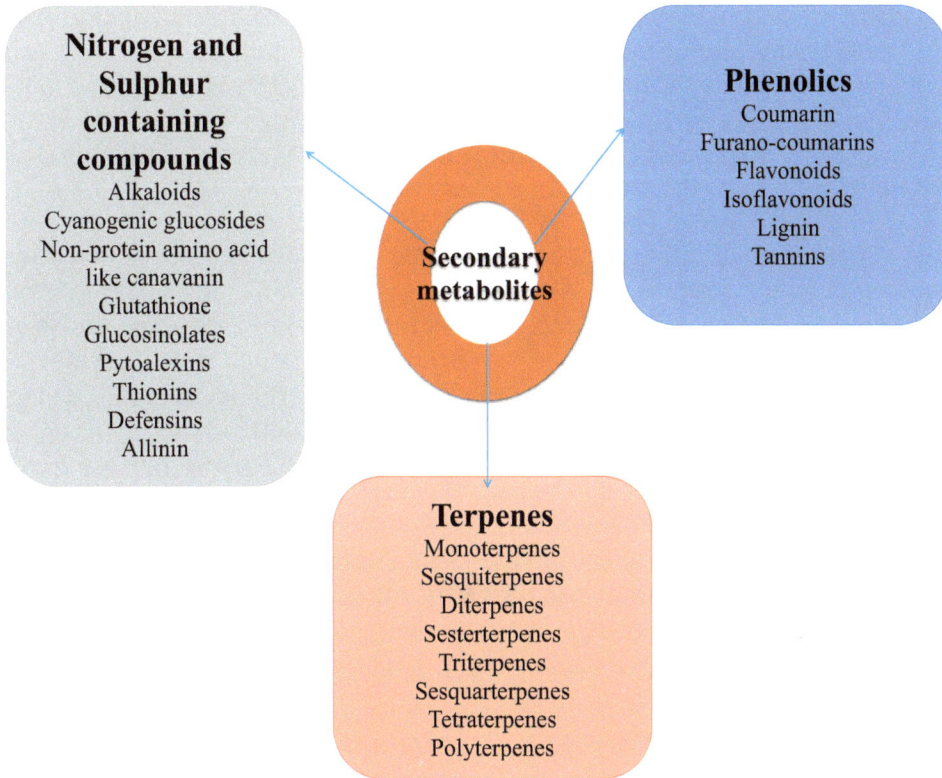

Nitrogen and Sulphur containing compounds
Alkaloids
Cyanogenic glucosides
Non-protein amino acid like canavanin
Glutathione
Glucosinolates
Pytoalexins
Thionins
Defensins
Allinin

Secondary metabolites

Phenolics
Coumarin
Furano-coumarins
Flavonoids
Isoflavonoids
Lignin
Tannins

Terpenes
Monoterpenes
Sesquiterpenes
Diterpenes
Sesterterpenes
Triterpenes
Sesquarterpenes
Tetraterpenes
Polyterpenes

Fig. (2). Types of secondary metabolites.

Phenolics

Plants produce several secondary products having phenol groups bearing one or more hydroxyl groups [33]. Polyphenols include flavonoids, phenolic acids, tannins, lignans, coumarins, *etc.* They are naturally found in vegetables, fruits, cereals, roots, and leaves and have several health benefits. Plants utilize phenols in reproduction, growth, and defense against stress [33]. They also perform several other functions like photosynthesis, enzyme activity, protein synthesis, nutrient uptake, *etc.* Phenolics have several health benefits, which are mainly linked to direct (free-radical scavenging ability) and indirect (stimulating activity of antioxidant enzymes) antioxidant properties. These properties help them to prevent chronic and oxidative stress, such as cancer, cardiovascular and neurodegenerative disease [34, 35].

Nitrogen and Sulphur-containing Compounds

This group includes nitrogen-containing compounds such as alkaloids, glucosinolates, cyanogneic glycosides, and nonprotein amino acids (NPAAs). Alkaloids are synthesized from amino acids such as lysine, tyrosine, and tryptophan [36] and have significant importance in the medicinal sector. These nitrogen-containing secondary metabolites help in the plant's defense mechanism and the plant's response to the incompatible interaction [37]. Nitrogen-containing secondary metabolites are used as antiarrhythmic, anticholinergic, antitumor, vasodilating, antihypertensive, anesthetic, analgesic, antipyretic, antimalarial, and vasodilator [38].

Sulphur containing compounds is a relatively small group of secondary metabolites obtained from plants. Glucosinolates and alliins are two main groups of sulphur containing secondary metabolites [39]. They are relatively physiologically inert and are separated from their hydrolyzing enzymes, the myrosinases, and alliinases. These compounds are useful in treating oxidative stress, inflammation, and apoptosis [40]. These metabolites have a formidable wall of defense against pathogens and pests [41]. These compounds are used in oxidative stress, inflammation, and apoptosis [40].

INFLUENCE OF PGRs ON SECONDARY METABOLITES PRODUCTION OF MEDICINAL PLANTS IN PLANT TISSUE CULTURE

Plant growth regulators, change in basal medium components, carbon source, and elicitors can alter the growth and production of secondary metabolites in plant tissue culture. Several studies have evaluated the potential of plant growth regulators for the alteration of secondary metabolites (Table **2**).

Table 2. List of plants showing alterations in the production of secondary metabolites by Plant Growth Regulators.

PGRs	Plant Species	Secondary Metabolites	Major Class	References
Cytokinins	*Mentha spicata*	1–8, Cineole	Terpenes	[46]
-	*Eucomis autumnalis*	Iridoids	Terpenes	[43]
-	*Mentha×piperita*	Menthone, Menthol	Terpenes	[45]
-	*Artemisia annua*	Artemisinin	Terpenes	[44] [47]
-	*Rubia akane*	Anthraquinone	Phenolics	[42]
BAP	*Ammi majus*	Coumarins	Phenolics	[51]
-	*Ammi majus*	Umbelliferone	Phenolics	[51]

PGRs	Plant Species	Secondary Metabolites	Major Class	References
-	*Oxalis linearis*	Anthocyanin	Phenolics	[52]
-	*Vinca major*	Vincamine	NCSM	[53]
KN	*Nicotiana tabacum*	Chlorogenic acid	Phenolics	[48]
-	*Nicotiana tabacum*	Scopoletin	Phenolics	[48]
-	*Cinchona ledgeriana*	Quinine	NCSM	[75]
-	*Agave amanuensis*	Saponin	NCSM	[76]
Auxins (2, 4-D)	*Gymnema sylvestre*	Gymnemic acid	Terpenes	[77]
-	*Centella asiatica*	Asiaticoside	Terpenes	[78, 79]
-	*Anchusa officinalis*	Rosmarinic acid	Phenolics	[80]
-	*Rubia tinctorum*	Anthraquinone	Phenolics	[81]
-	*Daucus carota*	Anthocyanin	Phenolics	[82]
-	*Oxalis reclinata*	Anthocyanin	Phenolics	[83]
-	*Cinchona ledgeriana*	Quinine	NCSM	[84, 85]
-	*Bupleurum falcatum*	Saikosaponins	NCSM	[86]
IBA	*Taxus wallichiana*	Taxol	Terpenes	[87]
-	*Panax ginseng*	Saponin	Terpenes	[79]
IAA	*Papaver somniferum*	Thebaine	NCSM	[88]
-	*Rauvolfia serpentina*	Reserpine	NCSM	[89]
-	*Corydalis ambigua*	Corydaline	NCSM	[90]
NAA	*Fagopyrum esculentum*	Rutin	Phenolics	[91]
GA	*Salvia officinalis*	1, 8-Cineole	Terpenes	[61]
GA3	*Digitalis lanata*	Anthocyanin	Phenolics	[60]
-	*Vitis rotundifolia*	Anthocyanin	Phenolics	[62]
-	*Petunia hybrid*	Anthocyanin	Phenolics	[63]
-	*Catharanthus roseus*	Vincristine	NCSM	[59]
ABA	*Taxus chinensis*	Paclitaxel	Terpenes	[92]
-	*Lactuca sativa*	Carotenoids	Terpenes	[93]
-	*Salvia miltiorrhiza*	Salvianic acid A, Salvianolic acid B	Phenolics	[94]
-	*Lactuca sativa*	Anthocyanin	Phenolics	[93]
-	*Vitis rotundifolia*	Anthocyanin	Phenolics	[95]
Auxins + Auxins	-	-	-	-
2, 4-D+IAA	*Gymnema sylvestre*	Gymnemic acid	Terpenes	[6]
IAA+NAA	*Astragalus mongholicus*	Cycloartane	Terpenes	[96]

(Table 2) cont.....

PGRs	Plant Species	Secondary Metabolites	Major Class	References
2, 4-D+NAA	*Camellia chinensis*	Flavonol	Phenolics	[97]
2, 4-D+NAA	*Camellia chinensis*	Flavones	Phenolics	[97]
Auxins+ Cytokinin	-	-	-	-
IAA+KN	*Centranthes ruber*	Valepotriates	Terpenes	[98]
IAA+KN	*Artemisia annua*	Artemisinin	Terpenes	[99]
IAA+KN	*Coleus forskohlii*	Forskolin	Terpenes	[100]
IAA+KN	*Zataria multiflora*	Rosmarinic acid	Phenolics	[101]
IAA+KN	*Withania somnifera*	Withanoloid A	Phenolics	[14]
NAA+KN	*Artemisia annua*	Artemisinin	Terpenes	[102]
NAA+KN	*Cruciata glabra*	Anthraquinone	Phenolics	[103]
2, 4-D+KN	*Citrullus colocynthis*	Cucurbitacin-E, Cucurbitacins	Terpenes	[104]
2, 4-D+KN	*Centella asiatica*	Asiaticoside	Terpenes	[105]
2, 4-D+KN	*Citrus species*	Limonin	Terpenes	[106]
2, 4-D+KN	*Agastache rugose*	Rosmarinic acid	Phenolics	[91]
2, 4-D+KN	*Aralia cordata*	Anthocyanin	Phenolics	[107]
2, 4-D+KN	*Aconitum heterophyllum*	Aconites	NCSM	[108]
2, 4-D+KN	*Capsicum annum*	Capsaicin	NCSM	[109, 110]
2, 4-D+KN	*Coffea Arabica*	Caffeine	NCSM	[111]
2, 4-D+KN	*Cryptolepis buchanani*	Cryptosin	NCSM	[55]
2, 4-D+BA	*Taxus species*	Taxol	Terpenes	[112]
IAA+BA	*Salvia officinalis*	Carnosic acid, carnosol	Terpenes	[113]
IAA+BA	*Centella asiatica*	Asiaticoside	Terpenes	[78, 79]
IAA+BA	*Gymnema sylvestre*	Gymnemic acid	Terpenes	[114]
IAA+BA	*Salvia officinalis*	Rosmarinic acid	Phenolics	[115]
IAA+BA	*Hypericum perforatum*	Hypericin	Phenolics	[116]
IBA+BA	*Thymus vulgaris*	Carotenoids	Terpenes	[50]
IBA+BA	*Rheum ribes*	Catechin	Phenolics	[117]
NAA+BA	*Pluchea lanceolata*	Quercetin	Phenolics	[118]
NAA+BA	*Vitis vinifera*	Anthocyanin	Phenolics	[119]
IAA+ TDZ	*Cassia obtusifolia*	Anthraquinone	Phenolics	[120]
IAA+TDZ	*Saponaria officinalis*	Saponin	NCSM	[121]
NAA+TDZ	*Frangula alnus*	Anthraquinone	Phenolics	[122]

(Table 2) cont.....

PGRs	Plant Species	Secondary Metabolites	Major Class	References
Other combinations GA+ Auxins	-	-	-	-
GA3 +IAA	*Cinchona succirubra*	Anthraquinone	Phenolics	[123]
GA3 +NAA	*Hypericum perforatum*	Hypericin	Phenolics	[124]
GA3 +IAA	*Corydalis cava*	Corydaline	NCSM	[125]
IBA+ Cytokinin	-	-	-	-
IBA+BA	*Thymus vulgaris*	Carotenoids	Terpenes	[50]
2, 4-D+KIN+GA3	*Taxus baccata*	Taxol baccatin III	Terpenes	[126]
2, 4-D+BA+2, 4-D	*Diocorea doryophora, Dioscorea deltoidea*	Diosgenin	Terpenes	[127] [128]
BAP+NAA+KIN+2, 4-D	*Momordica harantia*	Kaempferol, Quercetin, Luteiolin	Phenolics	[129]
2, 4-D+KIN+IAA	*Catharanthus roseus*	Vincristine, Vinblastine	NCSM	[130]

Effects of Cytokinins on the Alteration of Secondary Metabolites Production

Cytokinins have been tested to enhance the production of secondary metabolites. Species like *Mentha* spp., *Eucomis autumnalis*, *Artemisia annua*, and *Rubia akane* accumulates secondary metabolites in culture medium when supplemented with cytokinins [42 - 47]. Kinetin improved the concentration of lignin in the callus tissue of *Nicotiana tabacum* [48]. In *Brassica rapa* hairy roots KN enhanced glucosinolate [49]. BA enhanced the flavonoids production in *Thymus vulgaris* [50]. BA resulted in the accumulation of Umbelliferone, Anthocyanin, and Vincamine in the culture of *Amni majus*, *Oxalis linerasis* and *Vinca major*, respectively [51 - 53]. Likewise, several reports are available for the alteration of secondary metabolites production in a culture medium by cytokinins (Table **2**).

Effects of Auxins on the Alteration of Secondary Metabolites Production

Several plants have shown the accumulation of secondary metabolites by the use of auxins in the culture medium (Table **2**). The effects of auxins on the production of secondary metabolites depend on the auxins type, concentration, and interaction with other plant hormones. The hairy root culture of *Lactuca virosa* resulted in the induction of sesquiterpene with the treatment of 2,4 D [54]. Callus culture of *Eucalyptus terticornis* treated with 2,4 D stimulated the sterols and phenolic compounds [55]. Other hormones, such as IAA, are known to stimulate flavonoids content in *Scutellaria baicalensis* [56], alkaloid content in root culture of *Cephaelis ipecacuanha* [57], and *Fumaria capreolata* [58].

Effects of GA on the Alteration of Secondary Metabolites Production

GA is known to alter the secondary metabolites production in *Salvia officinalis*, *Digitalis lanata*, *Vitis rotundifolia*, *Petunia hybrid*, *Catharanthus roseus* [59 - 63]. A lower concentration of GA3 enhanced the lignin synthesis in *Nicotiana tabacum* [64]. GA3 has shown enhancement of steroidal alkaloids accumulation in *Solanum aviculare* [65].

Effects of ABA on the Alteration of Secondary Metabolites Production

ABA is the principal hormone in the plant's responses to stress [66, 67]. It has been utilized successfully to enhance the terpenoids production in *Cannabis sativa* [68], phenolic and flavonoids in *Orthosiphon stamineus* [69], and several other secondary metabolites (Table **2**).

Effects of Combinations on the Alteration of Secondary Metabolites Production

Several combinations of hormones are known to alter the secondary metabolites production in plant tissue culture (Table **2**). The combination of cytokinins and auxins stimulates the production of flavonoids in the cell suspension culture of *Digitalis lanata* [70]. Callus culture of *Eriobotrya japonica* stimulated triterpenes production with the use of NAA and BA [71]. Tannin content was found to improve in the hairy root culture of *Geranium thunbergii* with the implementation of 2,4 D and BA [72]. An increase in essential oil content was reported in *Cymbopogon citratus* treated with IAA and GA3 [73]. Indole alkaloids were stimulated in the cell culture of *Cinchona ledgeriana* with the implementation of 2,4 D, IAA, and NAA [74].

CONCLUDING REMARKS

The present chapter summarizes the types of plant growth regulators and their major role in plant tissue culture, with particular emphasis on the production of secondary metabolites. Plant growth regulators influence secondary metabolites production in different cultures. The response of PGRs depends on their type, concentration, and combination. Production of secondary metabolites under in-vitro conditions has an advantage in the controlled production of quality material. Although several reports are available on the production of secondary metabolites by tissue culture, intensive research is needed to optimize the conditions, such as medium concentration, the use of plant growth regulators, and other environmental variables. Advancements in plant tissue culture techniques, along with molecular and fermentation technology, can replace the traditional practice of obtaining secondary metabolites from wild plants.

REFERENCES

[1]   World Health Organization. Connecting global priorities: Biodiversity and human health. World Health Organization and Secretariat of the Convention on Biological Diversity. 2015.

[2]   Barata AM, Rocha F, Lopes V, Carvalho AM. Conservation and sustainable uses of medicinal and aromatic plants genetic resources on the worldwide for human welfare. Ind Crops Prod 2016; 88: 8-11.
        [http://dx.doi.org/10.1016/j.indcrop.2016.02.035]

[3]   Negi VS, Kewlani P, Pathak R, *et al.* Criteria and indicators for promoting cultivation and conservation of medicinal and aromatic plants in western himalaya, india. Ecol Indic 2018; 93: 434-46.
        [http://dx.doi.org/10.1016/j.ecolind.2018.03.032]

[4]   Lange D. Trade figures for botanical drugs world-wide. Med Plant Conserv 1997; 3: 16-7.

[5]   Asl Roosta R, Moghaddasi R, Hosseini SS. Export target markets of medicinal and aromatic plants. J Appl Res Med Aromat Plants 2017; 7: 84-8.
        [http://dx.doi.org/10.1016/j.jarmap.2017.06.003]

[6]   Ahmed AB, Rao AS, Rao MV. *In vitro* production of gymnemic acid from *Gymnema sylvestre* (Retz) R. Br. ex roemer and schultes through callus culture under abiotic stress conditions. Protocols for *In Vitro* In: Jain SM, Saxena PK, Eds. Cultures and Secondary Metabolite Analysis of Aromatic and Medicinal Plants. Totowa, NJ: Humana Press 2009; pp. 93-105.
        [http://dx.doi.org/10.1007/978-1-60327-287-2_8]

[7]   Schippmann UW, Leaman D, Cunningham AB. A comparison of cultivation and wild collection of medicinal and aromatic plants under sustainability aspects. In: Bogers RJ, Craker LE, Lange D, Eds. Medicinal and Aromatic Plants. Netherlands: Springer 2006; pp. 75-95.
        [http://dx.doi.org/10.1007/1-4020-5449-1_6]

[8]   Wink M. Modes of action of herbal medicines and plant secondary metabolites. Medicines 2015; 2(3): 251-86.
        [http://dx.doi.org/10.3390/medicines2030251] [PMID: 28930211]

[9]   Hadacek F. Secondary metabolites as plant traits: Current assessment and future perspectives. Crit Rev Plant Sci 2002; 21(4): 273-322.
        [http://dx.doi.org/10.1080/0735-260291044269]

[10]   Giri CC, Zaheer M. Chemical elicitors versus secondary metabolite production *in vitro* using plant cell, tissue and organ cultures: Recent trends and a sky eye view appraisal. Plant Cell Tissue Organ Cult 2016; 126(1): 1-18.
        [http://dx.doi.org/10.1007/s11240-016-0985-6]

[11]   Song MC, Kim EJ, Kim E, Rathwell K, Nam SJ, Yoon YJ. Microbial biosynthesis of medicinally important plant secondary metabolites. Nat Prod Rep 2014; 31(11): 1497-509.
        [http://dx.doi.org/10.1039/C4NP00057A] [PMID: 25072622]

[12]   Abdin MZ, Zhu Y, Tan B, Bay B, Liu C. Enhancing bioactive molecules in medicinal plants. In: Zhu Y, Tan B, Bay B, Liu C, Eds. Natural Products-Essential resources for human survival. Singapore: World Scientific Publishing Co. Pvt. Ltd. 2007; pp. 45-57.
        [http://dx.doi.org/10.1142/9789812707444_0004]

[13]   Matkowski A. Plant *in vitro* culture for the production of antioxidants : A review. Biotechnol Adv 2008; 26(6): 548-60.
        [http://dx.doi.org/10.1016/j.biotechadv.2008.07.001] [PMID: 18682287]

[14]   Murthy HN, Dijkstra C, Anthony P, *et al.* Establishment of *Withania somnifera* hairy root cultures for the production of withanolide A. J Integr Plant Biol 2008; 50(8): 975-81.
        [http://dx.doi.org/10.1111/j.1744-7909.2008.00680.x] [PMID: 18713347]

[15]   Jeong GT, Park DH. Enhanced secondary metabolite biosynthesis by elicitation in transformed plant root system: Effect of abiotic elicitors. Appl Biochem Biotechnol 2006; 130(1-3): 436-46.

[http://dx.doi.org/10.1385/ABAB:130:1:436] [PMID: 16915660]

[16] Neljubow D. Uber die horizontale nutation der stengel von *Pisum Sativum* und einiger anderen planzen. Bot Centralbl 1901; (10)128-39.

[17] Bartholomew DP. History and perspectives on the role of ethylene in pineapple flowering. InXII International Symposium on Plant Bioregulators in Fruit Production. 269-84.

[18] Rademacher W. Plant growth regulators: Backgrounds and uses in plant production. J Plant Growth Regul 2015; 34(4): 845-72.
[http://dx.doi.org/10.1007/s00344-015-9541-6]

[19] Jiang Z, Li J, Qu L. Auxins. In: Li J, Li C, Smith SM, Eds. Hormone metabolism and signaling in plants. Academic Press 2017; pp. 39-65.
[http://dx.doi.org/10.1016/B978-0-12-811562-6.00002-5]

[20] Simon S, Petrášek J. Why plants need more than one type of auxin. Plant Sci 2011; 180(3): 454-60.
[http://dx.doi.org/10.1016/j.plantsci.2010.12.007] [PMID: 21421392]

[21] Gao X, Zhang Y, He Z, Fu X. Gibberellins. In: Li J, Li C, Smith SM, Eds. Hormone metabolism and signaling in plants. Academic Press 2017.
[http://dx.doi.org/10.1016/B978-0-12-811562-6.00004-9]

[22] Hao D, Sun X, Ma B, Zhang J, Guo H. Hormone metabolism and signaling in plants. In: Li J, Li C, Smith SM, Eds. Academic press 2017; pp. 203-41.
[http://dx.doi.org/10.1016/B978-0-12-811562-6.00006-2]

[23] VanEtten H, Temporini E, Wasmann C. Phytoalexin (and phytoanticipin) tolerance as a virulence trait: Why is it not required by all pathogens? Physiol Mol Plant Pathol 2001; 59(2): 83-93.
[http://dx.doi.org/10.1006/pmpp.2001.0350]

[24] Gershenzon J, Croteau R. Terpenoids. In: Rosenthal GA, Berenbaum MR, Eds. Herbivores their interaction with secondary plant metabolites : The chemical participants. 2nd. San Diego: Academic Press 1991; 1: pp. 165-219.

[25] Roberts SC. Production and engineering of terpenoids in plant cell culture. Nat Chem Biol 2007; 3(7): 387-95.
[http://dx.doi.org/10.1038/nchembio.2007.8] [PMID: 17576426]

[26] Jamwal K, Bhattacharya S, Puri S. Plant growth regulator mediated consequences of secondary metabolites in medicinal plants. J Appl Res Med Aromat Plants 2018; 9: 26-38.
[http://dx.doi.org/10.1016/j.jarmap.2017.12.003]

[27] Aldred EM. Pharmacology E-Book: A handbook for complementary healthcare professionals. Elsevier Health Sciences 2008.

[28] Davis EM, Croteau R. Cyclization enzymes in the biosynthesis of monoterpenes, sesquiterpenes, and diterpenes. Top Curr Chem 2000; 209: 53-95.
[http://dx.doi.org/10.1007/3-540-48146-X_2]

[29] Boutanaev AM, Moses T, Zi J, *et al.* Investigation of terpene diversification across multiple sequenced plant genomes. Proc Natl Acad Sci 2015; 112(1): E81-8.
[http://dx.doi.org/10.1073/pnas.1419547112] [PMID: 25502595]

[30] Specter M. A Life of Its Own Where will synthetic biology lead us? 2009.https://www.newyorker.com/magazine/2009/09/28/a-life-of-its-own

[31] Cox-Georgian D, Ramadoss N, Dona C, Basu C. Therapeutic and medicinal uses of terpenes. In: Joshee N, Dhekney SA, Parajuli P, Eds. Medicinal Plants from Farm to Pharmacy. Cham: Springer 2019; pp. 333-59.
[http://dx.doi.org/10.1007/978-3-030-31269-5_15]

[32] Franklin LU, Cunnington GD, Young DE. inventors; XiMed group plc, assignee terpene based pesticide treatments for killing terrestrial arthropods including, amongst others, lice, lice eggs, mites

and ants. US 6130253, 2000.

[33]   Achakzai AK, Achakzai P, Masood A, Kayani SA, Tareen RB. Response of plant parts and age on the distribution of secondary metabolites on plants found in Quetta. Pakistan. J Bot 2009; 41(5): 2129-35.

[34]   Cosme P, Rodríguez AB, Espino J, Garrido M. Plant phenolics: Bioavailability as a key determinant of their potential health-promoting applications. Antioxidants 2020; 9(12): 1263.
[http://dx.doi.org/10.3390/antiox9121263] [PMID: 33322700]

[35]   Park ES, Moon WS, Song MJ, Kim MN, Chung KH, Yoon JS. Antimicrobial activity of phenol and benzoic acid derivatives. Int Biodeterior Biodegradation 2001; 47(4): 209-14.
[http://dx.doi.org/10.1016/S0964-8305(01)00058-0]

[36]   Taiz L, Zeiger E. Plant Physiology. Sunderland, Massachusetts: Sinauer Associates, Inc. Publisher 2002.

[37]   Dixon RA. Natural products and plant disease resistance. Nature 2001; 411(6839): 843-7.
[http://dx.doi.org/10.1038/35081178] [PMID: 11459067]

[38]   Kaur R, Arora SA. Alkaloids-important therapeutic secondary metabolites of plant origin. Journal of Critical Reviews 2015; 2(3): 1-8.

[39]   Burow M, Wittstock U, Gershenzon J. Sulfur-containing secondary metabolites and their role in plant defense. In: Hell R, Dahl C, Knaff D, Leustek T, Eds. Sulfur metabolism in phototrophic organisms. Dordrecht: Springer 2008; pp. 201-22.
[http://dx.doi.org/10.1007/978-1-4020-6863-8_11]

[40]   Venditti A, Bianco A. Sulfur-containing secondary metabolites as neuroprotective agents. Curr Med Chem 2020; 27(26): 4421-36.
[http://dx.doi.org/10.2174/0929867325666180912105036] [PMID: 30207214]

[41]   Nwachukwu ID, Slusarenko AJ, Gruhlke MC. Sulfur and sulfur compounds in plant defence. Natural Product Communications 2012; 7(3).
[http://dx.doi.org/10.1177/1934578X1200700323]

[42]   Jin JH, Shin JH, Kim JH, Chung IS, Lee HJ. Effect of chitosan elicitation and media components on the production of anthraquinone colorants in madder (*Rubia akane* Nakai) cell culture. Biotechnol Bioprocess Eng 1999; 4(4): 300-4.
[http://dx.doi.org/10.1007/BF02933757]

[43]   Masondo NA, Aremu AO, Finnie JF, Van Staden J. Plant growth regulator induced phytochemical and antioxidant variations in micropropagated and acclimatized Eucomis autumnalis subspecies autumnalis (Asparagaceae). Acta Physiol Plant 2014; 36(9): 2467-79.
[http://dx.doi.org/10.1007/s11738-014-1619-4]

[44]   Sa G, Mi M, He-chun Y, Ben-ye L, Guo-feng L, Kang C. Effects of ipt gene expression on the physiological and chemical characteristics of *Artemisia annua* L. Plant Sci 2001; 160(4): 691-8.
[http://dx.doi.org/10.1016/S0168-9452(00)00453-2] [PMID: 11448744]

[45]   Santoro MV, Nievas F, Zygadlo J, Giordano W, Banchio E. Effects of growth regulators on biomass and the production of secondary metabolites in peppermint (*Mentha piperita*) micropropagated *in vitro*. Am J Plant Sci 2013; 4(5): 49-55.
[http://dx.doi.org/10.4236/ajps.2013.45A008]

[46]   Stoeva T, Iliev L. Influence of some phenylurea cytokinins on spearmint essential oil composition. Bulg J Plant Physiol 1997; 23(3-5): 66-71.

[47]   Weathers PJ, Bunk G, McCoy MC. The effect of phytohormones on growth and artemisinin production in *Artemisia annua* hairy roots. *In Vitro* Cell Dev Biol Plant 2005; 41(1): 47-53.
[http://dx.doi.org/10.1079/IVP2004604]

[48]   Bergmann L. The effect of kinetin on the metabolism of plant tissue cultures. In: White PR, Grove AR, Eds. Plant tissue culture. 1965; pp. 171-80.

[49]   Kastell A, Smetanska I, Ulrichs C, Cai Z, Mewis I. Effects of phytohormones and jasmonic acid on glucosinolate content in hairy root cultures of *Sinapis alba* and *Brassica rapa*. Appl Biochem Biotechnol 2013; 169(2): 624-35.
[http://dx.doi.org/10.1007/s12010-012-0017-x] [PMID: 23269631]

[50]   Karalija E, Paric A. The effect of BA and IBA on the secondary metabolite production by shoot culture of *Thymus vulgaris* L. Biol Nyssana 2011; 2(1): 29-35.

[51]   Królicka A, Kartanowicz R, Wosiński SA, Szpitter A, Kamiński M, Łojkowska E. Induction of secondary metabolite production in transformed callus of *Ammi majus* L. grown after electromagnetic treatment of the culture medium. Enzyme Microb Technol 2006; 39(7): 1386-91.
[http://dx.doi.org/10.1016/j.enzmictec.2006.03.042]

[52]   Meyer HJ, Van Staden J. The *in vitro* production of an anthocyanin from callus cultures of *Oxalis linearis*. Plant Cell Tissue Organ Cult 1995; 40(1): 55-8.
[http://dx.doi.org/10.1007/BF00041119]

[53]   Tanaka N, Takao M, Matsumoto T. Vincamine production in multiple shoot culture derived from hairy roots of *Vinca minor*. Plant Cell Tissue Organ Cult 1995; 41(1): 61-4.
[http://dx.doi.org/10.1007/BF00124087]

[54]   Kisiel W, Stojakowska A, Malarz J, Kohlmüzer S. Sesquiterpene lactones in *Agrobacterium rhizogenes*—Transformed hairy root culture of *Lactuca virosa*. Phytochemistry 1995; 40(4): 1139-40.
[http://dx.doi.org/10.1016/0031-9422(95)00433-8]

[55]   Venkateswara R, Sankara Rao S, Vaidyanathan CS. Phytochemical constituents of cultured cells of *Eucalyptus tereticornis* SM. Plant Cell Rep 1986; 5(3): 231-3.
[http://dx.doi.org/10.1007/BF00269127] [PMID: 24248141]

[56]   Zhou Y, Hirotani M, Yoshikawa T, Furuya T. Flavonoids and phenylethanoids from hairy root cultures of *Scutellaria baicalensis*. Phytochemistry 1997; 44(1): 83-7.
[http://dx.doi.org/10.1016/S0031-9422(96)00443-8]

[57]   Teshima D, Ikeda K, Satake M, Aoyama T, Shimomura K. Production of emetic alkaloid by *in vitro* culture of *cephaelis ipecacuanha* A. Richard. Plant Cell Rep 1988; 7(4): 278-80.
[http://dx.doi.org/10.1007/BF00272542] [PMID: 24241766]

[58]   Tanahashi T, Zenk MH. Isoquinoline alkaloids from cell suspension cultures of *Fumaria capreolata*. Plant Cell Rep 1985; 4(2): 96-9.
[http://dx.doi.org/10.1007/BF00269216] [PMID: 24253694]

[59]   Masidur Alam M, Naeem M, Idrees M, Masroor M, Khan A, Moinuddin . Augmentation of photosynthesis, crop productivity, enzyme activities and alkaloids production in Sadabahar (*Catharanthus roseus* L.) through application of diverse plant growth regulators. J Crop Sci Biotechnol 2012; 15(2): 117-29.
[http://dx.doi.org/10.1007/s12892-011-0005-7]

[60]   Ohlsson AB, Björk L. Effects of gibberellic acid on cardenolide accumulation by *Digitalis lanata* tissue cultures grown in light and darkness. J Plant Physiol 1988; 133(5): 535-8.
[http://dx.doi.org/10.1016/S0176-1617(88)80003-8]

[61]   Schmiderer C, Grausgruber-Gröger S, Grassi P, Steinborn R, Novak J. Influence of gibberellin and daminozide on the expression of terpene synthases and on monoterpenes in common sage (Salvia officinalis). J Plant Physiol 2010; 167(10): 779-86.
[http://dx.doi.org/10.1016/j.jplph.2009.12.009] [PMID: 20163890]

[62]   Teszlák P, Gaál K, Pour Nikfardjam MS. Influence of grapevine flower treatment with gibberellic acid (GA₃) on polyphenol content of *Vitis vinifera* L. wine. Anal Chim Acta 2005; 543(1-2): 275-81.
[http://dx.doi.org/10.1016/j.aca.2005.04.013]

[63]   Weiss D, van Tunen AJ, Halevy AH, Mol JNM, Gerats AGM. Stamens and gibberellic acid in the regulation of flavonoid gene expression in the corolla of *Petunia hybrida*. Plant Physiol 1990; 94(2):

511-5.
[http://dx.doi.org/10.1104/pp.94.2.511] [PMID: 16667742]

[64]   Li HC, Rice EL, Rohrbaugh LM, Wender SH. Effects of abscisic acid on phenolic content and lignin biosynthesis in tobacco tissue culture. Physiol Plant 1970; 23(5): 928-36.
[http://dx.doi.org/10.1111/j.1399-3054.1970.tb06490.x]

[65]   Subroto MA, Doran PM. Production of steroidal alkaloids by hairy roots of *Solanum aviculare* and the effect of gibberellic acid. Plant Cell Tissue Organ Cult 1994; 38(2-3): 93-102.
[http://dx.doi.org/10.1007/BF00033866]

[66]   Bari R, Jones JDG. Role of plant hormones in plant defence responses. Plant Mol Biol 2009; 69(4): 473-88.
[http://dx.doi.org/10.1007/s11103-008-9435-0] [PMID: 19083153]

[67]   Ton J, Flors V, Mauch-Mani B. The multifaceted role of ABA in disease resistance. Trends Plant Sci 2009; 14(6): 310-7.
[http://dx.doi.org/10.1016/j.tplants.2009.03.006] [PMID: 19443266]

[68]   Mansouri H, Asrar Z, Szopa J. Effects of ABA on primary terpenoids and Δ9-tetrahydrocannabinol in *Cannabis sativa* L. at flowering stage. Plant Growth Regul 2009; 58(3): 269-77.
[http://dx.doi.org/10.1007/s10725-009-9375-y]

[69]   Ibrahim M, Jaafar H. Abscisic acid induced changes in production of primary and secondary metabolites, photosynthetic capacity, antioxidant capability, antioxidant enzymes and lipoxygenase inhibitory activity of *Orthosiphon stamineus* Benth. Molecules 2013; 18(7): 7957-76.
[http://dx.doi.org/10.3390/molecules18077957] [PMID: 23884129]

[70]   Bota C, Deliu C. Effect of plant growth regulators on the production of flavonoids by cell suspension cultures of *Digitalis lanata.* Farmacia 2015; 63(5): 716-9.

[71]   Taniguchi S, Imayoshi Y, Kobayashi E, *et al.* Production of bioactive triterpenes by *Eriobotrya japonica* calli. Phytochemistry 2002; 59(3): 315-23.
[http://dx.doi.org/10.1016/S0031-9422(01)00455-1] [PMID: 11830140]

[72]   Ishimaru K, Shimomura K. Tannin production in hairy root culture of *Geranium thunbergii.* Phytochemistry 1991; 30(3): 825-8.
[http://dx.doi.org/10.1016/0031-9422(91)85260-7]

[73]   Quiala E, Barbón R, Jimenez E, *et al.* Biomass production of *Cymbopogon citratus* (D.C.) stapf., a medicinal plant, in temporary immersion systems. *In Vitro* Cell Dev Biol Plant 2006; 42(3): 298-300.
[http://dx.doi.org/10.1079/IVP2006765]

[74]   Harkes PAA, Krijbolder L, Libbenga KR, Wijnsma R, Nsengiyaremge T, Verpoorte R. Influence of various media constituents on the growth of *Cinchona ledgeriana* tissue cultures and the production of alkaloids and anthraquinones therein. Plant Cell Tissue Organ Cult 1985; 4(3): 199-214.
[http://dx.doi.org/10.1007/BF00040194]

[75]   Kueh JSH, MacKenzie IA, Pattenden G. Production of chrysanthemic acid and pyrethrins by tissue cultures of *Chrysanthemum cinerariaefolium.* Plant Cell Rep 1985; 4(3): 118-9.
[http://dx.doi.org/10.1007/BF00571294] [PMID: 24253739]

[76]   Sri Andrijany V, Indrayanto G, Adi Soehono L. Simultaneous effect of calcium, magnesium, copper and cobalt ions on sapogenin steroids content in callus cultures of *Agave amaniensis.* Plant Cell Tissue Organ Cult 1998; 55(2): 103-8.
[http://dx.doi.org/10.1023/A:1006119600153]

[77]   Ahmad S, Othman N. Strategic planning, issues, prospects and the future of the Malaysian herbal industry. Int J Acad Res AccFin Manag Sci 2013; 3(4): 91-102.

[78]   Kim OT, Kim MY, Hong MH, Ahn JC, Hwang B. Stimulation of asiaticoside accumulation in the whole plant cultures of *Centella asiatica* (L.) Urban by elicitors. Plant Cell Rep 2004; 23(5): 339-44.
[http://dx.doi.org/10.1007/s00299-004-0826-7] [PMID: 15316748]

[79]   Kim Y, Hahn E, Murthy HN, Paek K. Adventitious root growth and ginsenoside accumulation in *Panax ginseng* cultures as affected by methyl jasmonate. Biotechnol Lett 2004; 26(21): 1619-22. [http://dx.doi.org/10.1007/s10529-004-3183-2] [PMID: 15604808]

[80]   De-Eknamkul W, Ellis BE. Effects of macronutrients on growth and rosmarinic acid formation in cell suspension cultures of *Anchusa officinalis*. Plant Cell Rep 1985; 4(2): 46-9. [http://dx.doi.org/10.1007/BF00269203] [PMID: 24253681]

[81]   Sato K, Yamazaki T, Okuyama E, Yoshihira K, Shimomura K. Anthraquinone production by transformed root cultures of *Rubia tinctorum*: Influence of phytohormones and sucrose concentration. Phytochemistry 1991; 30(5): 1507-9. [http://dx.doi.org/10.1016/0031-9422(91)84198-2]

[82]   Narayan MS, Thimmaraju R, Bhagyalakshmi N. Interplay of growth regulators during solid-state and liquid-state batch cultivation of anthocyanin producing cell line of *Daucus carota*. Process Biochem 2005; 40(1): 351-8. [http://dx.doi.org/10.1016/j.procbio.2004.01.009]

[83]   Makunga NP, Van Staden J, Cress WA. The effect of light and 2, 4-D on anthocyanin production in *Oxalis reclinata* callus. Plant Growth Regul 1997; 23(3): 153-8. [http://dx.doi.org/10.1023/A:1005966927813]

[84]   Hamill J, Robins R, Rhodes M. Alkaloid production by transformed root cultures of *Cinchona ledgeriana*. Planta Med 1989; 55(4): 354-7. [http://dx.doi.org/10.1055/s-2006-962027] [PMID: 17262435]

[85]   Schripsema J, Ramos-Valdivia A, Verpoorte R. Robustaquinones, novel anthraquinones from an elicited *Cinchona robusta* suspension culture. Phytochemistry 1999; 51(1): 55-60. [http://dx.doi.org/10.1016/S0031-9422(98)00470-1]

[86]   Wang PJ, Huang CI. Production of saikosaponins by callus and redifferentiated organs of Bupleurum falcatum L. Fujiwara A. Plant tissue culture: proceedings, 5th International Congress of Plant Tissue and Cell Culture. Tokyo and Lake Yamanake, Japan. 1982.

[87]   Datta MM, Majumder A, Jha S. Organogenesis and plant regeneration in *Taxus wallichiana (Zucc.)*. Plant Cell Rep 2006; 25(1): 11-8. [http://dx.doi.org/10.1007/s00299-005-0027-z] [PMID: 16240121]

[88]   Furuya T, Ikuta A, Syōno K. Alkaloids from callus tissue of *Papaver somniferum*. Phytochemistry 1972; 11(10): 3041-4. [http://dx.doi.org/10.1016/0031-9422(72)80101-8]

[89]   Nurcahyani N, Solichatun S, Anggarwulan E. The reserpine production and callus growth of indian snake root (*Rauvolfia serpentina* (L.) benth. Ex Kurz) culture by addition of Cu2+. Biodiversitas 2008; 9(3): 177-9. [http://dx.doi.org/10.13057/biodiv/d090305]

[90]   Hiraoka N, Bhatt ID, Sakurai Y, Chang JI. Alkaloid production by somatic embryo cultures of *Corydalis ambigua*. Plant Biotechnol 2004; 21(5): 361-6. [http://dx.doi.org/10.5511/plantbiotechnology.21.361]

[91]   Lee SY, Cho SI, Park MH, Kim YK, Choi JE, Park SU. Growth and rutin production in hairy root cultures of buckwheat (*Fagopyrum esculentum* M.). Prep Biochem Biotechnol 2007; 37(3): 239-46. [http://dx.doi.org/10.1080/10826060701386729] [PMID: 17516253]

[92]   Luo J, Liu L, Wu CD. Enhancement of paclitaxel production by abscisic acid in cell suspension cultures of *Taxus chinensis*. Biotechnol Lett 2001; 23(16): 1345-8. [http://dx.doi.org/10.1023/A:1010597802741]

[93]   Li Z, Zhao X, Sandhu AK, Gu L. Effects of exogenous abscisic acid on yield, antioxidant capacities, and phytochemical contents of greenhouse grown lettuces. J Agric Food Chem 2010; 58(10): 6503-9. [http://dx.doi.org/10.1021/jf1006962] [PMID: 20420437]

[94]   Hao G, Ji H, Li Y, *et al.* Exogenous ABA and polyamines enhanced salvianolic acids contents in hairy root cultures of *Salvia miltiorrhiza* Bge. f. alba. Plant Omics 2012; 5(5): 446.

[95]   Sandhu AK, Gray DJ, Lu J, Gu L. Effects of exogenous abscisic acid on antioxidant capacities, anthocyanins, and flavonol contents of muscadine grape (*Vitis rotundifolia*) skins. Food Chem 2011; 126(3): 982-8.
[http://dx.doi.org/10.1016/j.foodchem.2010.11.105] [PMID: 25212327]

[96]   Ionkova I, Kartnig T, Alfermann W. Cycloartane saponin production in hairy root cultures of *Astragalus mongholicus.* Phytochemistry 1997; 45(8): 1597-600.
[http://dx.doi.org/10.1016/S0031-9422(97)00247-1]

[97]   Nikolaeva TN, Zagoskina NV, Zaprometov MN. Production of phenolic compounds in callus cultures of tea plant under the effect of 2,4-D and NAA. Russ J Plant Physiol 2009; 56(1): 45-9.
[http://dx.doi.org/10.1134/S1021443709010075]

[98]   Gränicher F, Christen P, Kapétanidis I. Production of valepotriates by hairy root cultures of *Centranthus ruber* DC. Plant Cell Rep 1995; 14(5): 294-8.
[http://dx.doi.org/10.1007/BF00232031] [PMID: 24186763]

[99]   Rao VK, Venkanna N, Lakshmi Narasu M. *Agrobacterium rhizogenes* mediated transformation of *Artemisia annua.* J Sci Ind Res 1998; 57(10-11): 773-6.

[100] Sasaki K, Udagawa A, Ishimaru H, *et al.* High forskolin production in hairy roots of *Coleus forskohlii.* Plant Cell Rep 1998; 17(6-7): 457-9.
[http://dx.doi.org/10.1007/s002990050425] [PMID: 30736619]

[101] Françoise B, Hossein S, Halimeh H, Fallah Zah N. Growth optimization of *Zataria multiflora* Boiss. tissue cultures and rosmarinic acid production improvement. Pak J Biol Sci 2007; 10(19): 3395-9.
[http://dx.doi.org/10.3923/pjbs.2007.3395.3399] [PMID: 19090157]

[102] Baldi A, Dixit VK. Enhanced artemisinin production by cell cultures of *Artemisia annua.* Curr Trends Biotechnol Pharm 2008; 2: 341-8.

[103] Dörnenburg H, Knorr D. Semicontinuous processes for anthraquinone production with immobilized *Cruciata glabra* cell cultures in a three-phase system. J Biotechnol 1996; 50(1): 55-62.
[http://dx.doi.org/10.1016/0168-1656(96)01549-0] [PMID: 8672285]

[104] Hegazy AK, Mohamed AA, Sakere MM. Enhancement of callus induction and cucurbitacin content in *Citrullus colocynthis* L. (Schrad) using plant growth regulators. J Ala Acad Sci 2010; 81(1): 23-35.

[105] Maziah Mahmood , Mahmood M, Fadzillah NM, Daud SK. Effects of precursor supplementation on the production of triterpenes by *Centella asiatica* callus culture. Pak J Biol Sci 2005; 8(8): 1160-9.
[http://dx.doi.org/10.3923/pjbs.2005.1160.1169]

[106] Barthe GA, Jourdan PS, McIntosh CA, Mansell RL. Naringin and limonin production in callus cultures and regenerated shoots from Citrus sp. J Plant Physiol 1987; 127(1-2): 55-65.
[http://dx.doi.org/10.1016/S0176-1617(87)80041-X]

[107] Sakamoto K, Iida K, Sawamura K, *et al.* Anthocyanin production in cultured cells of *Aralia cordata* Thunb. Plant Cell Tissue Organ Cult 1994; 36(1): 21-6.
[http://dx.doi.org/10.1007/BF00048311]

[108] Giri A, Banerjee S, Ahuja PS, Giri CC. Production of hairy roots in *Aconitum heterophyllum* wall. using *Agrobacterium rhizogenes*. In Vitro Cell Dev Biol Plant 1997; 33(4): 280-4.
[http://dx.doi.org/10.1007/s11627-997-0050-6]

[109] Umamaheswa A, Lalitha V. *In vitro* effect of various growth hormones in *Capsicum annum* L. on the callus induction and production of Capsiacin. J Plant Sci 2007; 2(5): 545-51.
[http://dx.doi.org/10.3923/jps.2007.545.551]

[110] Johnson TS, Ravishankar GA, Venkataraman LV. *In vitro* capsaicin production by immobilized cells and placental tissues of *Capsicum annuum* L. grown in liquid medium. Plant Sci 1990; 70(2): 223-9.

[http://dx.doi.org/10.1016/0168-9452(90)90137-D]

[111] Waller GR, MacVean CD, Suzuki T. High production of caffeine and related enzyme activities in callus cultures of *Coffea arabica* L. Plant Cell Rep 1983; 2(3): 109-12.
[http://dx.doi.org/10.1007/BF00269330] [PMID: 24257975]

[112] Wu J, Wang C, Mei X. Stimulation of taxol production and excretion in Taxus spp cell cultures by rare earth chemical lanthanum. J Biotechnol 2001; 85(1): 67-73.
[http://dx.doi.org/10.1016/S0168-1656(00)00383-7] [PMID: 11164964]

[113] Grzegorczyk I, Wysokińska H. Antioxidant compounds in *Salvia officinalis* L. shoot and hairy root cultures in the nutrient sprinkle bioreactor. Acta Soc Bot Pol 2011; 79(1): 7-10.
[http://dx.doi.org/10.5586/asbp.2010.001]

[114] Devi CS, Murugesh S, Srinivasan VM. Gymnemic acid production in suspension cell cultures of *Gymnema sylvestre.* J App Sci 2006; 6(10): 2263-8.
[http://dx.doi.org/10.3923/jas.2006.2263.2268]

[115] Grzegorczyk I, Wysokińska H. Liquid shoot culture of *Salvia officinalis* L. for micropropagation and production of antioxidant compounds; effect of triacontanol. Acta Soc Bot Pol 2011; 77(2): 99-104.
[http://dx.doi.org/10.5586/asbp.2008.013]

[116] Kornfeld A, Kaufman PB, Lu CR, *et al.* The production of hypericins in two selected *Hypericum perforatum* shoot cultures is related to differences in black gland structure. Plant Physiol Biochem 2007; 45(1): 24-32.
[http://dx.doi.org/10.1016/j.plaphy.2006.12.009] [PMID: 17300946]

[117] Sepehr MF, Ghorbanli ZM. Formation of catechin in callus cultures and micropropagation of *Rheum ribes* L. Pak J Biol Sci 2005; 8(10): 1346-50.
[http://dx.doi.org/10.3923/pjbs.2005.1346.1350]

[118] Arya D, Patni V, Kant U. *In vitro* propagation and quercetin quantification in callus cultures of Rasna (*Pluchea lanceolata* Oliver & Hiern.). Indian J Biotechnol 2008; 7: 383-7.

[119] Qu JG, Yu XJ, Zhang W, Jin MF. Significant improved anthocyanins biosynthesis in suspension cultures of *Vitis vinifera* by process intensification. Sheng Wu Gong Cheng Xue Bao 2006; 22(2): 299-305.
[PMID: 16607960]

[120] Ko KS, Ebizuka Y, Noguchi H, Sankawa U. Production of polyketide pigments in hairy root cultures of *Cassia* plants. Chem Pharm Bull 1995; 43(2): 274-8.
[http://dx.doi.org/10.1248/cpb.43.274]

[121] Fulcheri C, Morard P, Henry M. Stimulation of the growth and the triterpenoid saponin accumulation of *Saponaria officinalis* cell and *Gypsophila paniculata* root suspension cultures by improvement of the mineral composition of the media. J Agric Food Chem 1998; 46(5): 2055-61.
[http://dx.doi.org/10.1021/jf970627+]

[122] Kovačević N, Grubišić D. *In vitro* cultures of plants from the rhamnaceae: Shoot propagation and anthraquinones production. Pharm Biol 2005; 43(5): 420-4.
[http://dx.doi.org/10.1080/13880200590963691]

[123] Khouri HE, Ibrahim RK, Rideau M. Effects of nutritional and hormonal factors on growth and production of anthraquinone glucosides in cell suspension cultures of *Cinchona succirubra.* Plant Cell Rep 1986; 5(6): 423-6.
[http://dx.doi.org/10.1007/BF00269632] [PMID: 24248396]

[124] Hohtola A, Jalonen J, Tolnen A, *et al.* Natural product formation by plants, enhancement, analysis, processing and testing. In: Jalkanen A, Nygren P, Eds. Sustainable use renewable natural resources–from principles to practices. University of Helsinki Publication 2005; pp. 34-69.

[125] Rueffer M, Bauer W, Zenk MH. The formation of corydaline and related alkaloids in *Corydalis cava in vivo* and *in vitro.* Can J Chem 1994; 72(1): 170-5.

[http://dx.doi.org/10.1139/v94-026]

[126] Cusidó RM, Palazón J, Navia-Osorio A, *et al.* Production of Taxol® and baccatin III by a selected Taxus baccata callus line and its derived cell suspension culture. Plant Sci 1999; 146(2): 101-7. [http://dx.doi.org/10.1016/S0168-9452(99)00093-X]

[127] Huang WW, Cheng CC, Yeh FT, Tsay HS. Tissue culture of *Dioscorea doryophora* HANCE 1. Callus organs and the measurement of diosgenin content. Chin Med Coll J 1993; 2(2): 151-60.

[128] Kaul B, Staba EJ. *Dioscorea* tissue cultures. I. Biosynthesis and isolation of diosgenin from *Dioscorea deltoidea* callus and suspension cells. Lloydia 1968; 31(2): 171.

[129] Agarwal M, Kamal R. Studies on flavonoid production using *in vitro* cultures of *Momordica charantia* L. Indian J Biotechnol 2007; 6: 277-9.

[130] Ataei-Azimi A, Hashemloian BD, Ebrahimzadeh H, Majd A. High *in vitro* production of ant-canceric indole alkaloids from periwinkle (*Catharanthus roseus*) tissue culture. Afr J Biotechnol 2008; 7(16): 2834-9.

CHAPTER 7

Hassawi Rice (*Oryza Sativa* L.) Nutraceutical Properties, *In Vitro* Culture and Genomics

Muneera Q. Al-Mssallem[1,*], Krishnananda P. Ingle[2], Gopal W. Narkhede[3], S. Mohan Jain[4], Penna Suprasanna[5], Gholamreza Abdi[6] and Jameel M. Al-Khayri[7]

[1] *Department of Food Science and Nutrition, College of Agriculture and Food Sciences, King Faisal University, Al-Ahsa 31982, Saudi Arabia*

[2] *Biotechnology Centre, Department of Agricultural Botany, Post Graduate Institute, Dr. Panjabrao Deshmukh Krishi Vidyapeeth, Krishi Nagar, Akola, Maharashtra, India*

[3] *Department of Agricultural Botany (Genetics and Plant Breeding), Vasantrao Naik Marathwada Krishi Vidyapeeth, Parbhani-431402, Maharashtra, India*

[4] *Department of Agricultural Sciences, PL-27, University of Helsinki-00014, Helsinki, Finland*

[5] *Nuclear Agriculture and Biotechnology Division, Bhabha Atomic Research Centre, Trombay, Mumbai, MS, India*

[6] *Department of Biotechnology, Persian Gulf Research Institute, Persian Gulf University, Bushehr-7516913817, Iran*

[7] *Department of Agricultural Biotechnology, College of Agriculture and Food Sciences, King Faisal University, Al-Ahsa 31982, Saudi Arabia*

Abstract: An indigenous reddish-brown landrace rice of the *indica* variety known as Hassawi rice (*Oryza sativa* L.) is cultivated in Saudi Arabia. This rice variety has both nutritive and non-nutritive bioactive components that have therapeutic potential and promote favorable metabolic profiles. Hassawi rice has health advantages that should be further investigated, especially for the treatment of diabetes and obesity. There is a direct need for the conservation and improvement of this important germplasm source. Breeding efforts are limited, although a couple of hybrids were developed. Biotechnology approaches offer effective tools for crop genetic improvement. In this direction, *in vitro* regeneration of this crop has been developed that enabled the evaluation of abiotic stress factors. Furthermore, recent genomic studies revealed that Hassawi rice harbors novel alleles for salinity tolerance. This chapter reviews the research carried out on Hassawi rice in relation to nutritional and health benefits as well as secondary metabolites bioactivity and progress made on *in vitro* culture and genomics.

* **Corresponding author Muneera Q. Al-Mssallem:** Department of Food Science and Nutrition, College of Agriculture and Food Sciences, King Faisal University, Al-Ahsa 31982, Saudi Arabia; E-mails: sjkaur@rediffmail.com; mmssallem@kfu.edu.sa

Keywords: Abiotic stress, Anti-diabetes, Anti-obesity, Breeding, Genomics, Nutrients, Secondary metabolites.

INTRODUCTION

Rice is one among the foremost important cereal crops and widely used for genetic studies. *Indica* and *japonica* are the two main subspecies of *Oryza sativa* L [1]. The cultivation of Hassawi rice began in Al-Ahsa oasis in Saudi Arabia, where it orginates from the wild-type of *indica* variety [2]. Its major characteristics are wide adaptability to drought and soil salinity [3]. However, it is susceptible to lodging, photoperiod sensitivity, and delayed maturity. Therefore, a breeding program was initiated to produce improved rice varieties by overcoming undesirable traits Two hybrids, Hassawi-1 and Hassawi-2, were developed by crossing local Hassawi rice and a Chinese inbred ancestor (IR1112) [2, 4]. The organelle genome sequences of Hassawi rice are very useful for understanding the inheritance of cultivars and their forthcoming breeding studies. There have been several publications on the whole genomes of the chloroplasts and mitochondria of indica and japonica plants [1, 5 - 7]. Comparative study revealed that many cp genomes had substantially conserved gene order and critical gene content. Two Hassawi rice cultivars' genomes were sequenced using next-generation sequencing technologies, according to Zhang *et al.* [2] (both cp and mt genomes). Hassawi-1, Hassawi-2, indica 93-11, and japonica Nipponbare all had single-nucleotide polymorphisms (SNPs), insertions or deletions (InDels), reverse complementary variation (RCV), simple sequence repeats (SSRs), and repeats in their genomes, according to a comparative analysis of the organellar genomes [2]. Hassawi rice, an underutilized food resource, is classified as pigmented rice and is characterized by its brown reddish color (Fig. **1**). It has lower carbohydrate and higher protein contents and also possesses considerable amounts of non-starch polysaccharides and phenolic compounds [8]. This characteristic of Hassawi rice points to its potential as a functional food that effectively supports and safeguards the human body against several chronic disorders. Therefore, Hassawi rice has significant potential economic benefits as well as nutritional value.

This chapter discusses nutritional and functional properties, beneficial health impact on the human body, *in vitro* culture, and genomics of Hassawi rice.

NUTRITIONAL COMPOSITION OF HASSAWI RICE

Both macro- and micronutrients of Hassawi rice have been studied and compared with the most commonly consumed rice types, such as Basmati rice and long grain white rice. Details on the macro- and micronutrients of Hassawi rice are presented in Table **1**.

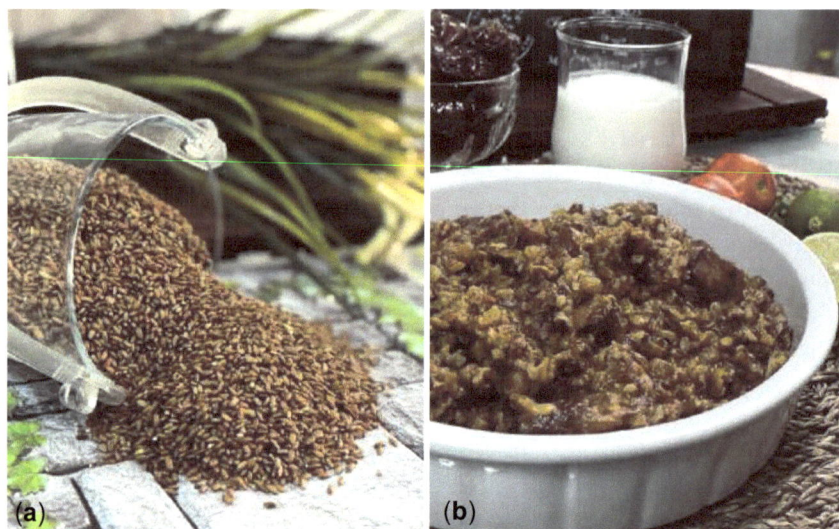

Fig. (1). Uncooked Hassawi rice grains (**a**) and cooked Hassawi rice in the popular local dish known as Kabsa (**b**). (Photos by Shareefa Q. Al-Mssallem).

Table 1. Nutritional composition of raw Hassawi rice, brown rice, long grain rice, and white Basmati rice size.

Components	Brown Rice	Long Grain White Rice	Hassawi Rice	White Basmati Rice
Nutrients (g/100g)				
Total carbohydrates	76.74	80.66	66.82	78.68
Non-starch polysaccharides	4.06	1.64	3.84	2.30
Total protein	8.22	6.90	10.49	7.97
Total fat	2.80	0.56	1.99	1.66
Macroelements (μg/g)				
Calcium, Ca	300.60	285.00	126.52	57.71
Phosphorus, P	3193.00	1130.00	1856.77	1250.53
Potassium, K	2515.33	1150.00	1522.65	1342.75
Sodium, Na	124.00	50.00	79.14	11.91
Microelements (μg/g))				
Zinc, Zn	23.00	10.90	39.04	15.58
Iron, Fe	14.57	7.78	13.25	8.93

(Table 1) cont.....

Components	Brown Rice	Long Grain White Rice	Hassawi Rice	White Basmati Rice
Copper, Cu	3.28	2.2	3.46	1.63
Selenium, Se	0.17	0.15	0.16	0.20
Boron, B	n/a	n/a	1.66	4.00
Water-soluble vitamins (mg/100g)				
Thiamine (B1)	0.55	0.07	0.55	0.18
Riboflavin (B2)	0.21	0.04	0.16	0.08
Niacin (B3)	4.38	1.6	0.74	1.20

Sources: This table was constructed based on data presented by [4, 8 - 11].

Macronutrients

Unlike most other rice, Hassawi rice has higher total protein and fat contents than the most commonly consumed long-grain white rice [9]. This is also applicable to the non-starch polysaccharides (NSPs) content of Hassawi rice, which is significantly higher than that of brown and white long grain rice [8, 9] and has a lower total carbohydrate content [9].

Micronutrients

Despite the fact that Hassawi rice is unprocessed and non-fortified rice, its content of some water-soluble vitamins such as thiamine and riboflavin is high (Table **1**). The most abundant macro-mineral in Hassawi rice is phosphorus and potassium. However, zinc is the highest micro-mineral in Hassawi rice, followed by iron (Table **1**). This indicates the importance of Hassawi rice as a source of macro- and micro-minerals without fortification with any kind of nutrients.

SECONDARY METABOLITES

Plants, fungi, and bacteria all naturally create secondary metabolites. In actuality, the normal growth, development, and reproduction of the organism do not directly depend on secondary metabolites [12]. Moreover, they are not involved in the daily functioning of the organism but are implicated in the overall maintenance of the organism, such as the excretion of waste and toxic products from the human body [13].

Classification

Most of the secondary metabolites can be categorized based on their biosynthetic origin. Plant secondary metabolites can be classified based on their chemical structure into phenolics, glycosides, terpenes, and alkaloids. Phenolics are the most abundant secondary metabolites, ranging from phenolic acids to tannins [14,

15]. Glycosides are the largest compounds presented in nature and consist of glycone (carbohydrate) bound to aglycone (non-carbohydrate) by a glycosidic bond. Therefore, glycosides can be classified based on their glycone, aglycone, and glycosidic bond. For pharmaceutical and biochemical purposes, the most appropriate classification of glycosides is based on the chemical nature of the aglycone, such as coumarin glycosides, steroidal glycosides, and flavonoid glycosides [16]. Alkaloids are nitrogen-containing compounds and the main alkaloids in rice are phenylamides and accumulated due to a pathogen attack. Examples of alkaloids in whole grain rice include 2-Acetyl-1-pyrroline, *N-trans*-Cinnamoyltyramine, and Indole 3-acetic acid [17]. In fact, 2-Acetyl-1-pyrroline gives aromatic rice its distinctive flavor. Additionally, some of these alkaloids in rice possess antimicrobial properties against plant pathogens [17]. Similarly, terpenes have nitrogen-containing constituents and are favorably useful in biotechnological, nutraceutical and pharmaceutical applications [18 - 20].

Biological Functions

Secondary metabolites provide useful substances which can be efficiently used in medicinal and pharmaceutical products for preventing some human diseases. In general, secondary metabolites exert antioxidant activity and play an important role in scavenging free radicals and inhibiting oxidative activity. Some secondary metabolites exhibit antimicrobial activity, anticancer, anti-inflammatory, antidiabetic and cholesterol-lowering properties [17, 21, 22].

Secondary metabolites are also beneficial to plants by developing an essential defense strategy against herbivorous insects and pathogenic fungi [23]. They may also suppress the development of competitor plants and protect the plants from external abiotic and biotic factors [24]. In actuality, exposure to numerous environmental variables, including drought, salt, UV radiation, and severe temperatures, causes the formation of secondary metabolites in plants [25]. Some secondary metabolites build up as a defence against pathogen assault [17]. Secondary metabolites also act as signal components during plant pollination and dispersion of seeds, where their pigments and odors attract pollinators. Plants can protect themselves from their competitors by producing anti-microbial components. Moreover, some sulfur- and nitrogen-containing compounds of secondary metabolite provide distinctive flavors and aroma to aromatic rice [17, 21].

Secondary Metabolites in Rice

Rice produces several secondary metabolites, including phenolic acids, flavonoids, tocopherols and tocotrienols, anthocyanins and proanthocyanidins, phytic acid, and γ-oryzanol [26]. These compounds play important physiological and biological functions. and beneficial impact on human health through their antioxidant activity in rice [17, 26].

Secondary metabolites are significantly accumulated in Hassawi rice (Table **2**). Hassawi rice has much greater total phenolic acid and flavonoid levels than Basmati rice (118 vs. 31 GAE mg/g and 61 vs. 8 CE mg/g, respectively). Prior to and following germination, Hadid and Elsheikh (2012) measured the levels of phytic acid, -tocopherol, and -oryzanol in Hassawi rice [27]. Furthermore, compared to Basmati rice, Hassawi rice had the highest free-radical scavenging activity at 76.4% [8]. It is generally known that the presence of phenolic chemicals, namely phenolic acids, has a high correlation with rice's natural antioxidant potential [28].

Table 2. Secondary metabolites percentages in raw Hassawi rice and Basmati rice (mg/100g) and their functions.

Secondary Metabolites Components	Hassawi Rice (%)	Basmati Rice (%)	Functions
Phenolic acids	11.8	3.1	• Antioxidant activity • Allelopathic effect
Flavonoids	6.1	0.8	• Allelopathic effect • Antioxidant activity
α-Tocopherols	0.4	7.2	• Antioxidant activity • Antihypercholesterolemic activity • Anticancer activity • Neuroprotective activity
γ-Oryzanol	85.0	30.4	• Antioxidant activity • Anti-inflammatory activity • Antimutagenic activity • Cholesterol-lowering activity • Anti-cancer activity • Anti-diabetic activity
Phytic acid	1.3	1.6	• Antioxidant activity

Sources: This table was constructed based on data presented by Al-Mssallem and Alqurashi; Al-Bahrani; Hadid and Elsheikh [8, 17, 27].

MEDICINAL AND PHARMACEUTICAL PROPERTIES

Bioactive substances that are both nutritive and non-nutritive may have an effect when combined with Hassawi rice. NSPs, vitamin E precursors, and selenium all contribute to the nutritional bioactive components in Hassawi rice [8, 27]. However, other nutritive bioactive constituents, such as tocotrienols, have yet to be determined. Phenolic compounds such as phenolic acid, flavonoids, γ-oryzanol and phytic acid in Hassawi rice are considered as non-nutritive bioactive substances [8, 27]. All these compounds possess medicinal and pharmaceutical properties.

Antidiabetic Properties

Clinical research using measurements of the glycaemic and insulinemic indices of Hassawi rice has examined the effect of its ingredients in managing diabetes [9]. The presence of phenolic compounds and NSPs may be responsible for this anti-diabetic effect of Hassawi rice components [8, 27]. According to Ranilla *et al.* [29], it is clear that phenolic compounds contribute to the inhibition of α-glucosidase and α-amylase activity. This decreases the amount of glucose that can be absorbed from the small intestine and, as a result, lessens the plasma glucose response to carbs [30]. Additionally, the significant amount of NSPs present in Hassawi rice is crucial in reducing the glycaemic response [31]. Dietary NSPs have been linked to a lower risk of developing diabetes in several studies [32 - 36]. Additionally, Hassawi rice has a low glycemic load and an insulinaemic index [9]. Hassawi rice's decreased glycaemic and insulinaemic effects may help control and prevent type 2 diabetes.

Anti-Obesity and Gastrointestinal Activities

Hassawi rice, as a whole unprocessed wild rice, is rich in nutrients such as NSPs, mostly insoluble. Indeed, high NSPs foods are substantially recommended for maintaining a healthy body weight. Decreased appetite and increased satiety are among the many health benefits that insoluble NSPs possess [37]. Thus, enhancing satiety encourages regulating energy intake and lowers the chance of becoming overweight and obese [38]. Hassawi rice plays an important role as a functional food as it is a good source of NSPs. From Table **1**, we can conclude that the serving size of cooked Hassawi rice (150 g) can provide 2.16 g NSPs, and this contributes to approximately 8.6% of the recommended daily intake of NSPs for healthy adults (Table **1**). The NSPs exert an important role in improving gastrointestinal functions, and thus Hassawi rice can be used as natural laxatives to regulate intestinal transit and promote regular bowel movements [31].

BREEDING APPROACHES

Cultivation and Limitations

Hassawi rice is a wild local rice native to the Eastern Providence of Saudi Arabia. Hassawi rice is consumed in its entire structure, which implies the external bran layers are not removed. Hassawi rice is utilized generally to provide strength to unfit individuals. The rice is planted after the late spring during September-October [39].

The continuous interest in developing improved rice varieties applies biotechnological tools alongside biotic and abiotic restrictions. Biotic stress (weeds, pests and diseases), abiotic (scarcity of good quality water, salt burdens, soil nutrient limitations and climatic components), and financial factors present obstacles to higher potential yields and limit rice selection efficiency for genetic enhancement.

Breeding Objectives

The most popular food in India and other Asian countries, including China, Japan, Vietnam, Thailand, and Bangladesh, is rice. This crop develops in a variety of agro-climatic environments, including flooded rice, upland rice, swamp rice, and deep-water rice. Goals identified with reproducing for protection from different contagious and bacterial diseases were recognized as the top needs for rice. Stem borer (*Scirpophaga* sp., *Chilo* sp., *Sesamia inferens* Walker) and brown plant hopper (*Nilaparvata lugens* Stål) cause broad yield losses in rice and need consideration. In this way, the improvement of transgenics for protection from biotic stresses should be given the most elevated need. Breeding for better return through the exploitation of heterosis was likewise recognized as a significant test. Heterosis breeding cold resistance at development in blustery season yield and cold resilience as a rule for 'boro rice' were viewed as significant. Herbicide tolerance was proposed to be especially significant for upland rice and for permitting direct seeding to supplant the act of enormous scope transplantation. Quality improvement by the consolidation of characters' fragrance and grain length was referenced, despite the fact that it is not obvious from the overview whether this should be cultivated through the advancement of transgenics or whether it tends to be accomplished by regular breeding. To put it plainly, biotic stress takes the most noteworthy need in rice breeding, followed by abiotic stresses like dry spells and flooding. For creating safe rice assortments for both biotic and abiotic stresses, this review underlined the utilization of transgenic advances [40].

Heterosis Breeding

Heterosis breeding is the superiority of hybrid over the average performance of parents in yield and yield attributing traits. The difference between the crossbred and inbred means is used to compute it:

$$\text{Hybrid vigor} = \{[F_1-(P1+P2)/2]/[P1+P2)/2]\}$$

The estimate is usually calculated as a percentage [41].

Several scientists have proposed and evaluated the genetic underpinnings of heterosis. To explain the genetic basis of heterosis, two traditional hypotheses, dominance and over dominance, have been put forth. The accumulation of advantageous dominant alleles and the epistatic effects of harmful recessive alleles at various loci are factors in the dominance hypothesis' contribution to heterosis in the hybrid [42 - 44]. According to the over-dominance theory, heterozygous allele combinations at one or more loci in a hybrid are preferable to either of the homozygous allele combinations in the parental inbreds [45]. To explain heterosis at the molecular level, two hypotheses have been put forth [46]. According to the first hypothesis, the hybrid's heterosis is caused by the several genes' combined allelic expression. According to the second hypothesis, heterosis results from the interaction of several alleles inside the hybrid, which alters gene expression and produces a departure from the mid-parent values. Allelic interaction between regulatory genes may be the cause of this condition. In addition to these two models, altered gene regulation may be caused by variations in the expression of particular transcription factors [47], altered regulation [48], and a variety of transcriptional and post-transcriptional regulatory processes as well as epigenetic changes like DNA methylation, histone acetylation, and chromatin remodulation [49]. The development of molecular biology has made it feasible to explore the heterosis phenomena in more detail [50].

Hybridization

According to the reproducing record, Hassawi-1 and Hassawi-2 are the results of local Hassawi rice's hybridization with a Chinese inbred progenitor (IR1112) [4]. The genetic history of the two Hassawi rice cultivars has received less attention in the literature. Hasswi-1 and Hassawi-2 shared a common indica ancestor, which was closely linked to O. Nivara, according to a molecular phylogenetic study based on entire cp genomes of five rice cultivars, including broad rice Oryza nivara [51]. Further research into the resequencing of 50 varieties of domesticated and wild rice revealed that indica was closely connected to Oryza nivara, whilst japonica was more closely related to Oryza rufipogon and paternal from O. nivara [52]. While the nuclear genome is acquired by biparental reproduction, the chloroplasts and mitochondria of higher plants are maternally acquired and have their own copies and DNA fix frameworks [53, 54]. Organellar genomes are frequently used for tracking evolutionary relationships when there is a uniparental legacy [54]. Hassawi-1 and IR1112 are independently the mother and paternal parents of Hassawi-2, and both the mt and cp genomes of Hassawi-2 are acquired from Peta in remote origin, according to the analysis of the diversity in both the cp and mt genomes between Hassawi-1 and Hassawi-2. We propose that the wild-type Hassawi rice is a descendant of Peta, which had adapted to the current or similar environment some hundreds or even thousands of years ago. It would be interesting to know the specific history and origin of the Hassawi rice for the sake of both science and civilization studies. This is because the divergence of rice organellar genomes among all the analysed indica or japonica varieties and between Hassawi-1 and Hassawi-2 (Fig. **2**).

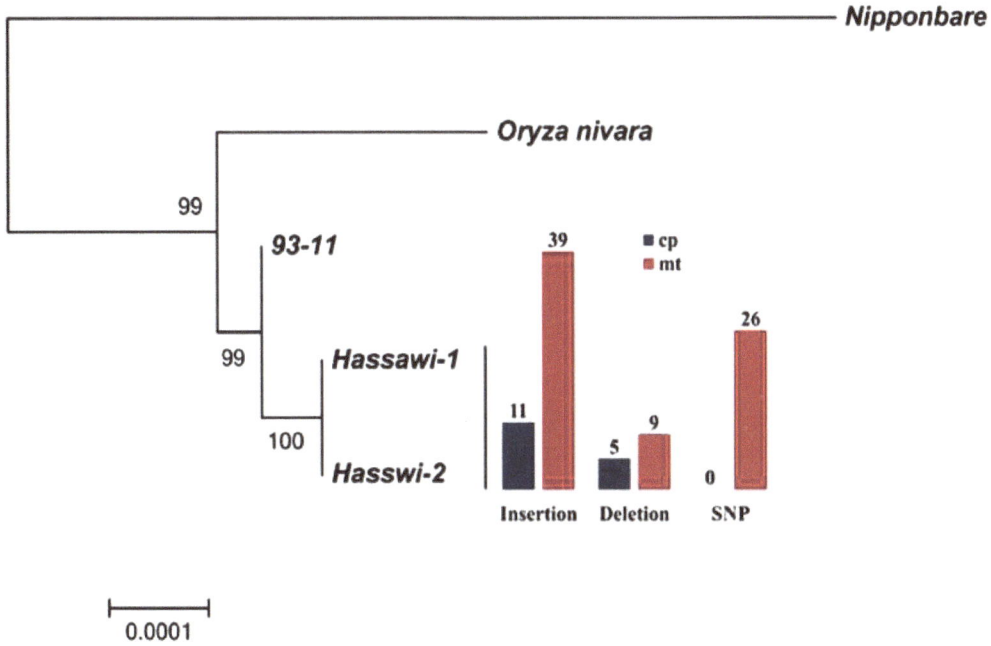

Fig. (2). Hassawi rice origins and its hybrid. The Indonesian variant is the source of wild-type Hassawi rice. Blue line represents Peta (Source [2]).

Molecular Breeding Potential

Marker-Assisted- Selection for Genetic Improvement

Plant breeders regularly transpose certain traits of economic importance, such as biotic stress tolerance, from one varietal framework to another. Most features are not easily transferable from one variety to another. Screening techniques are cumbersome, expensive, and call for a sizable field. A "tag" that may be used to indirectly choose the gene(s) in the breeding programme is an atomic marker strongly linked to the objective quality [55]. When screening for field-based traits, molecular markers have given scientists useful tools for phenotypic selection [56]. For instance, root morphology and other drought-associated features were used to filter mapping populations in order to find quantitative trait loci (QTLs) that may be used in MAS to enhance rice varieties [57]. The authors isolated a major QTL, which controlled deep rooting using the recombinant inbred lines between cv. IR64 and cv. Kinandang Patong. The Dro1 QTL has the potential to be used for screening for drought tolerance based on root growth traits. Rice being glycophytes, is salt sensitive. Using salt tolerant cv. Pokkali, Bonilla *et al.* (2002) identified a major QTL, referred to as Saltol, which confers salinity tolerance at the vegetative stage [58]. In a recent study, Marker Assisted Backcross Breeding using the major QTL Saltol QTL has been done to incorporate the trait into high yielding mega rice varieties (Pusa44 and Sarjoo52) [59]. Yeo *et al.* (2015) discovered a QTL qHTSF4.1 as a source of heat tolerance at the flowering stage, and this was found to be present in rice of all genetic backgrounds [60].

Marker assisted selection has also been successfully employed in rice breeding programmes aimed at disease resistance. Functional markers like xa13-prom and xa5FM, along with Xa21 (pTA248), were employed to distinguish rice germplasm in a multiplex PCR based screening of major resistance genes, and the technique found good applicability for screening a segregating population [61]. Using 10 SSR markers linked to blast resistance genes (Pi-9, Pi-1, Pi5-(t), Piz-5, Pi-b, Pi-ta, Pi33, Pi-27(t), Pitp(t), and Pikh), Singh *et al.* (2015) developed screening for rice blast disease, indicating that these linked markers could be used in the molecular screening of rice blast resistance genes [62]. Pyramiding of genes/QTLs for other quality attributes, such as resistance to biotic and abiotic stressors, has also been used to enhance rice [63]. MAS has been used to create a number of rice varieties [64] (Fig. **3**).

Potential Impact

New potential to improve the effectiveness of both the evolutionary and assessment phases of rice breeding is presented by recent developments in the cellular and molecular biology of rice. The breeding of rice is increasingly using biotechnology. Plant breeders now frequently utilise anther culture to fix recombinants, accelerate the breeding cycle for the creation of new rice varieties, and overcome sterility in crossbreeds. For mapping agronomic traits, including QTL, multiplied haploid populations are important. The labelling of diverse traits for resistance to significant biotic and abiotic challenges has been inspired by sub-atomic markers. For pyramiding attributes, transferring traits from one varietal foundation to the next, and advancing hardy pest-resistant cultivars, MAS has emerged as a key strategy in rice breeding. Pyramid QTLs for resistance to significant abiotic stresses should be made possible by fine QTL mapping. With the use of guide-based cloning, it is now possible to separate desirable traits with important agronomic properties and combine these traits into elite rice cultivars through mutation. The genetic diversity of rice has increased due to developments in tissue culture and the development of subatomic markers, which have also increased the efficiency with which beneficial traits from other species may be introduced across ability borders [55]. The introduction of cloned unique traits into rice through change has been promoted by advancements in hereditary construction. The function of rice genes. Identification of genes and their manipulation present another major breakthrough in rice genetics and breeding. As discussed above, many rice cultivars have been developed through the application of biotechnology tools. Many more will be forthcoming. The availability of rice cultivars with increased production potential, long-lasting resistance to diseases and insects, tolerance to abiotic stressors, and higher levels of micronutrients in the grain will be crucial for future food and nutritional security. These difficulties will be overcome with the use of biotechnology and conventional breeding techniques.

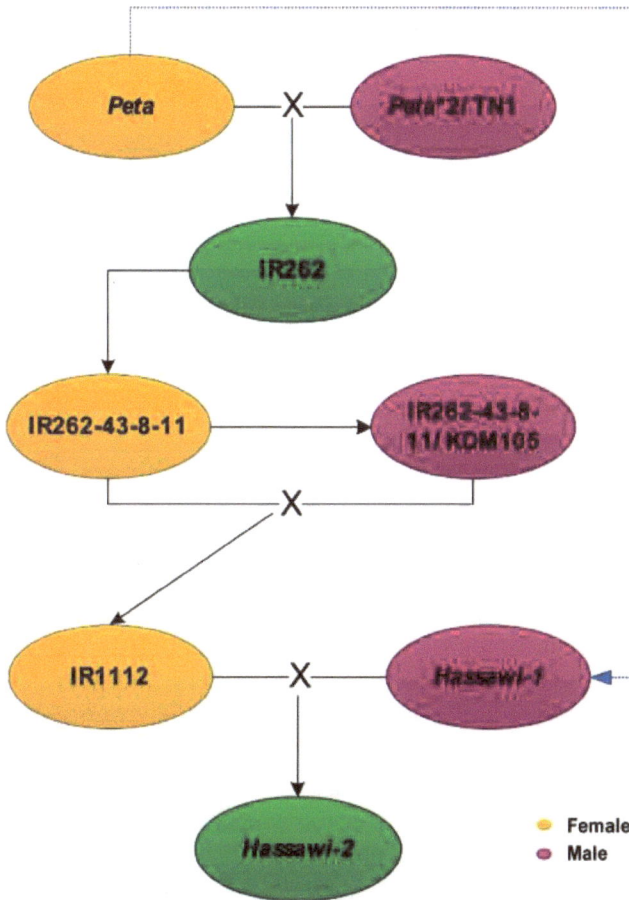

Fig. (3). Five rice varieties' phylogenetic relationships are determined by whole cp genomes. The maximum probability bootstrap support values for nodes are displayed. The scale bar indicates substitutions per site. The variations (Insertion, deletion, and SNP) in the cp genomes of Hassawi-1 and Hassawi-2 are shown in the histogram. (Source [2]).

TISSUE CULTURE APPLICATIONS

Mutation

Induced genetic variability using physical and chemical mutagens has been the basis for crop improvement through mutation induction and selection [65, 66]. Currently, there are 3275 mutant varieties developed in different crops and of these, 823 mutants have been reported in rice (FAO/IAEA 2019). It is also estimated that China and Japan together account for 50% of the mutant resource [67]. Among the chemical mutagens, Ethyl methanesulfonate has shown high potential for inducing mutations for higher yield and stress tolerance, besides several morphological and agronomic traits development [67]. On the other hand, gamma rays have been the most sought-after physical mutagen, and almost 90% of rice mutants have been developed using gamma irradiation. It is suggested that this mutagen majorly induces small deletions (1–16 bp) in rice, but large deletions have also been reported [68].

Despite considerable success with rice mutation breeding, one of the constraints remains to be achieved and is the large-scale screening of the mutant population. In this context, *in vitro* cultures can be mutagenized, followed by selection under *in vitro* conditions and plant regeneration from mutant cells [69]. *In vitro* cultures can be established from a wide variety of explants to induce callus and, subsequently somatic embryos and to establish cell suspension cultures [70]. Since rice suspension cultures have small cell clusters, they are amenable to chemical mutagenesis [71]. An efficient EMS based mutagenesis has been reported by using cell suspension cultures in rice, and it has been possible to achieve high mutagenesis efficiency for important agronomic traits [71, 72].

In Vitro Response to Stress

Agricultural biotechnology's main objective is to increase crop resistance to osmotic stressors, and using biochemical markers like proline analysis can help with this. This is dependent on the plant's capacity to collect non-toxic solutes, which are mostly found in the cytoplasm. A key component of an overproduction mechanism to maintain turgor and the driving gradient for water intake under osmotic stressors is to increase osmotic pressure [73]. In cell and callus cultures, accumulation of proline in osmotically stressed plant tissues has been discovered [74 - 77]. Al-Bahrany (2002) showed that proline accumulation rose gradually in response to rising PEG-induced water pressure in the Hassawi rice callus. In order to identify rice varieties with dry season tolerant cell lines, polyethylene glycol (PEG) 70 g l^{-1} has been used as the fundamental inhibitory threshold [10]. For the purpose of identifying drought-tolerant calli, 1-month-old calli that had been widely multiplied were also transferred to MS medium supplemented with PEG

(MW 6000) at 10, 20, 30, 40, 50, 60, and 70 g l^{-1}. Using developing plant parts as explants, Joshi *et al.* (2011) pioneered *in vitro* testing of rice calli for dry spell tolerance. Currently, showed that PEG treatment-induced expanding water pressure produced a dynamic reduction in calli volume in all genotypes [78]. Rice was subjected to an *in vitro* screening for enhanced dry season resistance by Biswas *et al.* in 2002. With an increase in PEG emphasis, callus volume decreased and total proline content was seen to have increased. By acting as a non-entering osmotic operator and reducing the medium's water capacity, they showed that PEG causes water stress in the medium. This might advance the development of a suitable determination method, appropriate genotypes, and the optimal PEG concentration to produce dry spell-tolerant lines. To determine the extent and limits of stress resilience that may be used in explaining the resistance tools at the cell level, further correlation of such tolerant cell lines with the PEG calm medium was also examined. This system's suitability, as stated earlier by Siddeswar and Kavikishore (1989) in advancing dry season tolerant lines in indica rice, was confirmed by the creation of putative dry season tolerant plantlets by *in vitro* screening that included embryogenic callus [79]. They believed that developing lines of indica rice that are tolerant to dry spells would be a good use of *in vitro* screening with the acceptance of the substance dry season and PEG (molecular weight - 6000) to modify dry season resilience. Plant cell and tissue culture strategies offer an intense apparatus for creating salt tolerant lines [79]. *In vitro* screening for salt resilience can fill in as a snappy system in the starter screening of genotypes. Early stage calli determined by refined in Murashige and Skoog (MS) media enhanced with 2,4-Dichlorophenoxyacetic corrosive (2,4-D) with or without the expansion of cytokinins and added substances have been used to screen for salt resistance. Crisp or dry load of calli, multiplication of calli, days to callus enlistment, callus morphology, aggregation of osmolytes like proline, centralization of cellualr particles like Na^+ and K^+, protein content and so on; have been utilized as records to quantify salt resilience.

In vitro tissue culture could be an important method for improving harvest resistance capacity. The percent callus acceptance was found to diminish with an expansion in salt convergence of the medium and the days taken for callus enlistment expanded with an increment in salt centralization of the medium. NaCl in the development medium adversely influenced the enlistment of rice callus and its consequent development. Genotypic constitution assumes a significant job in callus advancement. The decrease in the development of callus in the NaCl condition was because of the preoccupation of some quantum of vitality for development and metabolism.

Proline has a significant role in salt resistance instruments in many plant species, including rice. Hassawi rice is described as tolerant to high saltiness. A higher proline level in salt adjusted callus might be because of an expanded pace of amalgamation or diminished pace of oxidation of this compound [80]. Summart *et al.* (2010) announced that the proline content expanded impressively with an increment in salt grouping of the development medium [81]. Htwe *et al.* (2011) evaluated significant levels of proline in the media enhanced with expanded degree of NaCl and recommended as a factor giving salt resilience [82].

Bal and dutt (1986) revealed that salt tolerant rice assortments collects lesser Na^+ and higher K^+ than defenseless assortments [83]. Lower Na^+:K^+ proportion has been seen as qualities of saline resilience in rice. Raised degrees of Na^+ can induce insufficiency of the fundamental components K^+ and actuate pernicious changes in protein compliance [84]. Proline, sucrose, polyols, trehalose, and quaternary ammonium mixtures (QACs, such as glycine betaine, alinine betaine, proline betaine, and pipecolate betaine) are compatible solutes that accumulate under pressure [85, 86]. By enhancing cell osmotic change, reactive oxygen species detoxification, confirmation of the veracity of the film, and compound/protein stability, they protect plants from stress [87-89]. Proline, an amino corrosive, assumes an exceptionally useful job in plants presented to different pressure conditions. It acts as a metal chelator, an antioxidative guard atom and a flagging particle [90]. *In vitro* screening method with various grouping of NaCl stress could likewise be utilized as goof screening procedure for salt resilience as opposed to the field screening due to less time, little space and less work and the outcomes additionally exceptionally precise than the field screening. The genotypes performed better recovery recurrence in control recovery media yet the recovery recurrence diminished with expanded salt fixation. In prior reports, it was discovered that salt pre-treatment had beneficial outcome on plant recovery [91].

GENOMICS

Genetic Diversity

The key to breeding initiatives for rice and other crops is genetic diversity of agronomic traits. Various top strains and rice cultivars with increased nutritional quality and tolerance to abiotic stress have been created through a traditional breeding method. Special collections collected through genetics and genetic research have been used as a basis for studies on evolution or taxonomy, gene manipulation, whole chromosomes or genomes and incorporation of genes in crops from related weeds or related species. Breeders consequently look for hereditary changeability in other genetic stocks including wild family members of *Oryza* and new strategies are applied for the creation of new lines through somaclonal variety and hereditary breeding [55].

Genetic Engineering

Plant breeders are now able to achieve breeding goals that, just ten years ago, were not thought possible because of the entrance of alien genes from tiny organisms, diseases, parasites, critters, and, obviously, insignificant plants into crop species. Several methods are presently available for changing rice, including electroporation, microprojectile siege, polyethylene-glycol-initiated take-up of DNA into protoplasts, and, more recently, Agrobacterium-interceded alteration. Agronomically relevant traits in transgenic rice have been developed, including resistance to herbicides, protection from parasite diseases and stem borer. A few research institutions have successfully introduced transgenic rice, usually by DNA insertion into protoplasts, but also using microprojectile siege. Using Agrobacterium-intervened alteration, Hiei *et al.* (1994) and Cheng *et al.* (1998) obtained a large number of successful transgenic plants, and Cheng *et al.* (1998) created transgenic rice with several transgenes [41, 92]. After co-besieging embryogenic callus and cell suspensions with a combination of 14 different pUC-based plasmids, transgenic plants were produced. More than two of the objective traits were present in 85% and more than nine in 17% of the R0 plants.

Whole Genome Sequence

Many peruse the mt and cp genomes which can be collected inside complete genome successions autonomously, and can be found in the early unrefined information preceding whole genome shotgun sequencing projects [1, 93]. Total cp and mt genome arrangements of Boeahygrometrica were obtained using this method using the information obtained from the full genome sequencing [2]. The cp and mt genomes of Hassawi-1 and Hassawi-2 were both collected using a similar methodology. With 95% of the bases over Q40 and the highest median information grade of over 30 of both Hassawi-1 and Hassawi-2, the crude information grade obtained by the 454 sequencing stage was adequate. The collection of the mt genome required more complicated Roche Newbler software than the cp genome. Using all available sequencing raw data, 278498 and 235389 contigs with typical lengths of 1061 bp and 1417 bp in Hassawi-1 and Hassawi-2, respectively, were obtained. Along with a comparable method for compiling the Boeahygrometrica genome [2, 94], total 117 and 213 contigs, having respective all-out lengths of 454820 bp and 454894 bp, were created from Hassawi-1 and Hassawi-2. Mapping of 454 raw data and the SOLID mate pair with varied supplement sizes to the collected mt and cp genomes was done in order to evaluate the quality of the cp and mt gathering for both Hassawi-1 and Hassawi-2. The results showed that there were no gaps between any two associated contigs, and all contig requests were supported by mate pair readings (Fig. **4**).

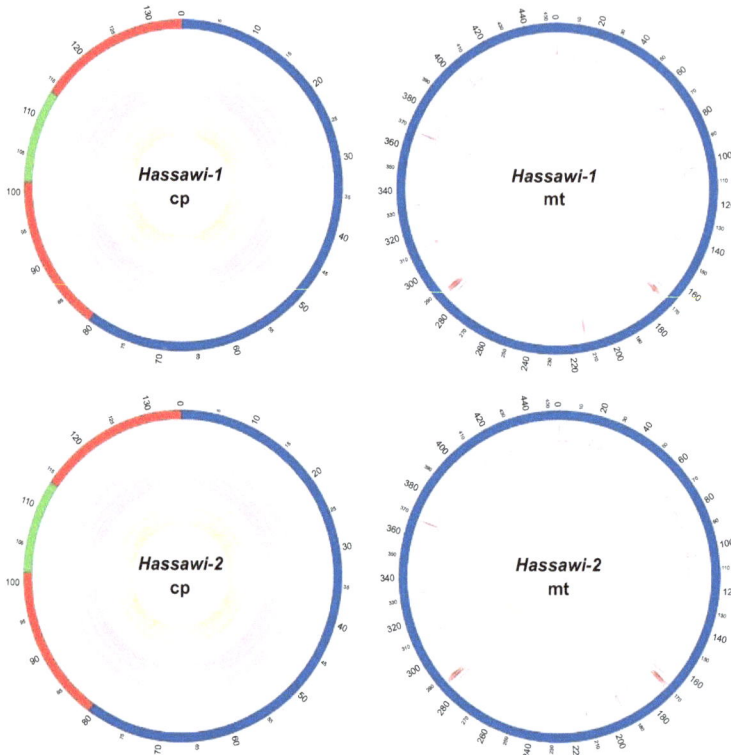

Fig. (4). The circular depiction of the Hassawi-1 and Hassawi-2 genome assemblies for the mitochondrial (mt) and chloroplast (cp) organelles. (From the outside) Circular display Physical map scale in kilobase pairs; read depths of the 454 sequencing data in plum (step size: 100 bp in cp genome and 200 bp in mt genome; cp assembly: range 200-1325 in Hassawi-1 and range 200-2230 in Hassawi-2; mt assembly: range 0-500); SOLiD mate-pair read validation with the 0.5-1 kb insert library in purple (insert size: 600 (4) Orange 1-3 kb library with insert sizes of 1400–1600 bp and steps of 150 bp in the cp assembly and 700 bp in the mt assembly. The sections of the mt genome with cp-derived sequences are the cause of the large read depth variance (Source [2]).

Chloroplast Genome

The tetrad structure of the chloroplast (cp) genome, which consists of a short single copy section (SSC) and a large single copy region (LSC), is segregated by two copies of inverted repeats (IRs). The IR regions are home to all 16 tRNA and rRNA characteristics (41590 bp, covering about 40 percent of the cp genome). The majority of NADH oxidoreductases are included in the SSC region (12345 bp, 9 percent). In contrast to atomic genomes, plant cp genomes have deeply preserved and continuously maternal heritage for quality substance, request, and association [95, 96]. Both varieties of Hassawi rice have the same gene number 136, rehash content (1.2 percent), and coding portion (55 percent). Arrangement of Hassawi-1 to 93–11 (indica) and Nipponbare represented superb collinearity (Fig. **5**).

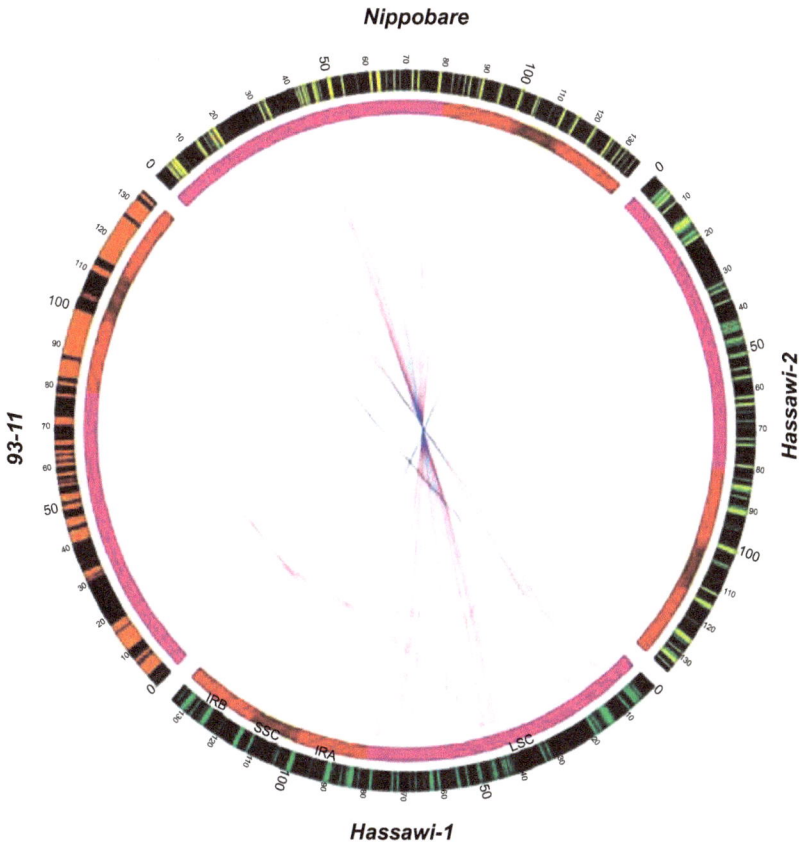

Fig. (5). Circos diagrams show the distributions of SNP and InDel in the cp genomes of Hassawi-1 and the other three cultivars. The first circle displays the genes (blocks) and genomes (color-coding) (from outside). The genetic regions SSC, LSC, IRA, and IRB are shown in the second circle. The connecting lines inside the circles represent the SNPs (blue) and InDels (red) between two genomes (Source [2]).

Contrasting cp genomes of Hassawi-1 and Hassawi-2, distinguished eleven addition and five erasure occasions identified, which brought about a 11-bp distinction in general. Among the 93–11 (indica) cp genomes and Hassawi-1, 37 out of 40 deletions are 1-bp erasures and the longest is a 6-bp one of every IRA locale. The greater part of them are interspecific cancellations. Combined length owing to InDels is forty nine base-pairs, which is predictable among the general length distinction between Hassaw-1 and 93–11 (indica) (Fig. **5**).

Mitochondrial Genome

Mitochondrial genomes of seed plants are abnormal in size at any rate in a request for size, and a lot of these varieties happen inside a solitary family [97]. The length of Hassawi mt genomes is clearly unique in relation to those of 93–11 (indica) and Nipponbare. Wildtype Hassawi rice holds roundabout DNA atom with 454,820 bp long, which is littler than both 93–11 (indica) (491,515 bp) and Nipponbare (490,520 bp). In any case, contrasted with 93–11 and Nipponbare, the mt genome of Hassawi-1 holds bigger coding district (16%) and littler recurrent locale (54%) (Fig. **5**). Dissimilar to cp genomes, most mt genomes has non-coding or practically obscure. Practical qualities in plant mt genomes are preserved among Hassawi and different assortments, for example, cytochrome c oxidase and NADH dehydrogenase. Hassawi-1 mt genomic structure is completely non-identical from that of 93–11 (indica) and Nipponbare. Arrangement plots among them in between, display numerous new combination occasions. Some huge rehashes (10 kb) present in the rice mt genomes were additionally found in other plant seeds [98, 99].

Quantitative Trait Loci

Although various significant characters are dictated by loci which affect phenotype, the most significant characteristics, for example, yield, quality and resilience to different abiotic stresses (dry spell, saltiness, submergence and so forth.), are of a quantitative sort. Hereditary contrasts influencing such characteristics (inside and between populaces) are constrained by a moderately enormous amount of loci, every one of which can make a little negative or positive commitment to the last phenotypic estimation of the attributes. Such loci are named quantitative trait loci (QTL). Qualities administering such characteristics called multiple genes or inconsiderable qualities - additionally go along with Mendelian legacy yet are enormously affected by nature. Coming of atomic markers has excelled conceivable to delineate a huge genotypic impact on phenotype. Atomic markers permit changes of QTL into Mendelian or semi-Mendelian substances, which may be controlled in traditional breeding projects. Linkage investigation of huge isolating populaces (polymorphic for sub-atomic markers and QTL for yield and yield parts) may resolve areas of the QTL. A few QTLs for qualities of financial significance, for example, atomic markers, were applied for mapping with impact obstruction, root characteristics, submergence resistance and yield parts [100 - 103]. Pi5 and Pi7 were mapped with respect to shoot opposition on linkage groups 4 and 11, individually [101]. Nine QTL with quantitative protection from separate PO6-6 of impact was additionally distinguished. Six QTL adding to protection from *Rhizoctonia solani* is recognized. QTL's are situated on six out of 12 rice chromosomes and represent 60 percent genotype constitution of variety in the cross Lemont x Tequing [104]. AFLP markers are recognized by four QTL for submergence resilience on rice linkage groups 6, 7, 11 and 12 [100]. Moreover, significant quality (Sub1) for submergence resilience was confined to linkage group 9. A sum of 68 huge quantitative trait loci was distinguished, and of these, 35 (51%) desirable QTLs regions were identified from the phenotypically mediocre *O. rufipogon* parent. Progressed backcross QTL investigation on *O. sativa* x *O. rufipogon* subsidiaries is utilized [105]. The authors concluded that specific locales of the rice genome harbor qualities that are helpful in a scope of situations. Atomic markers may utilize to distinguish QTL from wild species answerable for transgressive isolation. The productivity of mapping orthologous QTL has also increased because of relative mapping between different grains. The focus of future research should be on: identifying evidence of how QTL can be misapplied in various contexts; misappropriating integral QTL to exclude transgressive segregants, particularly from interspecific crosses; differentiating evidence of orthologous QTL among different species, as the protection of such QTL among species may open up new opportunities for the control of financial attributes; and high goals of QTL to determine whether QTL are single qualities or clusters of strongly connected qualities.

CONCLUSION AND PROSPECTS

Hassawi rice is a regional type that has been adapted to the environment of Saudi Arabia and is distinguished by its remarkable resilience to salt and drought. The genetic reservoir of Hassawi rice was in danger due to the notable decline in genetic variety. The Al-Ahsa region's rice germplasm has a high genetic diversity, which may be estimated with the use of marker-assisted breeding. Future breeding initiatives for creating new cultivars with valuable features, such as tolerance to abiotic stressors, high yielding varieties, and superior nutritional value compared to the present landraces, will utilise rice landraces in Saudi Arabia. Therefore, it is important to expedite national maintenance for the successful employment of genetic resources. Growers have accepted the inherent value of Hassawi rice for traits improvement of current cultivars. Another report on regeneration includes *in vitro* shoot regeneration of rice varieties under artificial drought stress. Further studies in the global rice community are directed to the allele mining of favorable genes from rice species. Indeed, Hassawi rice has had success introducing and identifying QTL boosting alleles for salt tolerance. Understanding heritable features requires the use of genetic markers, which act as landmarks for genes and their variants in Hassawi rice. The genetic foundation of contemporary cultivars can be expanded by using desired resources that are discovered and fully used through the genetic study of efficient genes. Due to its high concentration of nutritive and non-nutritive bioactive ingredients, such as non-starch polysaccharides and phenolic compounds, Hassawi rice may have used in nutraceuticals and pharmaceuticals in addition to its importance as a source of healthy carbohydrates and proteins. To examine the functional properties of the Hassawi rice ingredients and learn more about its antidiabetic, anticancer, and anti-obesity actions, more clinical investigations are necessary.

REFERENCES

[1] Tian X, Zheng J, Hu S, Yu J. The rice mitochondrial genomes and their variations. Plant Physiol 2006; 140(2): 401-10.
[http://dx.doi.org/10.1104/pp.105.070060] [PMID: 16384910]

[2] Zhang T, Hu S, Zhang G, *et al.* The organelle genomes of hassawi rice (*Oryza sativa* L.) and its hybrid in saudi arabia: Genome variation, rearrangement, and origins. PLoS One 2012; 7(7): e42041.
[http://dx.doi.org/10.1371/journal.pone.0042041] [PMID: 22870184]

[3] Bimpong IK, Manneh B, Diop B, *et al.* New quantitative trait loci for enhancing adaptation to salinity in rice from Hasawi, a Saudi landrace into three African cultivars at the reproductive stage. Euphytica 2014; 200(1): 45-60.
[http://dx.doi.org/10.1007/s10681-014-1134-0]

[4] Al-Mssallem IS, Al-Mssallem MQ. Study of glutelin (storage protein of rice) in Al-Hassawi rice grains. Arab Gulf J Sci Res 1997; 15: 633-46.

[5] Tang J, Xia H, Cao M, *et al.* A comparison of rice chloroplast genomes. Plant Physiol 2004; 135(1): 412-20.
[http://dx.doi.org/10.1104/pp.103.031245] [PMID: 15122023]

[6] Hiratsuka J, Shimada H, Whittier R, *et al.* The complete sequence of the rice (Oryza sativa) chloroplast genome: Intermolecular recombination between distinct tRNA genes accounts for a major plastid DNA inversion during the evolution of the cereals. Mol Gen Genet 1989; 217(2-3): 185-94.
[http://dx.doi.org/10.1007/BF02464880] [PMID: 2770692]

[7] Notsu Y, Masood S, Nishikawa T, *et al.* The complete sequence of the rice (Oryza sativa L.) mitochondrial genome: Frequent DNA sequence acquisition and loss during the evolution of flowering plants. Mol Genet Genomics 2002; 268(4): 434-45.
[http://dx.doi.org/10.1007/s00438-002-0767-1] [PMID: 12471441]

[8] Al-Mssallem MQ, Alqurashi RM. Nutrient components and antioxidant activity in hassawi rice and basmati rice varieties. Scienti J King Faisal Uni 2021; 22(1): 1442. In press.

[9] Al-Mssallem MQ, Hampton SM, Frost GS, Brown JE. A study of Hassawi rice (Oryza sativa L.) in terms of its carbohydrate hydrolysis *in vitro* and glycaemic and insulinaemic indices (*in vivo*). Eur J Clin Nutr 2011; 65(5): 627-34.
[http://dx.doi.org/10.1038/ejcn.2011.4] [PMID: 21364610]

[10] Al-Bahrany AM. Chemical composition and fatty acid analysis of saudi hassawi rice oryza sativa L. Pak J Biol Sci 2002; 5(2): 212-4.
[http://dx.doi.org/10.3923/pjbs.2002.212.214]

[11] USDA. National nutrient database for standard reference. us department of agriculture, agricultural research service. 2016. Available at:https://fdc.nal.usda.gov/fdc- app.html#/ (accessed on 23/12/2019)

[12] Verpoorte R, Alfermann AW. Secondary metabolism. In: Verpoorte R, Alfermann AW, Eds. Metabolic engineering of plant secondary metabolism. Dordrecht: Kluwer academic publishers 2000; p. 296.
[http://dx.doi.org/10.1007/978-94-015-9423-3_1]

[13] Pichersky E, Gang DR. Genetics and biochemistry of secondary metabolites in plants: An evolutionary perspective. Trends Plant Sci 2000; 5(10): 439-45.
[http://dx.doi.org/10.1016/S1360-1385(00)01741-6] [PMID: 11044721]

[14] Crozier A, Jaganath IB, Clifford MN. Phenols, polyphenols and tannins: An overview. wiley 2006.
[http://dx.doi.org/10.1002/9780470988558.ch1]

[15] D'Archivio M, Filesi C, Varì R, Scazzocchio B, Masella R. Bioavailability of the polyphenols: Status and controversies. Int J Mol Sci 2010; 11(4): 1321-42.
[http://dx.doi.org/10.3390/ijms11041321] [PMID: 20480022]

[16]   Gleadow RM, Møller BL. Cyanogenic glycosides: Synthesis, physiology, and phenotypic plasticity. Annu Rev Plant Biol 2014; 65(1): 155-85.
[http://dx.doi.org/10.1146/annurev-arplant-050213-040027] [PMID: 24579992]

[17]   Wang W, Li Y, Dang P, Zhao S, Lai D, Zhou L. Rice secondary metabolites: Structures, roles, biosynthesis, and metabolic regulation. Molecules 2018; 23(12): 3098.
[http://dx.doi.org/10.3390/molecules23123098] [PMID: 30486426]

[18]   Augustin JM, Kuzina V, Andersen SB, Bak S. Molecular activities, biosynthesis and evolution of triterpenoid saponins. Phytochemistry 2011; 72(6): 435-57.
[http://dx.doi.org/10.1016/j.phytochem.2011.01.015] [PMID: 21333312]

[19]   Pazouki L, Niinemets Ü. Multi-substrate terpene synthases: Their occurrence and physiological significance. Front Plant Sci 2016; 7: 1019.
[http://dx.doi.org/10.3389/fpls.2016.01019] [PMID: 27462341]

[20]   Thimmappa R, Geisler K, Louveau T, O'Maille P, Osbourn A. Triterpene biosynthesis in plants. Annu Rev Plant Biol 2014; 65(1): 225-57.
[http://dx.doi.org/10.1146/annurev-arplant-050312-120229] [PMID: 24498976]

[21]   Pagare S, Bhatia M, Tripathi N. Secondary metabolites of plants and their role: overview. Curr Trends Biotechnol Pharm 2015; 9(3): 293-304.

[22]   Reddy L, Odhav B, Bhoola KD. Natural products for cancer prevention: A global perspective. Pharmacol Ther 2003; 99(1): 1-13.
[http://dx.doi.org/10.1016/S0163-7258(03)00042-1] [PMID: 12804695]

[23]   Rhodes MJC. Physiological roles for secondary metabolites in plants: Some progress, many outstanding problems. Plant Mol Biol 1994; 24(1): 1-20.
[http://dx.doi.org/10.1007/BF00040570] [PMID: 8111009]

[24]   Shukla V, Upreti DK, Bajpai R. Secondary metabolites and its isolation and characterisation. In: Shukla V, Upreti DK, Bajpai R, Eds. Lichens to biomonitor the environment. New Delhi: Springer 2014; pp. 21-46.
[http://dx.doi.org/10.1007/978-81-322-1503-5_2]

[25]   Akula R, Ravishankar GA. Influence of abiotic stress signals on secondary metabolites in plants. Plant Signal Behav 2011; 6(11): 1720-31.
[http://dx.doi.org/10.4161/psb.6.11.17613] [PMID: 22041989]

[26]   Goufo P, Trindade H. Rice antioxidants: Phenolic acids, flavonoids, anthocyanins, proanthocyanidins, tocopherols, tocotrienols, γ-oryzanol, and phytic acid. Food Sci Nutr 2014; 2(2): 75-104.
[http://dx.doi.org/10.1002/fsn3.86] [PMID: 24804068]

[27]   Hadid ML, Elsheikh DM. Comparison of chemical composition, antioxidant, and bioactive compounds contents in different Hassawi and Basmati rice genotypes. Sci J King Faisal Univ 2012; 13(2): 1-23.

[28]   Adom KK, Liu RH. Antioxidant activity of grains. J Agric Food Chem 2002; 50(21): 6182-7.
[http://dx.doi.org/10.1021/jf0205099] [PMID: 12358499]

[29]   Ranilla LG, Kwon YI, Genovese MI, Lajolo FM, Shetty K. Antidiabetes and antihypertension potential of commonly consumed carbohydrate sweeteners using *in vitro* models. J Med Food 2008; 11(2): 337-48.
[http://dx.doi.org/10.1089/jmf.2007.689] [PMID: 18598178]

[30]   Phillips KM, Carlsen MH, Blomhoff R. Total antioxidant content of alternatives to refined sugar. J Am Diet Assoc 2009; 109(1): 64-71.
[http://dx.doi.org/10.1016/j.jada.2008.10.014] [PMID: 19103324]

[31]   Al-Mssallem MQ. The association between the glycaemic index of some traditional Saudi foods and the prevalence of diabetes in Saudi Arabia: A Review article. J Diabetes Metab 2014; 5(11): 452.

[32]   Anderson JW, Baird P, Davis RH Jr, *et al.* Health benefits of dietary fiber. Nutr Rev 2009; 67(4): 188-205.
[http://dx.doi.org/10.1111/j.1753-4887.2009.00189.x] [PMID: 19335713]

[33]   Meyer KA, Kushi LH, Jacobs DR Jr, Slavin J, Sellers TA, Folsom AR. Carbohydrates, dietary fiber, and incident type 2 diabetes in older women. Am J Clin Nutr 2000; 71(4): 921-30.
[http://dx.doi.org/10.1093/ajcn/71.4.921] [PMID: 10731498]

[34]   Schulze MB, Liu S, Rimm EB, Manson JAE, Willett WC, Hu FB. Glycemic index, glycemic load, and dietary fiber intake and incidence of type 2 diabetes in younger and middle-aged women. Am J Clin Nutr 2004; 80(2): 348-56.
[http://dx.doi.org/10.1093/ajcn/80.2.348]

[35]   Sluijs I, van der Schouw YT, van der A DL, *et al.* Carbohydrate quantity and quality and risk of type 2 diabetes in the European Prospective Investigation into Cancer and Nutrition–Netherlands (EPIC-NL) study. Am J Clin Nutr 2010; 92(4): 905-11.
[http://dx.doi.org/10.3945/ajcn.2010.29620] [PMID: 20685945]

[36]   Stevens J, Ahn K, Juhaeri , Houston D, Steffan L, Couper D. Dietary fiber intake and glycemic index and incidence of diabetes in African-American and white adults: The ARIC study. Diabetes Care 2002; 25(10): 1715-21.
[http://dx.doi.org/10.2337/diacare.25.10.1715] [PMID: 12351467]

[37]   Kumar V, Sinha AK, Makkar HPS, de Boeck G, Becker K. Dietary roles of non-starch polysaccharides in human nutrition: A review. Crit Rev Food Sci Nutr 2012; 52(10): 899-935.
[http://dx.doi.org/10.1080/10408398.2010.512671] [PMID: 22747080]

[38]   Kristensen M, Jensen MG. Dietary fibres in the regulation of appetite and food intake. Importance of viscosity 2011; 65: 65-70.

[39]   Fahad S, Adnan M, Noor M. Major constraints for global rice production advances in rice research for abiotic stress tolerance. Woodhead Publishing 2019; pp. 1-22.

[40]   Grover A, Pental D. Breeding objectives and requirements for producing transgenics for major field crops of India. Curr Sci 2003; 84(3): 310-20.

[41]   Burton GW, DeVane EH. Estimating heritability in tall fescue from replicated clonal material. Agron J 1953; 45: 478-81.
[http://dx.doi.org/10.2134/agronj1953.00021962004500100005x]

[42]   Davenport CB. Degeneration, albinism and inbreeding. Science 1908; 28(718): 454-5.
[http://dx.doi.org/10.1126/science.28.718.454.c] [PMID: 17771943]

[43]   Bruce AB. The mendelian theory of heredity and the augmentation of vigor. Science 1910; 32(827): 627-8.
[http://dx.doi.org/10.1126/science.32.827.627.b] [PMID: 17816706]

[44]   Keeble F, Pellew C. The mode of inheritance of stature and of time of flowering in peas (Pisum sativum). J Genet 1910; 1(1): 47-56.
[http://dx.doi.org/10.1007/BF02981568]

[45]   Shull GH. The composition of a field of maize. J Hered 1908; os-4(1): 296-301.
[http://dx.doi.org/10.1093/jhered/os-4.1.296]

[46]   Birchler JA, Yao H, Chudalayandi S, Vaiman D, Veitia RA. Heterosis. Plant Cell 2010; 22(7): 2105-12.
[http://dx.doi.org/10.1105/tpc.110.076133] [PMID: 20622146]

[47]   Osborn TC, Chris Pires J, Birchler JA, *et al.* Understanding mechanisms of novel gene expression in polyploids. Trends Genet 2003; 19(3): 141-7.
[http://dx.doi.org/10.1016/S0168-9525(03)00015-5] [PMID: 12615008]

[48]   Song R, Messing J. Gene expression of a gene family in maize based on noncollinear haplotypes. Proc

Natl Acad Sci 2003; 100(15): 9055-60.
[http://dx.doi.org/10.1073/pnas.1032999100] [PMID: 12853580]

[49] Yao Y, Ni Z, Zhang Y, *et al.* Identification of differentially expressed genes in leaf and root between wheat hybrid and its parental inbreds using PCR-based cDNA subtraction. Plant Mol Biol 2005; 58(3): 367-84.
[http://dx.doi.org/10.1007/s11103-005-5102-x] [PMID: 16021401]

[50] Rajendran A, Muthian A, Joel J, Shanmugasundaram P, Raju D. Heterotic grouping and patterning of quality protein maize inbreds based on genetic and molecular marker studies. Proc Natl Acad Sci 2014; 38: 10-20.

[51] Hiei Y, Ohta S, Komari T, Kumashiro T. Efficient transformation of rice (*Oryza sativa* L.) mediated by *Agrobacterium* and sequence analysis of the boundaries of the T-DNA. Plant J 1994; 6(2): 271-82.
[http://dx.doi.org/10.1046/j.1365-313X.1994.6020271.x] [PMID: 7920717]

[52] Xu X, Liu X, Ge S, *et al.* Resequencing 50 accessions of cultivated and wild rice yields markers for identifying agronomically important genes. Nat Biotechnol 2012; 30(1): 105-11.
[http://dx.doi.org/10.1038/nbt.2050] [PMID: 22158310]

[53] Tian X, Zheng J, Hu S, Yu J. The rice mitochondrial genomes and their variations. Plant Physiol 2006; 140(2): 401-10.
[http://dx.doi.org/10.1104/pp.105.070060] [PMID: 16384910]

[54] Nishikawa T, Vaughan DA, Kadowaki K. Phylogenetic analysis of *Oryza* species, based on simple sequence repeats and their flanking nucleotide sequences from the mitochondrial and chloroplast genomes. Theor Appl Genet 2005; 110(4): 696-705.
[http://dx.doi.org/10.1007/s00122-004-1895-2] [PMID: 15650813]

[55] Available at: http://www.fao.org/docrep/006/Y4751E/y4751e04.htm (23th - 26th July, 2002)

[56] Nogoy FM, Song JY, Ouk S, *et al.* Current applicable dna markers for marker assisted breeding in abiotic and biotic stress tolerance in rice (*Oryza sativa* L.). Plant Breed Biotechnol 2016; 4(3): 271-84.
[http://dx.doi.org/10.9787/PBB.2016.4.3.271]

[57] Uga Y, Okuno K, Yano M. Dro1, a major QTL involved in deep rooting of rice under upland field conditions. J Exp Bot 2011; 62(8): 2485-94.
[http://dx.doi.org/10.1093/jxb/erq429] [PMID: 21212298]

[58] Bonilla P, Dvorak J, Mackill D. RFLP and SSLP mapping of salinity tolerance genes in chromosome 1 of rice (*Oryza sativa* L.) using recombinant inbred lines. Philipp Agric Sci 2002; 85: 68-76.

[59] Krishnamurthy SL, Pundir P, Warraich AS, *et al.* Introgressed saltol QTL lines improves the salinity tolerance in rice at seedling stage. Front Plant Sci 2020; 11: 833.
[http://dx.doi.org/10.3389/fpls.2020.00833] [PMID: 32595689]

[60] Yeo AR, Yeo ME, Flowers SA, Flowers TJ. Screening of rice (*Oryza sativa* L.) genotypes for physiological characters contributing to salinity resistance, and their relationship to overall performance. Theor Appl Genet 1990; 79(3): 377-84.
[http://dx.doi.org/10.1007/BF01186082] [PMID: 24226357]

[61] Hajira SK, Sundaram RM, Laha GS, *et al.* A single-tube, functional marker-based multiplex PCR assay for simultaneous detection of major bacterial blight resistance genes Xa21, xa13 and xa5 in rice. Rice Sci 2016; 23(3): 144-51.
[http://dx.doi.org/10.1016/j.rsci.2015.11.004]

[62] Singh AK, Singh PK, Arya M, Singh NK, Singh US. Molecular screening of blast resistance genes in rice using SSR markers. Plant Pathol J 2015; 31(1): 12-24.
[http://dx.doi.org/10.5423/PPJ.OA.06.2014.0054] [PMID: 25774106]

[63] Das G, Patra JK, Baek KH. Insight into MAS: A molecular tool for development of stress resistant and quality of rice through gene stacking. Front Plant Sci 2017; 8: 985.

[http://dx.doi.org/10.3389/fpls.2017.00985] [PMID: 28659941]

[64] Das G, Rao GJN. Molecular marker assisted gene stacking for biotic and abiotic stress resistance genes in an elite rice cultivar. Front Plant Sci 2015; 6: 698.
[http://dx.doi.org/10.3389/fpls.2015.00698] [PMID: 26483798]

[65] Suprasanna P, Mirajkar SJ, Bhagwat SG. Induced mutations and crop improvement.Springer 2015; pp. 593-618.
[http://dx.doi.org/10.1007/978-81-322-2286-6_23]

[66] (a) Oladosu Y, Rafii MY, Abdullah N, *et al.* Principle and application of plant mutagenesis in crop improvement: A review. BiotechnolBiotechnol Equip 2016; 30: 1-16. (b) Redoña ED, Mackill DJ. Molecular mapping of quantitative trait loci in *japonica* rice. Genome 1996; 39: 395-403.

[67] Viana VE, Pegoraro C, Busanello C, Costa de Oliveira A. Mutagenesis in rice: The basis for breeding a new super plant. Front Plant Sci 2019; 10: 1326.
[http://dx.doi.org/10.3389/fpls.2019.01326] [PMID: 31781133]

[68] Morita R, Kusaba M, Iida S, Yamaguchi H, Nishio T, Nishimura M. Molecular characterization of mutations induced by gamma irradiation in rice. Genes Genet Syst 2009; 84(5): 361-70.
[http://dx.doi.org/10.1266/ggs.84.361] [PMID: 20154423]

[69] Jain SM, Suprasanna P. Induced mutations for enhancing nutrition for food production. Gene Conserve 2011; 40: 201-15.

[70] Gosal SS, Kang MS. Plant tissue culture and genetic transformation for crop improvement.In Improving Crop Resistance to Abiotic Stress. Tuteja N, Gill SS, Tiburcio AF, Tuteja R. Weinheim, Germany: wiley 2012; pp. 357-97.
[http://dx.doi.org/10.1002/9783527632930.ch16]

[71] Chen YL, Liang HL, Ma XL, *et al.* An efficient rice mutagenesis system based on suspension-cultured cells. J Integr Plant Biol 2013; 55(2): 122-30.
[http://dx.doi.org/10.1111/jipb.12000] [PMID: 23126685]

[72] Serrat X, Esteban R, Guibourt N, Moysset L, Nogués S, Lalanne E. EMS mutagenesis in mature seed-derived rice calli as a new method for rapidly obtaining TILLING mutant populations. Plant Methods 2014; 10(1): 5.
[http://dx.doi.org/10.1186/1746-4811-10-5] [PMID: 24475756]

[73] Hare PD, Cress WA, van Staden J. Proline synthesis and degradation: A model system for elucidating stress-related signal transduction. J Exp Bot 1999; 50(333): 413-34.
[http://dx.doi.org/10.1093/jxb/50.333.413]

[74] Hasegawa PM, Bressan RA, Sangita H, Handa AK. Cellular mechanisms of tolerance to water stress. HortScience 1984; 19(3): 371-7.
[http://dx.doi.org/10.21273/HORTSCI.19.3.371]

[75] Santos-Díaz MS, Ochoa-Alejo N. Effect of water stress on growth, osmotic potential and solute accumulation in cell cultures from chili pepper (a mesophyte) and creosote bush (a xerophyte). Plant Sci 1994; 96(1-2): 21-9.
[http://dx.doi.org/10.1016/0168-9452(94)90218-6]

[76] Heszky LE, Simon-Kiss I. "DAMA" the first plant variety of biotechnology origin in Hungary registered in 1992. Hung Agric Res 1992; 1: 30-2.

[77] Handa S, Handa AK, Hasegawa PM, Bressan RA. Proline accumulation and the adaptation of cultured plant cells to water stress. Plant Physiol 1986; 80(4): 938-45.
[http://dx.doi.org/10.1104/pp.80.4.938] [PMID: 16664745]

[78] Joshi R, Shukla A, Sairam RK. *In vitro* screening of rice genotypes for drought tolerance using polyethylene glycol. Acta Physiol Plant 2011; 33(6): 2209-17.
[http://dx.doi.org/10.1007/s11738-011-0760-6]

[79]   Siddeswar G, Kavikishore PB. Plant regeneration from polyethylene glycol adopted callus of rice. Curr Sci 1989; 58: 926-8.

[80]   Itai C, Paleg LG. Responses of water stressed *Hordeum distichum* L. and *Cucumis sativus* to proline and betaine. Plant Sci 1982; 25: 329-35.

[81]   Summart J, Thanonkeo P, Panichajakul S. Effect of salt stress on growth, inorganic ion and proline accumulation in Thai aromatic rice, Khao Dawk Mali 105, callus culture. Afr J Biotechnol 2010; 9(2): 145-52.

[82]   Htwe NN, Maziah M, Chai Ling H. Responses of some selected Malaysian rice genotypes to callus induction under *in vitro* salt stress. Afr J Biotechnol 2011; 10(3): 350-62.

[83]   Bal AR, Dutt SK. Mechanism of salt tolerance in wild rice (Oryza coarctata Roxb). Plant Soil 1986; 92(3): 399-404.
[http://dx.doi.org/10.1007/BF02372487]

[84]   Mahajan S, Tuteja N. Cold, salinity and drought stresses: An overview. Arch Biochem Biophys 2005; 444(2): 139-58.
[http://dx.doi.org/10.1016/j.abb.2005.10.018] [PMID: 16309626]

[85]   Rhodes D, Hanson AD. Quaternary ammonium and tertiary sulfonium compounds in higher plants. Annu Rev Plant Physiol Plant Mol Biol 1993; 44: 357-84.
[http://dx.doi.org/10.1146/annurev.pp.44.060193.002041]

[86]   Ashraf M, Harris PJC. Potential biochemical indicators of salinity tolerance in plants. Plant Sci 2004; 166(1): 3-16.
[http://dx.doi.org/10.1016/j.plantsci.2003.10.024]

[88]   Bohnert HJ, Jensen RG. Strategies for engineering water-stress tolerance in plants. Trends Biotechnol 1996; 14(3): 89-97.
[http://dx.doi.org/10.1016/0167-7799(96)80929-2]

[89]   Yancey PH. Compatible and counteracting solutes. Cell Plant Grow Reg 1994; 57: 271-80.

[90]   Hayat S, Hayat Q, Alyemeni MN, Wani AS, Pichtel J, Ahmad A. Role of proline under changing environments. Plant Signal Behav 2012; 7(11): 1456-66.
[http://dx.doi.org/10.4161/psb.21949] [PMID: 22951402]

[91]   Shanthi P, Jebaraj S, Geetha S. *In vitro* screening for salt tolerance in Rice (*Oryza sativa*). EJPB 2010; 1(4): 1208-12.

[92]   Cheng X, Sardana R, Kaplan H, Altosaar I. *Agrobacterium-* transformed rice plants expressing synthetic *cryIA(b)* and *cryIA(c)* genes are highly toxic to striped stem borer and yellow stem borer. Proc Natl Acad Sci 1998; 95(6): 2767-72.
[http://dx.doi.org/10.1073/pnas.95.6.2767] [PMID: 9501164]

[93]   Wang X, Shi X, Hao B. The transfer RNA genes in *Oryza sativa* L. ssp. indica. Sci China C Life Sci 2002; 45(5): 504-11.
[http://dx.doi.org/10.1360/02yc9055] [PMID: 18759038]

[94]   Zhang T, Zhang X, Hu S, Yu J. An efficient procedure for plant organellar genome assembly, based on whole genome data from the 454 GS FLX sequencing platform. Plant Methods 2011; 7(1): 38.
[http://dx.doi.org/10.1186/1746-4811-7-38] [PMID: 22126655]

[95]   Young HA, Lanzatella CL, Sarath G, Tobias CM. Chloroplast genome variation in upland and lowland switchgrass. PLoS One 2011; 6(8): e23980.
[http://dx.doi.org/10.1371/journal.pone.0023980] [PMID: 21887356]

[96]   Greiner S, Rauwolf U, Meurer J, Herrmann RG. The role of plastids in plant speciation. Mol Ecol 2011; 20(4): 671-91.
[http://dx.doi.org/10.1111/j.1365-294X.2010.04984.x] [PMID: 21214654]

[97] Alverson AJ, Wei X, Rice DW, Stern DB, Barry K, Palmer JD. Insights into the evolution of mitochondrial genome size from complete sequences of *Citrullus lanatus* and *Cucurbita pepo* (Cucurbitaceae). Mol Biol Evol 2010; 27(6): 1436-48.
[http://dx.doi.org/10.1093/molbev/msq029] [PMID: 20118192]

[98] Kubo T, Nishizawa S, Sugawara A, Itchoda N, Estiati A, Mikami T. The complete nucleotide sequence of the mitochondrial genome of sugar beet (Beta vulgaris L.) reveals a novel gene for tRNACys(GCA). Nucleic Acids Res 2000; 28(13): 2571-6.
[http://dx.doi.org/10.1093/nar/28.13.2571] [PMID: 10871408]

[99] Clifton SW, Minx P, Fauron CMR, *et al.* Sequence and comparative analysis of the maize NB mitochondrial genome. Plant Physiol 2004; 136(3): 3486-503.
[http://dx.doi.org/10.1104/pp.104.044602] [PMID: 15542500]

[100] Nandi S, Subudhi PK, Senadhira D, Manigbas NL, Sen-Mandi S, Huang N. Mapping QTLs for submergence tolerance in rice by AFLP analysis and selective genotyping. Mol Gen Genet 1997; 255(1): 1-8.
[http://dx.doi.org/10.1007/s004380050468] [PMID: 9230893]

[101] Wang GL, Mackill DJ, Bonman JM, McCouch SR, Champoux MC, Nelson RJ. RFLP mapping of genes conferring complete and partial resistance to blast in a durably resistant rice cultivar. Genetics 1994; 136(4): 1421-34.
[http://dx.doi.org/10.1093/genetics/136.4.1421] [PMID: 7912216]

[102] Yadav R, Courtois B, Huang N, McLaren G. Mapping genes controlling root morphology and root distribution in a doubled-haploid population of rice. Theor Appl Genet 1997; 94(5): 619-32.
[http://dx.doi.org/10.1007/s001220050459]

[103] Zheng HG, Babu RC, Pathan MS, *et al.* Quantitative trait loci for root-penetration ability and root thickness in rice: Comparison of genetic backgrounds. Genome 2000; 43(1): 53-61.
[http://dx.doi.org/10.1139/g99-065] [PMID: 10701113]

[104] Li Z, Pinson SRM, Marchetti MA, Stansel JW, Park WD. Characterization of quantitative trait loci (QTLs) in cultivated rice contributing to field resistance to sheath blight (Rhizoctonia solani). Theor Appl Genet 1995; 91(2): 382-8.
[http://dx.doi.org/10.1007/BF00220903] [PMID: 24169789]

[105] Moncada P, Martínez CP, Borrero J, *et al.* Quantitative trait loci for yield and yield components in an Oryza sativa×Oryza rufipogon BC2F2 population evaluated in an upland environment. Theor Appl Genet 2001; 102(1): 41-52.
[http://dx.doi.org/10.1007/s001220051616]

CHAPTER 8

In Vitro Rapid Regeneration of Plantlets from Shoot Tip Explants of *Allamanda Cathartica* L. and Characterization of Phytochemicals in Regenerants

Mehrun Nisha Khanam[1,2,*] and **Mohammad Anis**[2]

[1] *University Centre for Research & Development, Chandigarh University, Mohali-140-413, Punjab, India*

[2] *Plant Biotechnology Laboratory, Department of Botany, Aligarh Muslim University, Aligarh-202-002, India*

Abstract: This study demonstrates a rapid, economic and efficient plantlet regeneration protocol for an exotic ornamental and medicinal plant *Allamanda cathartica* L. by using shoot tip explants. Interaction of various PGRs (mT, IAA, IBA or NAA) and sucrose was tested in MS medium to obtain maximum shoot regeneration from shoot tip explants. mT (3.0 µM) + NAA (0.5 µM) + 4% sucrose was found to be an optimum combination for maximum shoot proliferation with 20.80 mean shoot number and 7.60 cm mean shoot length after 12 weeks of culture based on 93.20% responsive explants. Microshoots (4-5 cm) showed maximum rhizogenic response as they produced 4.20 mean root number with 4.90 cm root length after 4 weeks of culture on ½ MS medium when supplemented with 0.5 µM NAA. Well-developed rooted plantlets were acclimatized successfully with a 96% survival rate. The primary phytochemical screening of aqueous leaf extract in the regenerants revealed the presence of proteins, carbohydrates, lipids, phenols, proteins, and saponins. Quantification of phytochemical constituents showed that the amount of phenols was highest, followed by lipids, proteins, carbohydrates, saponins and alkaloids in the micropropagated plants. These phyto-constituents are known to cure numerous ailments.

Keywords: Acclimatization, *In vitro* rooting, Micropropagation, PGRs, Sucrose.

INTRODUCTION

Ornate plants are grown worldwide for green industries, aesthetic values and decorative purposes in gardens and roadsides. The economic values of decorative plants have considerably increased over the last few decades and are expected to

* **Corresponding author Mehrun Nisha Khanam:** University Centre for Research & Development, Chandigarh University, Mohali-140-413, Punjab, India; & Plant Biotechnology Laboratory, Department of Botany, Aligarh Muslim University, Aligarh-202-002, India; E-mail: meherkhan680@gmail.com

continue further escalation in both domestic and international markets. The growth in floriculture cultivation has been phenomenal in the last decade, the area under flower cultivation has doubled in India [1]. One such potential plant is *Allamanda cathartica* (Apocyanaceae) which possesses both ornamental and medicinal values. It is a woody climber, grown for its attractive funnel shaped yellow colored flowers and is commonly known as the golden trumpet vine. It is native to South America and West Indies, distributed throughout the tropics [2]. The plant was introduced to many countries owing to its ornamental value. The leaves of the plant are of high medicinal importance due to the presence of various phytochemicals like alkaloids, carbohydrates, lipids, phenols, proteins and saponins. These phyto-constituents have displayed anti-inflammatory and healing activities [3]. Leaves are also used as an antidote and for relieving coughs and headaches. *A. cathartica* is widely cultivated in the gardens of Australia and some local businesses in the region even include it in their corporate identity. *Allamanda spp* regroups 15 valid species that grow up to 6m [4], some being utilized for ornamental or medicinal purposes. This plant species is reproduced by seeds and can also be propagated*via* stem segments. Under natural conditions, the plant has to cope up with numerous environmental challenges, particularly season dependency, heat, light, humidity and various other biotic and abiotic stresses. Besides these various factors, a major problem is the seed setting which does not take place in the regions of Uttar Pradesh, India. So the species is propagated through stem cutting, which takes a very long time to develop into an entire plant. Therefore, there is an urgent need to develop an alternative, efficient and cost-effective method to propagate this exotic ornamental plant on a mass scale.

Phytochemical screening is a significant source in identifying new medicinally and industrially important compounds like alkaloids, flavonoids, phenolic compounds, saponins, steroids, tannins, terpenoids *etc.* Due to recent advancements in the field of pharmacognosy, several methods have been developed for the standardization and identification of crude drugs. It has been emphasized that complete phytochemical investigations of medicinal plants are necessary because the secondary metabolites present in the plants are responsible for medicinal activity [5].

In the present study, an attempt has been made to test the response of cytokinins and auxins for developing a simple but rapid and efficient protocol for large scale propagation of *A. cathartica* from shoot tip explant of a 3-year-old plant and also the quantification in the leaf extracts.

MATERIALS AND METHODS

Explants Collection

Shoot tips of *A. cathartica* were collected in the month of July from a 3-year-old plant maintained at the botanical garden of the university in Aligarh, India.

Explant Preparation

Shoot tip explants were washed under running tap water for 20 min to remove the adherent dust particles prior to immersion in an aqueous solution of 5% (v/v) labolene detergent (Qualigens, India) for 10 min, followed by thorough washing with double distilled water (DDW). They were then surface sterilized by soaking in 0.1% (w/v) $HgCl_2$/water solution and rinsed 4-5 times with sterile DDW to remove the disinfectant. Under the laminar flow hood, shoot tip explants of 0.5 cm were excised and placed on shoot bud induction media in a vertical position.

Media and Culture Condition

All explants were cultured on MS medium [6] supplemented with organic components (Myo-inositol, Thiamine HCl, Pyridoxine HCl, Nicotinic acid and Glycine) containing 10-50 g/l sucrose with different concentrations of Benzyladenine (BA), Kinetin (Kn) meta-Topolin (mT) alone (Table 1) and in combination with auxins (Indole-3- acetic acid (IAA), Indole-3-butyric acid (IBA) or α-Naphthalene acetic acid (NAA). The pH was adjusted to 5.8 using 1N NaOH and the medium was gelled with 0.8% (w/v) bacteriological grade (Fischer Scientific, India) before autoclaving at 121°C for 15 min. Cultures were maintained at 25 ± 2°C under 16/8 light/dark photoperiodic cycles with light intensity of 50 $\mu molm^{-2}s^{-1}$ provided by cool white fluorescent lamps (2 x 40W, Philips, India).

Table 1. Effect of various cytokinins on multiple shoots regeneration from shoot tip explants in MS medium after 8 weeks of culture.

Cytokinins (µM)			Response (%)	No. of Shoots/Explant	Shoot Length (cm)
BA	Kn	*m*T	Mean ± SE	Mean ± SE	Mean ± SE
00	00	00	0.00 ± 0.00^k	0.00 ± 0.00^i	0.00 ± 0.00^i
1.0	-	-	0.00 ± 0.00^k	0.00 ± 0.00^i	0.00 ± 0.00^i
2.0	-	-	0.00 ± 0.00^k	0.00 ± 0.00^i	0.00 ± 0.00^i
3.0	-	-	11.20 ± 0.32^j	1.60 ± 0.16^g	1.35 ± 0.15^g
4.0	-	-	36.10 ± 0.23^g	2.50 ± 0.22^{ef}	2.30 ± 0.15^f
5.0	-	-	60.90 ± 0.23^c	4.60 ± 0.16^c	3.45 ± 0.13^c

(Table 1) cont.....

Cytokinins (µM)			Response (%)	No. of Shoots/Explant	Shoot Length (cm)
6.0	-	-	50.80 ± 0.35^c	2.40 ± 0.26^{ef}	1.40 ± 0.16^g
-	1.0	-	0.00 ± 0.00^k	0.00 ± 0.00^i	0.00 ± 0.00^i
-	2.0	-	0.00 ± 0.00^k	0.00 ± 0.00^i	0.00 ± 0.00^i
-	3.0	-	0.00 ± 0.00^k	0.00 ± 0.00^i	0.00 ± 0.00^i
-	4.0	-	0.00 ± 0.00^k	0.00 ± 0.00^i	0.00 ± 0.00^i
-	5.0	-	0.00 ± 0.00^k	0.00 ± 0.00^i	0.00 ± 0.00^i
-	6.0	-	0.00 ± 0.00^k	0.00 ± 0.00^i	0.00 ± 0.00^i
-	-	1.0	21.40 ± 0.37^i	2.20 ± 0.20^f	2.05 ± 0.15^f
-	-	2.0	53.20 ± 0.41^d	3.60 ± 0.16^d	2.80 ± 0.13^d
-	-	3.0	82.50 ± 0.26^a	6.30 ± 0.15^a	5.50 ± 0.16^a
-	-	4.0	64.00 ± 0.25^b	5.10 ± 0.17^b	4.40 ± 0.16^b
-	-	5.0	41.60 ± 0.33^f	2.80 ± 0.13^e	2.40 ± 0.16^{ef}
-	-	6.0	31.00 ± 0.29^h	1.00 ± 0.25^h	0.80 ± 0.20^h

Values represent mean ± standard error of 10 replicates per treatment in three repeated experiments. Means sharing the same letter within a column are not significantly different (P=0.05) using Duncan's multiple range test.

Shoot Induction and Multiplication

MS nutrients supplemented with various concentrations of BA, Kn or *m*T (1-6 µM) were used for bud breaking. Further experiment was done on optimized media (3.0 µM mT) amended with different concentrations of IAA, IBA or NAA for enhanced shoot proliferation. MS medium without any plant growth regulators served as control. Cultures were subcultured onto fresh medium after every 4 weeks.

Rooting and Acclimatization

Developed microshoots (4-5 cm) were excised and transferred to root induction media comprising ½ and full MS with various concentrations of auxins (IAA, IBA, NAA). Cultures were incubated under the same condition as mentioned above. The rooted shoots were washed gently to remove adherent media with tap water and transplanted to thermacol cups containing Soilrite™ (Keltech Pvt. Ltd. Banglore, India) and covered with plastic bags to maintain relative humidity.

Sample Collection and Preparation

Fresh leaf samples of all the treated/optimized (MS + *m*T 3.0 µM + NAA 0.5 µM + 40 g/l Sucrose) and control plants (natural source) of *A. cathartica* from 30-day-old acclimatized plants were collected and washed thoroughly under running tap water, and samples were air dried in the shade. The samples so prepared were subsequently used for phytochemical analysis.

Preparation of Leaf Extract

5 g of each leaf sample was ground separately in 25 ml DDW using a motar and pestle. All the samples were poured into a 50 ml conical flask separately, boiled at 60 °C for 30 min in a water bath, and filtered through Whatman filter paper No.1. Filtrate was centrifuged at 7000 rpm for 10 min, and filtrates were stored in sterile bottles at 4 °C for phytochemical analysis as per the methods of Harborne [7].

Statistical Analysis

All the experiments were set up in a completely randomized design and repeated three times with ten replicates for each treatment. The data was subjected to analysis of variance (ANOVA) to detect significant differences between means. Means differing significantly were compared using Duncan's multiple range test P = 0.05 (SPSS version 16.0).

RESULTS AND DISCUSSION

Plant growth regulators (PGRs) are significant factors for successful plant regeneration. For *in vitro* cultures of plant tissues, cytokinin and auxin are the most used PGRs [8]. Interaction between these two growth regulators is complex and depends on plant species and tissue types. These together control many aspects of growth and differentiation. The concentration and the ratio between cytokinin and auxin determine whether to act synergistically (cell regulation) or antagonistically (callus and root formation). Proliferation and multiplication of *in vitro* shoots are largely based on media formulations containing cytokinins as major plant growth regulators [9, 10].

Meta-Topolin is a new group of natural aromatic cytokinin which is majorly used in plant tissue and organ culture as an alternative to BA [11]. It promotes shoot development in plant tissue culture from explants tissues. It has been applied for the micropropagation of numerous ornamental plants [12].

Effect of Meta-topolin

Organogenesis was stimulated by adding meta-Topolin in the shoot induction medium. The applied cytokinin stimulated the growth of axillary bud into shoots and often induced the growth of additional subsidiary buds adjacent to the new axillary shoots. Regeneration was effectively elicited in all meta-Topolin concentrations except those inoculated on mT-free media. Among the different concentrations of mT tested, 3.0 μM was found to be more effective for bud breaking, shoot formation and elongation compared to lower or higher concentrations. Similar effect of Kn at the same concentration has also been reported in other plant species, such as *Allamanda cathartica* [13], *Pterocarpus marsupium* [14], *Sesamum indicum* [15], *Corylus colurna* [16]. mT at 3.0 µM concentration yielded 6.30 ± 0.15 mean number of shoots with 5.50 ± 0.16 cm mean shoot length with 82% percent response after 8 weeks of culture (Table **1**), (Fig. **1A**). Explants treated with a high concentration of mT, above 3.0 µM, produced small shoots from an axillary bud which at a later stage failed to develop.

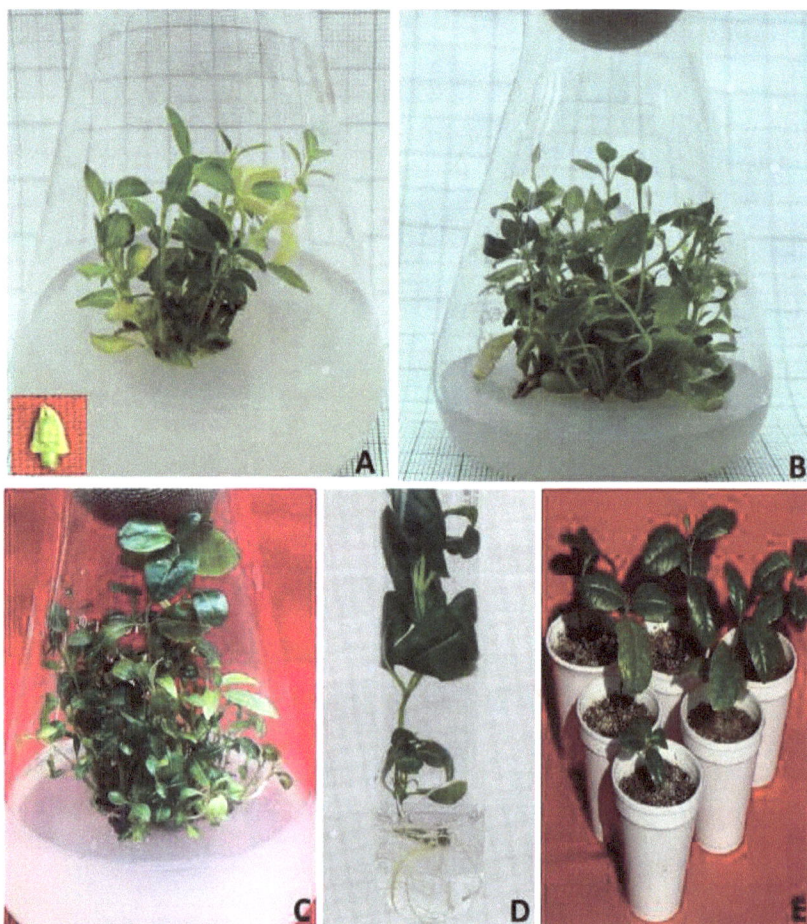

Fig. (1). (**A**): Aseptic nodal segment (inset), induction of multiple shoots on MS + 3.0 µM mT after 8 weeks of culture. (**B**): Elongation and proliferation of shoots on MS + 3.0 µM mT + 0.5 µM NAA after 12 weeks of culture. (**C**): Proliferation of shoots on optimized medium with 4% sucrose after 12 weeks of culture. (**D**): In vitro rooted shoot cultured on ½ MS + 0.5 µM NAA after 4 weeks of culture. (**E**): An acclimatized plantlet.

Cytokinin - Auxin Interaction on Shoot Proliferation

The interactive effect of auxin – cytokinin controls many aspects of cell regulation and proliferation. Auxin, though invariably used for rooting and callus formation, has been proven to be quite effective for promoting *in vitro* shoot growth in combination with cytokinin as well. The interactive effectiveness of auxin - cytokinin has been seen in many plants for promoting *in vitro* shoot proliferation, as in *Erythrina varigata* [17], *Mucuna pruriens* [18], and *Vitex trifolia* [19]. Various auxins (IAA, IBA & NAA) at different concentrations (0.1, 0.5 & 1.0 µM), when tested with optimum mT, resulted in an increase in shoot proliferation. The MS medium containing 3.0 µM mT in combination with 0.5 µM NAA produced a 15.00 ± 0.21 mean shoot number with 7.00 ± 0.21 cm shoot length in 86% of cultures, and this combination was found to be optimum after 12 weeks of culture (Table **2**), (Fig. **1B**). mT with IAA and IBA also yielded favorable results but with a statistically lower effect. Similar findings have been reported in plants such as *Maytenus emarginata* [20], *Vanilla planifolia* [21], *Tecoma stans* [22] and *Syzygium cumini* [23].

Table 2. Effect of different auxins amended with an optimal concentration of mT in MS medium on the proliferation of shoots originated from nodal explants after 8 and 12 weeks of culture.

IAA (µM)	IBA (µM)	NAA (µM)	Percent Response	Mean Number of Shoots	Mean Shoot Length (cm)	Mean Number of Shoots	Mean Shoot Length (cm)
-	-	-	-	8 weeks		12 weeks	
0.10	-	-	70.0±0.76^e	5.60±0.26^{ef}	5.30±0.21^b	6.60±0.16^f	5.30±0.15^c
0.50	-	-	76.0±0.57^c	6.20±0.24^e	5.70±0.21^b	7.50±0.16^e	6.20±0.13^b
1.00	-	-	60.0±0.76^h	3.70±0.21^g	4.00±0.14^c	4.90±0.23^g	4.20±0.20^d
-	0.10	-	66.0±0.47^f	7.00±0.21^d	5.50 ±0.16^b	8.50±0.16^d	5.70±0.15^c
-	0.50	-	73.0±0.66^d	7.80±0.32^c	5.40±0.16^b	9.60±0.16^c	5.60±0.16^c
-	1.00	-	55.0±0.47^j	5.40±0.22^f	3.80±0.20^{cd}	6.30±0.15^f	3.60±0.16^e
-	-	0.10	80.0±0.63^b	9.10±0.23^b	3.40±0. 16^d	12.00±0.21^b	4.50±0.16^d
-	-	0.50	86.0±0.47^a	13.10±0.27^a	6.50±0. 16^a	15.00±0.21^a	7.00±0.21^a
-	-	1.00	63.0±0.47^g	7.10±0.27^{cd}	2.80±0.24^e	7.60±0.16^e	3.30±0.15^e

Values represent mean ± standard error of 10 replicates per treatment in three repeated experiments. Means sharing the same letter within a column are not significantly different (P=0.05) using Duncan's multiple range test.

Effect of Sucrose

Sucrose is the main carbon source in the culture media utilized by the explants for energy requirements. Sucrose is hydrolysed into monosaccharides in culture media which can be further transported to plant cells [24]. The shoots developed in optimized media (MS + 3.0 µM mT + 0.5 µM NAA) with various concentrations of sucrose followed a variable pattern among them. The maximum number of shoots per explant was achieved in media containing 4 g/l sucrose with 20.80 ± 0.41 mean shoot number and 7.60 ± 0.16 cm mean shoot length (Table 3), (Fig. 1C). The effect of various concentrations of sucrose in shoot regeneration has been reported in *Toddalia asiatica* [25]. Low percentage of sucrose may not respond to regeneration due to the lesser amount of carbon present in the culture medium, and its high percentage may lead to osmotic stress that might suppress the growth of cultures [26].

Table 3. Effect of different sucrose concentrations in optimized medium on the proliferation of shoots originated from nodal explants after 12 weeks of culture.

Sucrose (g/l)	Percent Regeneration	Mean Number of Shoots	Mean Shoot Length (cm)
0	0.00±0.00^f	0.00±0.00^f	0.00±0.00^f
10	26.00±0.33^e	4.90±0.23^e	3.20±0.13^e
20	55.50±0.37^d	7.70±0.15^d	4.30±0.15^d
30	86.10±0.23^b	14.30±0.49^b	6.40±0.16^b
40	93.20±0.41^a	20.80±0.41^a	7.60±0.16^a
50	71.90±0.48^c	9.80±0.24^c	5.40±0.16^c

Values represent mean ± standard error of 10 replicates per treatment in three repeated experiments. Means sharing the same letter within a column are not significantly different (P=0.05) using Duncan's multiple range test.

Rooting and Acclimatization

In vitro, regenerated microshoots failed to produce root in MS and ½ MS media without any plant growth regulators even after 4 weeks of incubation. After 14 days of culture condition on ½ MS medium supplemented with auxins IAA, IBA & NAA at concentrations 0.1, 0.5 and 1.0 µM, root induction was observed from the cut end of microshoot at all tested auxins concentrations. The statistically best rooting was observed on ½ MS augmented with 0.5 µM NAA, which produced 4.20 ± 0.13 mean root number with 4.90 ± 0.08 cm root length after 4 weeks of culture (Table 4), (Fig. 1D). Similar effectiveness of NAA on rooting was also observed in *Vitex trifolia* [27], *Dianthus caryophyllous* [28] and *Withania somnifera* [29]. IBA and IAA also produced roots but were less effective than NAA. De Klerk [30] confirmed the positive influence of the tested auxins on microshoots rooting in various species, however, with different effects. Rooted microshoots with 4-5 leaves were transferred to plastic cups containing Soilrite™, moistened with water and covered with transparent plastic bags to maintain relative humidity (Fig. **1E**). After 4 weeks, the plastic bags were removed and the plantlets were transferred to pots containing garden soil and maintained in greenhouse under natural conditions with a survival rate of 96% (144 out of 150 plantlets). After the transfer of *in vitro* obtained plantlets to *in vivo* conditions, the plantlets have to adapt to various environmental stresses, and thus, the quality of developed roots is the major factor which affects the acclimatization of the plantlets. Generally, the fluctuating temperature, low humidity, air turbulence and irradiance are higher and the humidity of soil substrate is different as compared to *in vitro* conditions [31 - 33].

Table 4. Effect of various auxins on *in vitro* rooting of regenerated microshoots after 4 weeks of culture.

IAA (µM)	IBA (µM)	NAA (µM)	Percent Response	Mean Number of Roots	Mean Root Length (cm)
0.1	-	-	54.10±0.27[g]	1.80±0.13[e]	0.59±0.02[e]
0.5	-	-	63.00±0.42[e]	2.80±0.13[bc]	2.25±0.08[c]
1.0	-	-	46.10±0.34[i]	1.30±0.15[e]	1.38±0.03[d]
-	0.1	-	57.00±0.25[f]	2.40±0.16[d]	2.25±0.06[c]
-	0.5	-	67.80±0.24[d]	3.10±0.17[b]	3.18±0.05[b]
-	1.0	-	50.90±0.34[h]	0.50±0.16[f]	0.72±0.20[e]
-	-	0.1	73.90±0.37[b]	2.60±0.16[bc]	3.18±0.05[b]
-	-	0.5	80.10±0.27[a]	4.20±0.13[a]	4.90±0.08[a]
-	-	1.0	69.80±0.24[c]	1.30±0.30[e]	1.25±0.28[d]

Values represent mean ± standard error of 10 replicates per treatment in three repeated experiments. Means sharing the same letter within a column are not significantly different (P=0.05) using Duncan's multiple range test.

Phytochemical Screening

The phytochemical screening and quantitative estimation of aqueous leaf extract were conducted for various phytochemicals. The screening revealed that the leaves were rich in alkaloids, carbohydrates, lipids, phenols, proteins and saponins (Table **5**). The quantity of the carbohydrate was 0.072 mg/g and 0.065 mg/g in treated and control samples, respectively. Carbohydrates are the essential components of the building blocks of cells as they provide a high quantity of energy to cells. *A. cathartica* contains a high amount of lipid in the aqueous extract, which plays an important role in the formation of cellular structures. The lipid was found to be 0.850 mg/g and 0.920 mg/g in control and treated samples, respectively. It is a highly stable lubricant used by the industry as a renewable source of fuel. Phenols play an important role in the regulation of plant growth and development. Several types of phenolics have been shown to contain higher levels of antioxidant activities. The phenol content estimated was 1.801 mg/g in control and 1.910 mg/g in treated samples. The presence of higher protein level in the regenerated plants points towards their possible increase in protein-based bioactive compounds, which could also be isolated in the future. The amount of protein (0.120 mg/g) was slightly higher in the treated sample. Saponins are widely used as detergents and pesticides; their industrial applications as foaming and surface active agents are well-known and have beneficial health effects [34]. The amount of saponins recorded was 0.310 mg/g and 0.401 mg/g in control and treated samples, respectively. Similar phytochemical analysis in the leaf extract of *A. cathartica* has been reported by several workers [35, 36].

Table 5. Quantification of phytochemical constituents in the leaves of *A. cathartica*.

Metabolites	Control (mg/g)	Treated (mg/g)
Alkaloids	0.00	0.00
Carbohydrate	0.065	0.072
Lipid	0.850	0.920
Phenols	1.801	1.910
Proteins	0.081	0.150
Saponins	0.310	0.401

CONCLUSION

This study accentuates the use of plant tissue culture technique in developing a reproducible protocol for mass propagation of an exotic ornamental plant *A. cathartica* using nodal explants. The results showed the positive combined effect of kinetin and an auxin interaction on shoot proliferation and the phytochemical constituents. The aqueous leaf extract of the regenerants revealed various phytochemicals rich in carbohydrates, lipids, phenols, proteins, and saponins, which are known to possess various health-beneficial properties. Thus, the protocol developed can be exploited for rapid propagation of planting material of this ornamental plant for the need of floricultural praxis and utilization of the pharmacological properties of the active ingredients using the techniques like extraction, purification, separation, crystallization and identification.

ABBREVIATIONS

mT   meta-Topolin

DDW   Double Distilled Water

IAA   Indole-3- acetic acid

IBA   Indole-3-butyric acid

NAA α-Naphthalene acetic acid

PGR Plant Growth Regulators

MS Murashige and Skoog

REFERENCES

[1] Jain SM. Feeding the world with induced mutations and biotechnology. Proc Int Nuclear Conference, Global trends and Perspectives Seminar 1: agriculture and bioscience. Bangi, Malaysia: MINT. 2002; pp. 1-14.

[2] Wong SK, Lim YY, Chan EW. Botany, uses, phytochemistry and pharmacology of selected Apocynaceae species: A review. Pharmacogn Commun 2013; 3: 1-10.

[3] Góes JA. Preparações semissólidas contend extrato das flores de Allamandacathartica L. com potencial antioxidante e anti-inflamatório. Universidade do Vale do Itajaí, Itajaí 2011.

[4] Sharma KK, Saikia R, Kotoky J, Kalita JC, Das J. Evaluation of Antidermatophytic activity of Piper betle, *Allamanda cathartica* and their combination: an *in vitro* and *in vivo* study. Int J Pharm Tech Res 2011; 3: 644-51.

[5] Dubey NK, Kumar R, Tripathi P. Global promotion of herbal medicine: India's opportunity. Curr Sci 2004; 86: 37-41.

[6] Murashige T, Skoog F. A revised medium for rapid growth and bioassay with tobacco tissue culture. Physiol Plant 1962; 15(3): 473-97.
[http://dx.doi.org/10.1111/j.1399-3054.1962.tb08052.x]

[7] Harborne JB. Phytochemical methods :A guide to modern techniques of plant analysis. London: Chapman and Hall 1998.

[8] Eudes F, Acharya S, Laroche A, Selinger LB, Cheng KJ. Novel method to induce direct somatic embryogenesis, secondary embryogenesis and regeneration of fertile green cereal plants. Plant Cell Tissue Organ Cult 2003; 73(2): 147-57.
[http://dx.doi.org/10.1023/A:1022800512708]

[9] Mamidala P, Nanna RS. Efficient *in vitro* plant regeneration, flowering and fruiting of dwarf Tomato cv. Micro-Msk. Plant Omics 2009; 2: 98-102.

[10] Hoque ME. *in vitro* tuberization in potato (*Solanum tuberosum* L.). Plant Omics 2010; 3: 7-11.

[11] Aremu AO, Bairu MW, Szücová L, Doležal K, Finnie JF, Van Staden J. Assessment of the role of meta-topolins on *in vitro* produced phenolics and acclimatization competence of micropropagated 'Williams' banana. Acta Physiol Plant 2012; 34(6): 2265-73.
[http://dx.doi.org/10.1007/s11738-012-1027-6]

[12] Jain SM, Ochatt SJ. Protocols for *in vitro* propagation of ornamental plants. Springer protocols 2010; 589
[http://dx.doi.org/10.1007/978-1-60327-114-1]

[13] Khanam MN, Javed SB, Anis M, Alatar AA. meta-Topolin induced *in vitro* regeneration and metabolic profiling in *Allamanda cathartica* L. Ind Crops Prod 2020; 145: 111944.
[http://dx.doi.org/10.1016/j.indcrop.2019.111944]

[14] Ahmad A, Anis M. Meta-topolin Improves *in vitro* Morphogenesis, Rhizogenesis and Biochemical Analysis in *Pterocarpus marsupium* Roxb.: A Potential Drug-Yielding Tree. J Plant Growth Regul 2019; 38(3): 1007-16.
[http://dx.doi.org/10.1007/s00344-018-09910-9]

[15] Elayaraja D, Subramanyam K, Vasudevan V, *et al.* Meta-Topolin (mT) enhances the *in vitro* regeneration frequency of Sesamum indicum (L.). Biocatal Agric Biotechnol 2019; 21: 101320.
[http://dx.doi.org/10.1016/j.bcab.2019.101320]

[16]   Gentile A, Frattarelli A, Nota P, Condello E, Caboni E. The aromatic cytokinin meta-topolin promotes *in vitro* propagation, shoot quality and micrografting in Corylus colurna L. Plant Cell Tissue Organ Cult 2017; 128(3): 693-703. [PCTOC].
       [http://dx.doi.org/10.1007/s11240-016-1150-y]

[17]   Javed SB, Anis M. Cobalt induced augmentation of *in vitro* morphogenic potential in *Erythrina variegata* L.: A multipurpose tree legume. Plant Cell Tissue Organ Cult 2015; 120(2): 463-74.
       [http://dx.doi.org/10.1007/s11240-014-0613-2]

[18]   Faisal M, Siddique I, Anis M. *in vitro* rapid regeneration of plantlets from nodal explants of mucuna pruriens : A valuable medicinal plant. Ann Appl Biol 2006; 148(1): 1-6.
       [http://dx.doi.org/10.1111/j.1744-7348.2005.00034.x]

[19]   Ahmad N, Khan MI, Ahmed S, *et al.* Change in total phenolic content and antibacterial activity in regenerants of *Vitex negundo* L. Acta Physiol Plant 2013; 35(3): 791-800.
       [http://dx.doi.org/10.1007/s11738-012-1120-x]

[20]   Shekhawat JK, Rai MK, Shekhawat NS, Kataria V. Synergism of m-topolin with auxin and cytokinin enhanced micropropagation of *Maytenus emarginata*. in vitro Cell Dev Biol Plant 2021; 57(3): 418-26.
       [http://dx.doi.org/10.1007/s11627-020-10132-6]

[21]   Manokari M, Priyadharshini S, Jogam P, Dey A, Shekhawat MS. Meta-topolin and liquid medium mediated enhanced micropropagation *via ex vitro* rooting in Vanilla planifolia Jacks. ex Andrews. Plant Cell Tissue Organ Cult 2021; 146(1): 69-82.
       [http://dx.doi.org/10.1007/s11240-021-02044-z]

[22]   Hussain SA, Ahmad N, Anis M, Alatar AA. Influence of meta-topolin on *in vitro* organogenesis in *Tecoma stans* L., assessment of genetic fidelity and phytochemical profiling of wild and regenerated plants. Plant Cell Tissue Organ Cult 2019; 138(2): 339-51.
       [http://dx.doi.org/10.1007/s11240-019-01631-5]

[23]   Naaz A, Hussain SA, Anis M, Alatar AA. Meta-topolin improved micropropagation in *Syzygium cumini* and acclimatization to *ex vitro* conditions. Biol Plant 2019; 63(1): 174-82.
       [http://dx.doi.org/10.32615/bp.2019.020]

[24]   Taylor JLS, van Staden J. The effect of nitrogen and sucrose concentration on the growth of *Eucomis autumnalis* (Mill.) Chitt. plantlets *in vitro*, and on subsequent antiinflammatory activity in extracts prepared from the plantlets. Plant Growth Regul 2001; 34(1): 49-56.
       [http://dx.doi.org/10.1023/A:1013303624296]

[25]   Veeresham C, Praveena C. Multiple shoot regeneration and effect of sugars on growth and nitidine accumulation in shoot cultures of *Toddalia asiatica.* Pharmacogn Mag 2014; 10(39) (3): 480.
       [http://dx.doi.org/10.4103/0973-1296.139777] [PMID: 25298663]

[26]   Short KC, Warburton J, Roberts AV. *in vitro* hardening of cultured cauliflower and chrysanthemum plantlets to humidity. Acta Hortic 1987; (212): 329-34.
       [http://dx.doi.org/10.17660/ActaHortic.1987.212.50]

[27]   Ahmed MR, Anis M. Role of TDZ in the quick regeneration of multiple shoots from nodal explant of *Vitex trifolia* L.--an important medicinal plant. Appl Biochem Biotechnol 2012; 168(5): 957-66.
       [http://dx.doi.org/10.1007/s12010-012-9799-0] [PMID: 23065400]

[28]   Ahmad N, Srivastava R, Anis M. Improvement in Carnation Shoot Multiplication Using Thidiazuron. Propag Ornam Plants 2006; 6: 109-13.

[29]   Fatima N, Ahmad N, Anis M. Enhanced *in vitro* regeneration and change in photosynthetic pigments, biomass and proline content in *Withania somnifera* L. (Dunal) induced by copper and zinc ions. Plant Physiol Biochem 2011; 49(12): 1465-71.
       [http://dx.doi.org/10.1016/j.plaphy.2011.08.011] [PMID: 22078385]

[30]   Klerk G-J. Rooting of microcuttings: Theory and practice. *in vitro* Cell Dev Biol Plant 2002; 38(5):

415-22.
[http://dx.doi.org/10.1079/IVP2002335]

[31]   Preece JE, Sutter EG. Acclimatization of micropropagated plants to the greenhouse and field. In: Debergh PC, Zimmerman RH, Eds. Micropropagation Technology and Application. Dordrecht, Boston, London: Kluwer Academic Publishers 1991; pp. 71-93.
[http://dx.doi.org/10.1007/978-94-009-2075-0_5]

[32]   Pospíšilová J, Tichá I, Kadleček P, Haisel D, Plzáková Š. Acclimatization of micropropagated plants to *ex vitro* conditions. Biol Plant 1999; 42(4): 481-97.
[http://dx.doi.org/10.1023/A:1002688208758]

[33]   Rohr R, Iliev I, Scaltsoyinnes A, Tsoulpha P. Acclimatization of micropropagated forest trees. Acta Hortic 2003; (616): 59-69.
[http://dx.doi.org/10.17660/ActaHortic.2003.616.3]

[34]   Okwu DE, Okwu ME. Chemical composition of spondias mombin linn plant parts. J Sustain Agric Environ 2004; 6(2): 140-7.

[35]   Savithramma N, Linga Rao M, Suhrulatha D. Qualitative and quantification analysis of phytochemicals from leaf aqueous extract of allamanda cathartica L. and *Terminalia paniculata* Roth. Int J 2013; 1: 821-5.

[36]   Joselin J, Brintha TSS, Florence AR, Jeeva S. Screening of select ornamental flowers of the family apocynaceae for phytochemical constituents. Asian Pac J Trop Dis 2012; 2: S260-4.
[http://dx.doi.org/10.1016/S2222-1808(12)60162-5]

CHAPTER 9

Production of Secondary Metabolites from Endangered and Commercially Important Medicinal Plants Through Cell and Tissue Culture Technology

Fadime Karabulut[1]**, Mohammad Yaseen Mir**[2,*] and **Azra N. Kamili**[2]

[1] *Department of Biology, Firat University, Elazıg, India*

[2] *Centre of Research for Development, University of Kashmir, Hazratbal, Srinagar-190 006, (J&K), India*

Abstract: Pharmaceuticals such as alkaloids, terpenoids, steroids, saponins, monoterpenes, flavonoids and amino acids are now being produced using plant cell culture technologies. The standardization of plant metabolite processing technologies using *in vitro* cultures assists in the understanding of their biosynthesis and accumulation biology. The development of metabolites in plant cell cultures is affected by a number of factors, including physical, chemical, nutritional and genetic factors. The controlled production of plant metabolites in cell cultures is a viable alternative not only for reducing pressure on the natural habitats of plant species but also for providing year-round conditions for metabolite production. Exposure of cultured cells to biotic and abiotic elicitors increased the production of plant metabolites. Hairy root induction has recently been discovered to be effective in the production of metabolites synthesized in various parts of plants.

Keywords: Callus cultures, Elicitation, Hairy root cultures, Suspension cultures, Secondary metabolites.

INTRODUCTION

Anthropogenic activities, which increase with the rapid increase in the world population, are rapidly increasing the destruction of the natural habitat of many plant species. It also affects the ecosystem negatively. Many commercially used medicinal and endemic plants endanger the extinction of plants due to over-collection from their habitats. The production of plants by traditional methods brings with it many restrictions. Most plants grown from seed are highly heterozy-

* **Corresponding author Mohammad Yaseen Mir:** Centre of Research for Development, University of Kashmir, Hazratbal, Srinagar-190 006, (J&K), India; E-mail: yaseencord36@gmail.com

Mohammad Anis & Mehrun Nisha Khanam (Eds.)

gous and can vary greatly in growth and yield. In addition, the production of desired varieties is limited as many of the plants are not suitable for vegetative propagation by cutting and grafting. One of the most important methods to deal with this alarming situation is plant tissue culture, which is a biotechnological application [1]. People have been using plants for various purposes for ages. Primary metabolite needs such as carbohydrates, proteins and fats are met by plants. In addition to these primary metabolites, which are of great importance to humans, there are some substances that do not have a direct role in transport, energy, growth and differentiation events in the plant, but provide the social communication of the plant. These substances are called secondary metabolites. Secondary metabolites are chemicals that enable the plant to adapt to its environment and to be aware of its environment. Secondary metabolites in plants have important ecological functions such as resisting environmental stress factors such as drought, salinity, UV, protecting the plant against herbivores and microorganisms, pollination and seed dispersal. Plant secondary metabolites are generally classified according to their biosynthetic production pathways [2]. According to these pathways, secondary metabolites are; They are classified into three main families: phenolic compounds, terpenes and alkaloids. The largest group is phenolic compounds. Alkaloids are less common in the plant kingdom than phenolics. These chemicals, which differ in terms of amount and composition in plants, have led to the emergence of the disciplines of chemical taxonomy and chemical ecology [3]. These metabolites have very important benefits in the fields of food, cosmetics, agriculture and medicine. Perhaps the most important of these areas is the use of secondary metabolites in medicine, as it is very important for human health [2]. Plants from which drug-active ingredients are obtained are called medicinal plants. Many of the medicinal plants contain pharmaceutically highly active secondary compounds. *Betula lenta* L. plant is the source of aspirin, which is recommended because it provides blood thinner and protection against heart attack. *Hypericum perforatum* L. is a medicinal plant that is the source of hypericin, pseudohypericin, perforin, adiperforin active compounds and has an antidepressant effect. Before the chemistry of these compounds was known and their existence was revealed, people started to use plants to treat various diseases. This preference formed the basis for phytotherapy applications [2]. Plant tissue culture studies are of great importance in preventing the extinction of medicinal plants and reducing habitat destruction. In addition, many plants with secondary metabolites that the pharmaceutical industry is interested in are endangered plants due to the rapid consumption of natural populations. For this reason, it is imperative to find new approaches for the sustainable production of high-value molecules [4].

Micropropagation is a popular biotechnological method based on direct or indirect methods of reproduction, rooting and then growing of immature or mature plant parts [5]. This technique exhibits high potential for rapid propagation from plants and the production of high-quality products. Therefore, in *in vitro* culture, it is possible to increase and produce the desired compounds in line with consumer needs in controlled and sterile conditions independent of the environment. In recent years, micropropagation has been used for rapid and mass reproduction of medicinal plants through tissue culture, year-round production, pathogen-free production, increased productivity and yield, conservation of endangered species, and *in vitro* production of secondary metabolites [6]. In conventional production, many plants do not sprout, bloom, produce seeds in certain climatic conditions, or have long growth and reproduction times. Micropropagation can provide a steady supply of plants using minimal space and time. The benefits of *in vitro* micropropagation of the plant to the plant are listed below [7, 8]:

• To increase the plant's reproduction rate.

• To ensure the production of secondary metabolites.

• Meeting the needs of the plant for its controlled production.

• Ensuring that the plant reproduces independently of seasonal changes through-out the year.

• Production of clones with desired characteristics.

• Production of plants by ensuring their genetic development.

• To ensure the reproduction and protection of endangered plant species.

• To ensure the preservation of genetic material by cryopreservation.

As the need for medicinal plants increases, some of their natural habitats are more threatened [9]. Due to their medicinal use in the Ayurvedic, Unani and Siddha systems of medicine, the collection of wild plants from their native habitat has led to the species' extinction. Therefore, this study describes an alternative *in vitro* culture approach for the isolation and characterization of plant secondary metabolites [10]. A multi-dimensional approach is required for the selection of higher quality genotypes and *ex-situ*, as well as for the maintenance of *in-situ* conservation and subsequent reproduction by both conventional and biotechnological methods that can provide a solution to the current problem. *In vitro* plantlet regeneration is an effective method for plant protection [11]. Many techniques of somatic haploid embryos are needed in academic and applied plant science.

Studies on plant tissue culture techniques have increased in many countries. Advances in this technique contribute to the solution of problems related to subjects such as physiology, biochemistry, cytology, genetics and molecular biology in plants [12]. In recent years, plant tissue culture techniques have gained industrial importance in plant reproduction, conservation of plant resources and production of secondary metabolites. These techniques offer new and sustainable opportunities for solving numerous problems in plant breeding and conservation biology in medicine [13]. In plants, secondary metabolites are not a direct product of metabolism, but are seen as a by-product. They are compounds produced by plants that are not directly related to the primary metabolism of the plant, but are produced for the benefit of the organism and have a very important role in plants. Secondary metabolites have an ecological role in nature, protecting plants against microorganisms, insects, herbivores and even other plants. They act as secretion, aromatic odorants that attract animals that aid pollination or seed dispersal [14]. Medicinal and aromatic endemic plants are used in agriculture, pharmaceutics, bio pesticides and food additives, as well as the main substances that constitute an important source of secondary metabolites.

Some anticancer drugs are commercially produced from herbal sources [15, 16]. When the production amounts of medicinal and aromatic plants around the world are examined, garlic, ginger, anise, badian, fennel, and coriander take first place. Among the producing countries, India and China, which are rich in biodiversity, come to the fore.

IN VITRO CULTURE AS A SUBSTİTUTE SYSTEM FOR ENHANCEMENT OF PLANT SECONDARY METABOLİTES

Plant secondary metabolites appear to be important as a raw material or part of the final product for flavors, food additives, pharmaceuticals and many industrial products. Polyphenols from different secondary metabolites constitute the main group of innate antioxidants [17]. Antioxidants such as phenolics and flavonoids have properties such as protection against cancer, aging, Parkinson's, Alzheimer's, cardiovascular diseases and brain dysfunctions [18]. It has important biological and pharmacological activities such as anti-oxidative, anticarcinogenic and secondary metabolites obtained from plants.Theoretically, tissue culture studies give successful results in increasing the amount of secondary metabolites obtained from the explant taken from the plant. Root, shoot and embryo cultures formed from plant explants are cultures that have been differentiated (Table **1**). Undifferentiated cultures are callus and cell suspension cultures [19]. It contributes significantly to an enormous commercial development with consistent production and high yields in secondary metabolite production [20, 21]. Traditional and metabolic engineering approaches are used to increase the yield and production of secondary metabolites [22].

Table 1. Some important examples of *in vitro* propagation of medicinal plants.

Species	Explant Used	Results	References
Atropa belladona	Axillary meristem	Multiple shoots, plantlet formation	[23]
Catharanthus roseus	Shoot tips	Multiple shoots, plantlet formation	[24]
Plantago ovata	Shoot tips	Multiple shoots, plantlet formation	[25]
Rauwolfia serpentina	Nodal and leaf explants	Multiple shoots, plantlet formation	[26]
Centella asiatica	Shoot tips	Callus, shoot bud, plantlet	[27]
Aloe vera	Shoot tips	Shoot, root and plantlet forming	[28]
Bergenia ciliata	Seeds and leaf explants	Multiple shooting, rooting and plantlet formation	[29]
Artemisia amygdalina	Leaf explants	Callus and suspension cultures	[30]
Hypericum perforatum	Nodal explants	Shoot, root and plantlet forming	[31]
Arnebia benthamii	Seeds	Multiple shooting, rooting and plantlet formation	[32]
Hyoscyamus niger	Seeds	Multiple shooting, rooting and plantlet formation	[33]

Traditional Strategies

Secondary metabolites are produced as a result of primary metabolism. It depends on the rate at which substrates are redirected from primary metabolic pathways to secondary biosynthetic pathways. The development and physiology of syntheses depend on biotic factors as well as abiotic factors (such as temperature, humidity, light intensity, *etc.*). The metabolic productivity of *in vitro* cultures depends on the composition of the culture medium, pH, temperature and light intensity [22, 34]. Therefore, these culture media need to be optimized to promote growth and metabolite productivity. The selection of the appropriate culture medium plays a vital role in the production of secondary metabolites. Components of the culture medium such as vitamins (such as vitamins B1-B12), carbohydrates (sucrose, glucose), amino acids, macro and micronutrients, and plant growth regulators such as cytokinins, gibberellins, auxins, salicylates and jasmonates contribute to metabolite production [12].

Metabolic Engineering

Metabolic engineering is used to produce metabolites of commercial importance. For metabolite production, metabolomics, genomics, proteomics, *etc.*, are considered. It is necessary to change the metabolic pathways in an organism with biotechnological tools [35]. Thus, through endogenous biochemical pathways and deflecting common precursors, enzymes, and regulatory proteins with the help of recombinant DNA technology, manipulation of metabolic pathways by overexpression or downregulation is allowed. Since the metabolites of plants are complex, there are many metabolic pathways responsible for their biosynthesis. These pathways can be reconstructed in heterologous hosts for isolation and overproduction of economically important plant metabolites. The biosynthetic pathways for the production of secondary metabolites originate from the shikimate, polyketide, and terpenoid pathways. In most of these, the shikimat tract has been preserved. However, the shikimate pathway also constitutes the main source of phenylpropanoids and aromatic compounds [36]. Since more than 30% of fixed carbon is expected to be fixed through, it is considered a major metabolic pathway for carbon flux in plants [37]. It is formed through the shikimate biosynthesis of phenolic and phenylalanine, which is a secondary metabolite in plants. Pcoumaroyl-CoA intermediate contains coumarins, vanillin, gallic acid, lignans, flavonoids, stilbenoids, betalains, catechins, *etc.*, as a source of metabolites.

In a study, it was determined that phenolic compounds, which are the secondary metabolite production of callus, shoot and cell suspension cultures of *C. polygonoides*, were determined by HPLC. The profiles and amounts of phenolics vary according to the differentiation of cultures. Undifferentiated callus and cell suspension cultures contain less phenolic compounds than differentiated shoots. The compounds in these regenerating multiple shoots are composed of catechin and kaempferol-3-O-glucuronide, while in the case of callus, the parent compounds catechin and kaempferol occur. In addition, it is observed that catechin and isocercitrin compounds are formed in a cell suspension culture that does not produce gallic acid, quercetin, kaempferol and taxifolin [38].

APPROACHES TO MANİPULATE THE CONTENTS OF PLANT SECONDARY METABOLİTES

Synthesis of secondary metabolites varies depending on chemical and physical conditions. Studies have shown that growth hormones, medium formulations, temperature and photoperiod manipulation have effects on increasing secondary products.

Carbon Source

Generally, sucrose is used as a carbon source. This carbon source is significantly effective in increasing the amount of metabolites in *in vitro* cultures. However, as sucrose levels increase, rosmarinic acid production also increases. In cell cultures of Podophyllum hexandrum, it was observed that podophyllotoxin production increased when glucose was used instead of sucrose in MS medium [8].

Media Formulation

It can decrease or increase the production of the active components of the secondary metabolites of the compounds used in the culture medium. For example, serpentine production was found to be more efficient in the suspension culture of *Catharanthus roseus* in MS medium. As a result, it varies according to plant species and environmental components.

Temperature

Significant differences in secondary metabolite production can be observed in the *in vitro* culture environment due to changes in temperature and, accordingly, photoperiod and pH [8]. *Podophyllum hexandrum*plants were grown in a culture medium, and cultures grown in the dark medium had higher podophyllotoxin production and better friable callus than those grown in light [39].

Agitation

Cells growing in the culture medium need to adjust their speed during mixing, because it has been found to affect cell viability and product synthesis. Cells of *Podophyllum hexandrum* grown *in vitro* showed much more damage at 200 rpm, and little damaged cells were found between 125-150 rpm [39].

Phosphate

Secondary metabolite production in plants grown in a cell culture medium was affected by phosphate level. In some plant cell cultures, it was observed that the metabolite level and cell growth increased when the phosphate amounts were decreased. As the phosphate level decreased, the production of ajmalisin and phenolics in *Cath roseus* and caffeoyl putrescines in *Nicotiana tabacum* increased [8].

Nitrogen

Production of protein or amino acid-containing metabolites is affected by nitrogen amounts in the culture medium. Various culture media (MS, LS or B5) constitute the nitrogen source.

Plant Growth Hormones

In vitro, secondary metabolite production is affected by the amounts of plant growth hormones. For example, while it was reported that 2,4-D stopped the production of secondary metabolites [8], it was found that metabolite synthesis increased with NAA or IAA, one of the plant growth regulators [40]. Callus formation is observed with the addition of auxin to the MS medium of *Catharanthus roseus*. In this plant, it was determined that the production of secondary metabolites increased with the presence of only cytokinins in the medium. Plant growth hormones, 2.5 mg.l^{-1} IBA and 0.1 mg.l^{-1} kinetin, were added to the culture medium, and the production of ginsenoside saponins in the *Panax quinquefolium* plant was found to be higher than in adult plants [8].

Gas Composition

In culture media, significant effects of gas compositions on the concentration ratio of the secondary metabolite were detected [40]. In the culture medium in a bioreactor for the *Panax ginseng* plant, 40% of the oxygen gave the highest saponin production, and the oxygen concentrations decreased by 50%, 20.8% and 30% [41].

Precursor Supplementation

Secondary metabolite production can be increased by supplementing with a compound in metabolite production. This is called pre-feeding. In studies, it was reported that the production of metabolites increased in cell culture [40].

Callus Culture System

In vitro plant cell culture starts with leaving the explant taken from the plant tissue in a previously sterilized container into the environment containing nutrients. The medium usually contains vitamins, macro salts, micro salts, myo-inositol, carbon source (sucrose), plant growth regulators, and, if it is a semi-solid medium, agar as a solidifying agent. Various culture media have been developed, which are the basis for the media used today. Each plant species, even each metabolite, requires its own specific environment. Cultures made in these different environments usually start with a callus culture. The starting point of cell suspension cultures is essentially callus culture [42]. Without microorganism contamination of *in vitro* culture, the next steps consist of the replication of cells, tissues, shoots and roots. These processes are important in terms of their economic applicability because of high cell and tissue production [12]. The explant taken from the mother plant produces morphologically undifferentiated cell groups as a result of a series of divisions in the medium carrying the plant growth regulator. Callus tissue is a tissue ready to be anything. Continuity depends on subculture. Also suitable for mass production. The most important disadvantage of callus tissues is that they cannot show genetic stability during culture. Somaclonal variations can be seen in cultures, which may adversely affect metabolite production. There are studies reporting secondary metabolite production in callus, but significant metabolite formation is seen in callus tissues that have differentiated to form any organ. When differentiation disappears, secondary metabolite yield decreases significantly [2]. Callus culture formed *in vitro* is a collection of undifferentiated plant cells containing auxin concentrations from plant growth hormones or a combination of auxin and cytokinin. This cell population develops either embryogenic or non-embryogenic. The somatic embryogenesis process begins in the embryogenic callus. In this process, it contains differentiated embryogenic cells that can form a complete plant. The resulting cells have become competent cells [43]. It also provides somatic embryogenesis, clonal propagation of plants, and regeneration of haploid or transgenic plants. Non-embryogenic callus culture contains more or less homogeneous clusters of undifferentiated cells. This callus culture is used for secondary metabolite production. It is frequently used, especially for the production of flavonoids.

In general, the callus cultures of the species were found to produce more isoflavones than the parent plants as they had lower genistein ester content than the plants. In a study by Tumova and colleagues, they determined that the amount of flavonoids in *Ononis arvensis* L. plant was less than the flavonoids in the callus culture. The effect on the production of flavonoids that are potential selectors (killed Pseudomonas aeruginosa, linoleic acid, chromium trichloride, yasminic acid, substituted pyrazine-2-carboxylic acids and iodoacetic acid anilides) to the culture medium was investigated. These elicitors were found to significantly increase the production of flavonoids compared to control [44, 45].

Cell Suspension Cultures

In general, the production of secondary metabolites is influenced by different environmental factors such as climate, diseases and pests. In all plants, cell suspension cultures are considered suitable as a technological method for product quantity and quality problems [40, 46]. In cell suspension cultures, friable calli growing in liquid media are formed *in vitro* when the cells are shaken continuously in the conical flask to maintain suspension. These flasks are used to create a large surface area to maintain continuous gas exchange and liquid medium. Suspension cultures are administered in two ways. First, batch cultures are made by removing a portion of the initial cell suspension and subculturing on fresh medium at regular intervals. The second is continuous cultures; fresh medium is added to the existing culture and excess cell suspensions are removed at regular intervals. Cell suspension cultures are widely used in the production of secondary metabolites. Bioreactors such as Chemostat have been specially designed for continuous culture application [8].

High production of secondary metabolites such as alkaloids and total phenols was achieved by using monochromatic lights for cell suspension culture *Celastrus paniculatus* [47]. It was observed that redifferentiated shoots contained higher amounts of phenolic compounds than undifferentiated callus and cell suspension cultures. In the *in vitro* conditions, the yield was increased by applying salicylic acid and yeast extract to increase the production of phenolic compounds in cell suspension culture [38]. In plant tissue culture techniques, Jasmonic acid has been used to modulate the production of various secondary metabolites. Total phenolic production was maximized in the callus cell suspension culture of *Celastrus paniculatus* when jasmonic acid was applied at concentrations of 250 µM, 250 µM and 50 µM for 24, 48 and 72 hours, respectively. In many plant species, it has been determined that the total phenolic production reaches the maximum level when salicylic acid at 100 µM, 250 µM and 50 µM concentrations is applied for 24, 48 and 72 hours, respectively, to improve *in vitro* regeneration [48].

Hairy Root Cultures

Hairy root phenotype is characterized by a lack of geotropism, rapid growth, genetic stability and side branching without hormones. Secondary metabolites produced in hairy roots of plant material by *Agrobacterium rhizogenes* are the same as those synthesized in intact rootstock [49]. This property grows rapidly without phytohormones and genetic stability, making them suitable for biochemical studies that cannot simply be performed with root cultures of an intact plant. Hairy roots grow rapidly and show plagiotropic growth. These roots are highly branched in the phytohormone-free environment [50]. Hairy roots originating from *Agrobacterium rhizogenes* can be applied in different areas. Hairy root cultures are of great importance in studies with root nodules for the production of plant secondary metabolites. Transformed roots were used in different plants for the production of secondary metabolites and artificial seeds. Hairy root cultures, secondary metabolites can be produced without losing their biosynthetic or genetic properties [51]. Transformed root cultures have studied many aspects of secondary metabolite biosynthesis [52]. There is an important and strong relationship between morphological differentiation and secondary metabolite production. Thus, it accelerates the application of organized cell cultures for the production of large amounts of phytochemicals. Biological transformation is also replaced locally in interorgan metabolite synthesis [51]. Moreover, the simultaneous production of two different secondary metabolites can be observed [53]. The great potential of hairy root cultures as a source of biologically active chemicals [54] has enabled the use of the *in vitro* system through scale-up in new bioreactors [55]. Hairy root cultures of adventitious roots of *Scopolia parviflora* [56], *Lithospermum erythrorhizon*, *Harpagophytum procumbens* [57] and *Panax ginseng* [58] are derived from alkaloids, harpagide, shikonin, and ginsenos, respectively. Bubble column bioreactors have been studied. Ginsenoside was also produced in a 5 L stirred tank bioreactor using a random root culture [58]. Current scale-up technology has necessitated the use of stainless steel tanks and in-ship bioreactors equipped with special hangers for the growth of plant cells on an industrial scale. These cultures are seen as a potential source for the continued production of compounds of high economic value. When compared with the production of Plant Derived Medicinal Compounds (PDMC) by cell, callus and shoot cultures in hairy root cultures, it was observed that besides the advantage for hairy roots, the genetic stability of hairy roots, the preservation of cell viability and the capacity to produce different PDMCs in high concentration were observed [59, 60]. Accordingly, the hairy root technique is a viable and suitable method for *in vitro* production of large-scale PDMC.

Organ Culture

Medicinal compounds can be propagated by root culture methods [61]. For example, most of the secondary compounds, such as the tropane alkaloids hyoscyamine and scopolamine, have been efficiently increased in root cultures [62]. Production of secondary metabolites can be grown in the root, shoot and leaf parts of the plant [63, 64]. Secondary metabolites produced *in vitro* from the shoot part of the plant are of great commercial importance [65]. It has also been used to induce somaclonal variation *in vitro* and to select clones with high secondary yields [66].

The biggest problem of organ cultures is large-scale cultures [67]. The bioreactors of the culture obtained from the roots and leaves of the plant are also different [68, 69]. Generally, organ cultures show a lower susceptibility to plant cutting stress than cell suspension cultures. However, they show heterogeneity for greater length in biomass production in organ culture. Bioreactors used for the production of plant secondary metabolites are economically costly. Since competition begins with the planting of plants, it is not economically viable in this process [70]. For example, secondary metabolite was obtained from Fritillaria unibracteata plant grown in *in vitro* organ culture. The cultured onion tuber is cultured after 50 days after adding 4.44 M BA and 5.71 M IAA to the medium. The growth rate was 30 times higher than normal. It has been determined that there are too many alkaloids and beneficial microelements in onions in the culture medium. Therefore, it is possible to scale-up for industrial production in future studies by creating a new process to produce this natural herbal medicine [71].

Elicitation: A Biotechnological Tool

In vitro conditions, with the supplementation of different natural or synthetic plant growth regulators, the growth of cells and organs, the accumulation of various metabolites and the change of morphogenetic structure are provided [72]. As a stimulant, elicitors are used to increase bioactive production in various chemical and physical substances [73]. In the production of secondary metabolites, first of all, the expression of the necessary gene must be initiated. The process of creating an artificial pathogen attack scenario by chemical means is called elicitation [8]. For example, glucan polymers, jasmonic acid, glycoproteins, UV irradiation, heavy metal salts, fungal cell materials and many other chemicals can be elicitors [74]. Secondary metabolites are produced by plants in defense against pathogen attack and occur in cultures that produce certain compounds [40]. Yeast extract (elicitor) production from Rauvofja catrescetrs and Eschscholtzia califtnica plants is of great importance. It has been observed that methyl jasmonate has similar effects on some plant species [8].

The hairy root culture method is most commonly used in plant cell cultures to increase secondary metabolite production. With this method, metabolites emerge with various biotic and abiotic elicitors. As the mass amount per unit of plant roots increases, the metabolite product yield also increases. And also, elicitors applied in culture media stimulate the flow of intracellular products or product recovery, which facilitates the purification of a desired compound. In the *in situ* metabolite product extraction method applied in hairy root cultures, the roots are kept immobile in the culture medium, so that the used liquid medium is withdrawn and fresh medium is added. Thus, this culture method with biotic interaction can be applied for the commercial production of low-volume pharmaceutically important secondary metabolites [75]. Important elicitors applied to stimulate secondary metabolite production in hairy root cultures include: Raw mushroom extracts or partially purified polysaccharide fractions from mushroom cells, UV radiation, Jasmonic acid, Methyl jasmonate, heavy metal ions, hyperosmotic stress, hormones, temperature change and some chemicals. Optimization of the amount and duration of elicitors used according to plant species and being specific to the biosynthetic pathway are very effective in the production of secondary metabolites. Thus, an elicitor may not stimulate a similar secondary metabolite in all species as well as for different groups of secondary metabolite production of the same species. The benefits of applying an elicitor in the culture medium are to increase the metabolite yield, recover the product and stimulate the flow of intracellular products, which make purification of the desired compound quite easy. In the future, it will help to better understand the regulation mechanisms of a particular biosynthesis pathway by initiating gene expression of the biosynthesis pathway in metabolic engineering [76].

The response of plants to abiotic stress factors consists of four stages. These stages are; we can list them as the first alarm phase, the adaptation phase, the maintenance phase and the exhaustion phase (Kapoor *et al* ., 2018). The plant's response to stress is a dynamic process that depends on the stress duration and stress intensity. The plant's response to stress is seen in several stages. The first stage is the shock effect, in which stress-sensitive signaling pathways in the plant are stimulated and the plant's stress tolerance level decreases. In the acclimation phase, the biosynthesis of various proteins that defend against stress occurs and the plant's stress tolerance increases. During the maintenance phase, homeostasis is maintained and the plant stress tolerance level remains constant. If the plant's stress tolerance level falls during the extinction stage and is exposed to stress, homeostasis in the plant continues.

CONCLUSİON AND FUTURE PROSPECTİVE

Generally, medicinal plants are the preferred herbal resources for a healthy life and are also used as preventive and therapeutic. Due to the low side effects of herbal medicines, the demand for herbal products has increased rapidly. Apart from medicine, most of the chemicals used in food and industry are of plant origin. Although endemic plants with high medical and economic value, which are endangered, are protected by *in vitro* reproduction, many plant species with medical importance are unconsciously consumed by the pharmaceutical industry. In order to reduce the pressure caused by the excessive collection and export of medicinal plants from nature and to produce effective metabolites, rapid cultivation and *in vitro* production studies of these plant species should be increased. *In vitro* propagation has significant potential for the continuity of the production of high-quality medicinal products, the reproduction of endemic species that are difficult to cultivate, and a reliable source of natural products. In addition, cell culture techniques are the biggest advantage of producing bioactive secondary metabolites synthesis content that works in a controlled environment regardless of climate and soil conditions. The use of *in vitro* plant cell culture for the production of chemicals and pharmaceuticals has made great advances in plant science. These results indicate that *in vitro* plant cell cultures have the potential for commercial production of secondary metabolites. The low crop yields and supply concerns of plant harvesting combined with the increasing level of natural products for medicinal purposes have rekindled interest in large-scale plant cell culture technology. However, tissue culture methods also play an important role in the conservation of biodiversity and the reproduction of rare endangered plant species.

REFERENCES

[1]   Sharma S, Rathi N, Kamal B, Pundir D, Kaur B, Arya S. Conservation of biodiversity of highly important medicinal plants of India through tissue culture technology: A review. Agric Biol J N Am 2010; 1(5): 827-33.
[http://dx.doi.org/10.5251/abjna.2010.1.5.827.833]

[2]   Vuran NE, Türker M. Applications to increase secondary metabolite amount in plant tissue cultures. Int J Adv Eng Pure Sci 2021; 33(3): 487-98.

[3]   Bourgaud F, Gravot A, Milesi S, Gontier E. Production of plant secondary metabolites: A historical perspective. Plant Sci 2001; 161(5): 839-51.
[http://dx.doi.org/10.1016/S0168-9452(01)00490-3]

[4]   Georgiev MIK-YP, Ed. Production of biomass and bioactive compounds using bioreactor technology. Springer 2014.

[5]   Babaoglu, M.; Yorgancılar, M.; Akbudak, M.A. Tissue Culture, Basic Laboratory Techniques, Plant Biotechnology I, Tissue Culture and Applications: Offset Preparation/Printing ISBN 975-6652-04-7, 2001.

[6]   Ayaz E, Memon A. Development of the aromatic medicinal plants, *Mentha* x *piperita* L. and *Mentha pulegium* L. through *in vitro* callus induction and micropropagation. TurkJAgriculFood Sci Techn 2021; 9(1): 159-65.
[http://dx.doi.org/10.24925/turjaf.v9i1.159-165.3774]

[7]   Sidhu Y. *In Vitro* micropropagation of medicinal plants by tissue culture. Plymouth Student Scientist 2010; 4(1): 432-49.

[8]   Sidhu Y. *In vitro* micropropagation of medicinal plants by tissue culture. Plymouth Student Scientist 2011; 4(1): 432-49.

[9]   Narasimhan S, Nair GM. Release of berberine and its crystallization in liquid medium of cell suspension cultures of *Coscinium fenestratum* (Gaertn.). Colebr Curr Sci 2004; 86: 1369-71.

[10]   Khan T, Krupadanam D, Anwar SY. The role of phytohormone on the production of berberine in the calli cultures of an endangered medicinal plant, turmeric (*Coscinium fenestratum* L.). Afr J Biotechnol 2008; 7(18).

[11]   Hussain M, Raja NI, Akram A, *et al.* A status review on the pharmacological implications of *Artemisia absinthium*: A critically endangered plant. Asian Pac J Trop Dis 2017; 7(3): 185-92.
[http://dx.doi.org/10.12980/apjtd.7.2017D6-385]

[12]   Cardoso JC, Oliveira MEBS, Cardoso FCI. Advances and challenges on the *in vitro* production of secondary metabolites from medicinal plants. Hortic Bras 2019; 37(2): 124-32.
[http://dx.doi.org/10.1590/s0102-053620190201]

[13]   Chandran H, Meena M, Barupal T, Sharma K. Plant tissue culture as a perpetual source for production of industrially important bioactive compounds. Biotechnol Rep 2020; 26(00450): e00450.
[http://dx.doi.org/10.1016/j.btre.2020.e00450] [PMID: 32373483]

[14]   Isah T. Stress and defense responses in plant secondary metabolites production. Biol Res 2019; 52(1): 39.
[http://dx.doi.org/10.1186/s40659-019-0246-3] [PMID: 31358053]

[15] Allkin B. Useful Plants–Medicines: At least 28,187 plant species are currently recorded as being of medicinal use.Royal Botanic Gardens. Kew, London 2017; pp. 22-9.

[16] Inoue M, Hayashi S, Craker LE. Role of medicinal and aromatic plants: Past, present, and future. In: Perveen S, Al-Taweel A, Eds. In Pharmacognosy-medicinal plants. London, UK: IntechOpen 2019; pp. 1-13.
[http://dx.doi.org/10.5772/intechopen.82497]

[17] Cieśla Ł, Kowalska I, Oleszek W, Stochmal A. Free radical scavenging activities of polyphenolic compounds isolated from medicago sativa and medicago truncatula assessed by means of thin-layer chromatography DPPH˙ rapid test. Phytochem Anal 2013; 24(1): 47-52.
[http://dx.doi.org/10.1002/pca.2379] [PMID: 22745039]

[18] Zaka M, Abbasi BH, Rahman L, Shah A, Zia M. Synthesis and characterisation of metal nanoparticles and their effects on seed germination and seedling growth in commercially important *Eruca sativa*. IET Nanobiotechnol 2016; 10(3): 134-40.
[http://dx.doi.org/10.1049/iet-nbt.2015.0039] [PMID: 27256893]

[19] Babaoglu M, McCabe MS, Power JB, Davey MR. Agrobacterium-mediated transformation of *Lupinus mutabilis* L. using shoot apical explants. Acta Physiol Plant 2000; 22(2): 111-9.
[http://dx.doi.org/10.1007/s11738-000-0064-8]

[20] Vijaya Sree N, Udayasri PVV, Aswani Kumar Y, Ravi Babu B, Phani Kumar Y, Vijay Varma M. Advancements in the production of secondary metabolites. J Nat Prod 2010; 3: 112-23.

[21] Gonçalves S, Romano A. Production of plant secondary metabolites by using biotechnological tools. In: Vijayakumar R, Raja SSS, Eds. Secondary Metabolites - Sources and Applications. Intech Open 2018.
[http://dx.doi.org/10.5772/intechopen.76414]

[22] Isah T, Umar S, Mujib A, *et al.* Secondary metabolism of pharmaceuticals in the plant *in vitro* cultures: Strategies, approaches, and limitations to achieving higher yield. Plant Cell Tissue Organ Cult 2018; 132(2): 239-65.
[http://dx.doi.org/10.1007/s11240-017-1332-2]

[23] Benjamin BD, Roja PC, Heble MR, Chadha MS. Multiple shoot cultures of *Atropabelladonna*. Effect of physicochemical factors on growth and alkaloid formation. J Plant Nutr 1987; 129: 129-35.

[24] Begum T, Mathur M. *In vitro* Regeneration of *Catharanthus roseus* and *Bacopa monnieri* and their survey around jaipur district. Int JPure AppBiosci 2014; 2: 210-21.

[25] Barna KS, Wakhlu AK. Axillary shoot induction and plant regeneration in plantago ovata forssk. Plant Cell Tissue Organ Cult 1988; 15(2): 169-73.
[http://dx.doi.org/10.1007/BF00035758]

[26] Khan S, Banu TA, Akter S, *et al. In vitro* regeneration protocol of *Rauvolfia serpentina* L. Bangladesh J Sci Ind Res 2018; 53(2): 133-8.
[http://dx.doi.org/10.3329/bjsir.v53i2.36674]

[27] Joshi VP, Kumar N, Singh B, Chamoli RP. Chemical composition of the essential oil of *Centella asiatica* (L.) Urb. from Western Himalaya. Nat Prod Commun 2007; 2(5): 1934578X0700200.
[http://dx.doi.org/10.1177/1934578X0700200515]

[28] Molsaghi M, Moieni A, Kahrizi D. Efficient protocol for rapid *Aloe vera* micropropagation. Pharm Biol 2014; 52(6): 735-9.
[http://dx.doi.org/10.3109/13880209.2013.868494] [PMID: 24405115]

[29] Rafi S, Kamili AN, Ganai BA, Mir MY, Parray JA. *In vitro* culture and biochemical attributes of *Bergenia ciliata* (Haw.) Sternb. Proc Natl Acad Sci, India, Sect B Biol Sci 2018; 88(2): 609-19.
[http://dx.doi.org/10.1007/s40011-016-0797-9]

[30] Mir MY, Kamili AN, Hassan QP, Tyub S. Effect of light and dark conditions on biomass

accumulation and secondary metabolite production in suspension cultures of *Artemisia amygdalina* Decne. J Himalayan Ecol Sustain Dev 2017; 12: 107-12.

[31]   Mir MY, Kamili AN, Hassan QP, Rafi S, Parray JA, Jan S. *In Vitro* regeneration and free radical scavenging assay of *Hypericum perforatum* L. Natl Acad Sci Lett 2019; 42(2): 161-7.
       [http://dx.doi.org/10.1007/s40009-018-0699-x]

[32]   Parray JA, Kamili AN, Jan S, *et al.* Manipulation of plant growth regulators on phytochemical constituents and DNA protection potential of the medicinal plant arnebia benthamii. Biomed Res Int 2018; 2018: 6870139.
       [http://dx.doi.org/10.1155/2018/6870139]

[33]   Shah D, Kamili AN, Wani AA, *et al.* Ems induced point mutations in 18s rRNA gene of hyoscyamus niger L. An important medicinal plant of Kashmir Himalaya. Pak J Bot 2019; 51(3): 949-55.
       [http://dx.doi.org/10.30848/PJB2019-3(19)]

[34]   Ochoa-Villarreal M, Howat S, Hong S, *et al.* Plant cell culture strategies for the production of natural products. BMB Rep 2016; 49(3): 149-58.
       [http://dx.doi.org/10.5483/BMBRep.2016.49.3.264] [PMID: 26698871]

[35]   DellaPenna D. Plant metabolic engineering. Plant Physiol 2001; 125(1): 160-3.
       [http://dx.doi.org/10.1104/pp.125.1.160] [PMID: 11154323]

[36]   Herrmann KM, Weaver LM. The shikimate pathway. Annu Rev Plant Physiol Plant Mol Biol 1999; 50(1): 473-503.
       [http://dx.doi.org/10.1146/annurev.arplant.50.1.473] [PMID: 15012217]

[37]   Maeda H, Dudareva N. The shikimate pathway and aromatic amino Acid biosynthesis in plants. Annu Rev Plant Biol 2012; 63(1): 73-105.
       [http://dx.doi.org/10.1146/annurev-arplant-042811-105439] [PMID: 22554242]

[38]   Owis A, Abdelwahab N, Abul-Soad A. Elicitation of phenolics from the micropropagated endangered medicinal plant Calligonum polygonoides L. (Polygonoaceae). Pharmacogn Mag 2016; 12(47) (4): 465.
       [http://dx.doi.org/10.4103/0973-1296.191458] [PMID: 27761076]

[39]   Chattopadhyay S, Srivastava AK, Bhojwani SS, Bisaria VS. Production of podophyllotoxin by plant cell cultures of *Podophyllum hexandrum* in bioreactor. J Biosci Bioeng 2002; 93(2): 215-20.
       [http://dx.doi.org/10.1016/S1389-1723(02)80017-2] [PMID: 16233190]

[40]   Ramachandra Rao S, Ravishankar GA. Plant cell cultures: Chemical factories of secondary metabolites. Biotechnol Adv 2002; 20(2): 101-53.
       [http://dx.doi.org/10.1016/S0734-9750(02)00007-1] [PMID: 14538059]

[41]   Trung Thanh N, Niranjana Murthy H, Yu KW, Seung Jeong C, Hahn EJ, Paek KY. Effect of oxygen supply on cell growth and saponin production in bioreactor cultures of Panax ginseng. J Plant Physiol 2006; 163(12): 1337-41.
       [http://dx.doi.org/10.1016/j.jplph.2005.08.014] [PMID: 16488510]

[42]   Topcu Ş, Cölgecen H. Production of plant secondary metabolites in bioreactors. Turk J Scienti Rev 2015; 8(2): 9-29.

[43]   Ptak A, El Tahchy A, Skrzypek E, Wojtowıcz T, Laurаın-Mattar D. Influence of auxins on somatic embryogenesis and alkaloid accumulation in *Leucojum aestivum* callus. Cent Eur J Biol 2013; 8(6): 591-9.

[44]   Tůmová L, Tůma J, Doležal M, Danıelová B. Pyrazinecarboxylic acid derivatives as effective abiotic elicitors of isoflavonoids production. Ceska Slov Farm 2010; 59(3): 117-22. a

[45]   Tůmová L, Tůma J, Megušar K, Doležal M. Substituted pyrazinecarboxamides as abiotic elicitors of flavolignan production in *Silybum marianum* (L.) gaertn cultures *in vitro*. Molecules 2010; 15(1): 331-40. b
       [http://dx.doi.org/10.3390/molecules15010331] [PMID: 20110894]

[46] Yamamoto H, Zhao P, Inoue K. Origin of two isoprenoid units in a lavandulyl moiety of sophoraflavanone G from *Sophora flavescens* cultured cells. Phytochemistry 2002; 60(3): 263-7. [http://dx.doi.org/10.1016/S0031-9422(02)00111-5] [PMID: 12031444]

[47] Billore V, Khatediya L, Jain M. Sink? Source System of *In vitro* Suspension Culture of *Celastrus paniculatus* under Regulation of Monochromatic Lights. Plant Tissue Cult Biotechnol 2016; 26(2): 175-85. [http://dx.doi.org/10.3329/ptcb.v26i2.30567]

[48] T S A, M v J, K K E. Callus induction and elicitation of total phenolics in callus cell suspension culture of *Celastrus paniculatus* – willd, an endangered medicinal plant in India. Pharmacogn J 2016; 8(5): 471-5. [http://dx.doi.org/10.5530/pj.2016.5.10]

[49] Sevón N, Oksman-Caldentey KM. Agrobacterium rhizogenes-mediated transformation: Root cultures as a source of alkaloids. Planta Med 2002; 68(10): 859-68. [http://dx.doi.org/10.1055/s-2002-34924] [PMID: 12391546]

[50] Hu ZB, Du M. Hairy root and its application in plant genetic engineering. J Integr Plant Biol 2006; 48(2): 121-7. [http://dx.doi.org/10.1111/j.1744-7909.2006.00121.x]

[51] Giri A, Narasu ML. Transgenic hairy roots. Biotechnol Adv 2000; 18(1): 1-22. [http://dx.doi.org/10.1016/S0734-9750(99)00016-6] [PMID: 14538116]

[52] Kuzovkina IN, Schneider B. Genetically transformed root cultures : Generation, properties and application in plant sciences. Prog Bot 2006; 67: 275-314. [http://dx.doi.org/10.1007/3-540-27998-9_13]

[53] Wu CH, Murthy HN, Hahn EJ, Paek KY. Establishment of adventitious root co-culture of Ginseng and Echinacea for the production of secondary metabolites. Acta Physiol Plant 2008; 30(6): 891-6. [http://dx.doi.org/10.1007/s11738-008-0181-3]

[54] Cetın B, Gurel A, Bedır E, Akkaya M, Ay G. Formation of *Agrobacterium rhizogenes*-mediated Transformed Hairy Root Cultures of *Rubia tinctorum* L. and Analysis of Secondary Metabolites. XIV. National Biotechnology Congress. 2005, August 31-September 2; 40-4.

[55] Mehrotra S, Kukreja AK, Singh Khanuja SP, Mishra BN. Genetic transformation studies and scale up of hairy root culture of *glycyrrhiza glabra* in bioreactor. Electron J Biotechnol 2008; 11(2): 0. [http://dx.doi.org/10.2225/vol11-issue2-fulltext-6]

[56] Min J, Jung H, Kang S, *et al.* Production of tropane alkaloids by small-scale bubble column bioreactor cultures of *Scopolia parviflora* adventitious roots. Bioresour Technol 2007; 98(9): 1748-53. [http://dx.doi.org/10.1016/j.biortech.2006.07.033] [PMID: 16965915]

[57] Ludwig-Müller J, Georgiev M, Bley T. Metabolite and hormonal status of hairy root cultures of Devil's claw (Harpagophytum procumbens) in flasks and in a bubble column bioreactor. Process Biochem 2008; 43(1): 15-23. [http://dx.doi.org/10.1016/j.procbio.2007.10.006]

[58] Jeong CS, Murthy HN, Hahn EJ, Paek KY. Improved production of ginsenosides in suspension cultures of ginseng by medium replenishment strategy. J Biosci Bioeng 2008; 105(3): 288-91. [http://dx.doi.org/10.1263/jbb.105.288] [PMID: 18397781]

[59] Thiruvengadam M, Rekha K, Chung IM. Induction of hairy roots by Agrobacterium rhizogenes - mediated transformation of spine gourd (Momordica dioica Roxb. ex. willd) for the assessment of phenolic compounds and biological activities. Sci Hortic 2016; 198: 132-41. [http://dx.doi.org/10.1016/j.scienta.2015.11.035]

[60] Thakore D, Srivastava AK, Sinha AK. Mass production of ajmalicine by bioreactor cultivation of hairy roots of *Catharanthus roseus*. Biochem Eng J 2017; 119: 84-91. [http://dx.doi.org/10.1016/j.bej.2016.12.010]

[61]   Pence VC. Evaluating costs for the *in vitro* propagation and preservation of endangered plants. *in vitro* Cell Dev Biol Plant 2011; 47(1): 176-87.
[http://dx.doi.org/10.1007/s11627-010-9323-6]

[62]   Fazilatun N, Nornisah M, Zhari I. Superoxide radical scavenging properties of extracts and flavonoids isolated from the leaves of Blumea balsamifera. Pharm Biol 2004; 42(6): 404-8.
[http://dx.doi.org/10.1080/13880200490885969]

[63]   Nogueira JMF, Romano A. Essential oils from micropropagated plants of *Lavandula viridis.* Phytochem Anal 2002; 13(1): 4-7.
[http://dx.doi.org/10.1002/pca.609] [PMID: 11899605]

[64]   Smith MAL, Kobayashi H, Gawienowski M, Briskin DP. An *in vitro* approach to investigate medicinal chemical synthesis by three herbal plants. Plant Cell Tissue Organ Cult 2002; 70(1): 105-11.
[http://dx.doi.org/10.1023/A:1016081913719]

[65]   Khanam N, Khoo C, Khan AG. Effects of cytokinin/auxin combinations on organogenesis, shoot regeneration and tropane alkaloid production in Duboisia myoporoides. Plant Cell Tissue Organ Cult 2000; 62(2): 125-33.
[http://dx.doi.org/10.1023/A:1026568712409]

[66]   Dhawan S, Shasany AK, Arif Naqvi A, Kumar S, Khanuja SPS. Menthol tolerant clones of Mentha arvensis: Approach for *in vitro* selection of menthol rich genotypes. Plant Cell Tissue Organ Cult 2003; 75(1): 87-94.
[http://dx.doi.org/10.1023/A:1024684605967]

[67]   Kaimoyo E, Farag MA, Sumner LW, Wasmann C, Cuello JL, VanEtten H. Sub-lethal levels of electric current elicit the biosynthesis of plant secondary metabolites. Biotechnol Prog 2008; 24(2): 377-84.
[http://dx.doi.org/10.1021/bp0703329] [PMID: 18331050]

[68]   Kašparová M, Siatka T, Dušek J. Production of isoflavonoids in the *Trifolium pratense* L. suspension culture. Ceska Slov Farm 2009; 58(2): 67-70.

[69]   Kim Y, Wyslouzil BE, Weathers PJ. Secondary metabolism of hairy root cultures in bioreactors. *in vitro* Cell Dev Biol Plant 2002; 38(1): 1-10.
[http://dx.doi.org/10.1079/IVP2001243]

[70]   Zhao JL, Zhou LG, Wu JY. Effects of biotic and abiotic elicitors on cell growth and tanshinone accumulation in Salvia miltiorrhiza cell cultures. Appl Microbiol Biotechnol 2010; 87(1): 137-44.
[http://dx.doi.org/10.1007/s00253-010-2443-4] [PMID: 20195862]

[71]   Gao SL, Zhu DN, Cai ZH, Jiang Y, Xu DR. Organ culture of a precious Chinese medicinal plant – *Fritillaria unibracteata.* Plant Cell Tissue Organ Cult 1999; 59(3): 197-201.
[http://dx.doi.org/10.1023/A:1006440801337]

[72]   Mir MY, Hamid S, Kamili AN, Hassan QP. Sneak peek of *Hypericum perforatum* L.: Phytochemistry, phytochemical efficacy and biotechnological interventions. J Plant Biochem Biotechnol 2019; 28(4): 357-73.
[http://dx.doi.org/10.1007/s13562-019-00490-7]

[73]   Murthy HN, Georgiev MI, Park SY, Dandin VS, Paek KY. The safety assessment of food ingredients derived from plant cell, tissue and organ cultures: A review. Food Chem 2015; 176(0): 426-32.
[http://dx.doi.org/10.1016/j.foodchem.2014.12.075] [PMID: 25624252]

[74]   Zhong JJ. Plant cell culture for production of paclitaxel and other taxanes. J Biosci Bioeng 2002; 94(6): 591-9.
[http://dx.doi.org/10.1016/S1389-1723(02)80200-6] [PMID: 16233355]

[75]   Halder M, Sarkar S, Jha S. Elicitation: A biotechnological tool for enhanced production of secondary metabolites in hairy root cultures. Eng Life Sci 2019; 19(12): 880-95.
[http://dx.doi.org/10.1002/elsc.201900058] [PMID: 32624980]

[76]   Kapoor S, Raghuvanshi R, Bhardwaj P, Sood H, Saxena S, Chaurasia OP. Influence of light quality on growth, secondary metabolites production and antioxidant activity in callus culture of *Rhodiola imbricata* Edgew. J Photochem Photobiol B 2018; 183: 258-65.
[http://dx.doi.org/10.1016/j.jphotobiol.2018.04.018] [PMID: 29747145]

CHAPTER 10

Antimicrobial Efficacy of *In Vitro* Cultures and their Applications

Nishi Kumari[1,*], **Pooja Jaiswal**[1], **Alpana Yadav**[1], **Ashish Gupta**[1] and **Brajesh Chandra Pandey**[1]

[1] *Department of Botany, Mahila Mahavidyalaya, Banaras Hindu University, Varanasi, India*

Abstract: Treatment of microbial infections has become more challenging with the evolution of antibiotic resistant microbes and indiscriminate use of antibiotics. Several phytochemicals have shown potential inhibitory action against such microbes. These antimicrobials have shown their efficacy in treating such infections. These natural products also played significant role in restoration of activity of less effective antibiotics, when used in combination with antibiotics. But still, scientists are facing some major challenges in using such metabolites for medicines- there is urgent need to explore more plants showing microbial inhibition activity, plant products from field grown plants are not sufficient to meet the growing demand and purification of antimicrobial compounds, so that dosage for patients can be finalized. Tissue culture has emerged as great technology not only in the conservation of such medicinal plants but it provides major application for the production of secondary metabolites. Various micropropagules such as calli, *in vitro* cultures, and cell suspensions have shown their potential for the production of pharmaceutically active compounds similar to mature plants. Production of such phytochemicals can be enhanced by manipulating media supplements, culture conditions and elicitations. As, in nature production of antimicrobials is the result of interaction between the plants and microbes, therefore, such interaction can be provided to *in vitro* cultures by biotic elicitation. *In vitro* production of antimicrobial compounds has been reported in many plants such as *Ricinus communis*, *Calendula officinalis*, *Abrus precatorius*, *etc*. Thus, plant tissue culture paves an efficient and feasible method of production of such natural compounds as an alternative of antibiotics.

Keywords: Antibiotic, Antimicrobial, Antioxidant, Elicitation, Inhibition, Metabolites, Micropropagules, Pathogenic, Precursor.

INTRODUCTION

Plant secondary metabolites display great applications in the field of human health, nutrition and many industries. Plant cell and organ culture systems have

* **Corresponding author Nishi Kumari:** Department of Botany, Mahila Mahavidyalaya, Banaras Hindu University, Varanasi, India; E-mail: nishi.kumari5@bhu.ac.in

Mohammad Anis & Mehrun Nisha Khanam (Eds.)
All rights reserved-© 2024 Bentham Science Publishers

become an effective means for the production of pharmaceutically important compounds, phytochemicals used as industrial products and food additives. Secondary metabolites are natural products synthesized by plants and microbes. Primary metabolites of plants are directly involved in their growth and development, whereas secondary metabolites or better termed specialized metabolites are required for their survival. These compounds develop defense mechanism in the plants to combat stress induced by pathogenic attack or environmental variations. Elicitation of *in vitro* cultures is nowadays being used as an efficient method for the production of secondary metabolite compounds. Elicitors promote secondary metabolite synthesis and their accumulation by *in vitro* cultures. Elicitors are the chemical compounds from abiotic and biotic sources that can stimulate stress responses in plants, leading to enhanced synthesis and accumulation of secondary metabolites or the induction of novel secondary metabolites. Elicitor type, dose, and treatment methods are major factors determining the production of secondary metabolites. Other important parameters, which affect the production of such compounds are duration of exposure to cell lines, nutrient composition, age or stage of the culture, *etc.* The collections of these compounds from field grown plants is unable to meet the growing demand of plant based pharmaceutical products, as the metabolites produced by an individual plant is very less. As, both quality and quantity of these compounds are not uniform in nature, it is difficult to fix the dosage for the patients. The production of novel antimicrobial agents is still highly dependent on the discovery of new natural products. At present, most antimicrobial drugs used in medicine are of natural origin.

Antibiotic-resistant microorganisms have emerged as a great challenge for the treatment of patients. Hence, several researchers are focusing their attention on the discovery of new antimicrobial compounds as efficient alternative of antibiotics. Although several plant secondary metabolites and their derivatives have been identified as possible antimicrobial agents, they are not enough and there is a need to explore more such compounds [1, 2]. Secondary metabolites such as alkaloids and polyphenols have shown strong antimicrobial activity [3]. Polyphenols are considered one of the most diverse groups of secondary metabolites. Their strong antioxidant efficacies also contribute antimicrobial effects. Similarly, many alkaloids have shown their antimicrobial potential. These phytochemicals have become greatest tool in overcoming the problem of antibiotic resistance. Several antimicrobials show wide spectrum antimicrobial function, thus they can serve as efficient alternative of antibiotics. To make it cost-effective and commercially feasible, there is a need to optimize various factors, and a standardized protocol can be used for enhanced production of these phytochemicals.

There are different steps:

Culture Initiation

There is a need to grow cells or tissues of medicinal plants. Development of their regeneration protocols is also required to provide a continuous source of materials. *In vitro* cultures are being grown in aseptic and fully controlled condition thus, it provides contamination-free and more uniform material. Secondary metabolite production from *in vitro* cultures at commercial level is feasible by using bioreactors. However, it requires optimization of various factors: growth and maintenance of cell lines or other *In vitro* cultures, identification of suitable elicitor, and extraction of metabolites [4]. The establishment of cultures for phytochemical production undergo mainly two phases- first proliferation and another production phase. After culture initiation, cultures are transferred on a favorable medium which supports the growth and multiplication, but less metabolites are produced by growing cultures. However, production medium favors secondary metabolite production, but not the growth of the cultures.

Type of Cultures

Generally, cell supensions or calli are used for the production of these compounds. But some phytochemicals are organ specific, and their synthesis take place from differentiated organs such as *in vitro* leaves, shoots, somatic embryos, roots, plantlets, *etc.* Among differentiated tissues, hairy root cultures (Fig. 1) are highly efficient in producing such metabolites at the commercial level [5]. Many researchers have observed the significant antimicrobial potential of different micropropagules of plants (Table 1). *In vitro* cultures of many plants have also shown their broad spectrum of action against several pathogenic microbes.

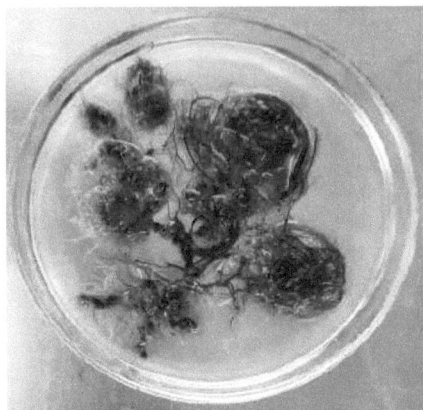

Fig. (1). Hairy root culture of *Wedelia chinensis*.

Table 1. Antimicrobial potential of micropropagules of some medicinal plants.

Name of Plant	Types of Micropropagules	Inhibition Against	References
Annona mucosa	Cell suspension	*Streptococcus pyrogenes* and *Bacillus thuringiensis*	[6]
Bacopa monniera	Fresh leaves of micropropagated plants	*Klebsiella pneumoniae, Escherichia coli, Bacillus subtilis, Staphylococcus aureus, Aspergillus fumigatus, Candida albicans*	[7]
Scutellaria orientalis	Callus	*Staphylococcus aureus, Bacillus subtilis*	[8]
Commiphora gileadensis	Callus	*Bacillus cereus, Phytophthora infestans, Staphylococcus aureus, Escherichia coli*	[9]
Lamium album	Micrpropagated plants	*Micrococcus luteus, Staphylococcus aureus, Staphylococcus epidermis, Bacillus subtilis, Pseudomonas aeruginosa, Enterobacter aerogenes, Klebsiella pneumoniae*	[10]
Cotyledon orbiculata	Callus, shoots and micropropagated plants	*Enterococcus faecalis, Micrococcus luteus, Staphylococcus aureus, Escherichia Coli, Klebsiella pneumoniae, Pseudomonas aeruginosa*	[11]
Thymus mastichina L	Micropropagated plant	Different species of *Fusarium*	[12]
Cleome rosea Vahl	Micropropagated plant, callus & cell suspension	*Bacillus thuringiensis, Bacillus subtilis, Micrococcus luteus, Staphylococcus simulans, Staphylococcus. saprophyticus, Staphylococcus xylosus, Staphylococcus hominis, Staphylococcus aureus Escherichia coli, Klebsiella pneumoniae*	[13]
Clitoria ternatea Linn	Callus & micropropagated plant	*Bacillus subtilis, Bacillus cereus, Staphylococcus aureus, Proteus vulgaris, Klebsiella pneumoniae, Salmonella typhi*	[14]

(Table 1) cont.....

Name of Plant	Types of Micropropagules	Inhibition Against	References
Tylophora indica	Micropropagated plant & leaf callus	*Staphylococcus aureus,* *Staphylococcus epidermidis,* *Bacillus subtilis,* *Escherichia coli,* *Klebsiella pneumoniae,* *Pseudomonas aeruginosa,* *Salmonella typhi,* *Shigella dysenteriae*	[15]
Petunia	Callus	*Baccilus subtilis,* *Streptococcus spp,* *Staphylococcus aureus* *Escherichia coli, Pseudomonas* *aeroginosa, Salmonella spp*	[16]
Asparagus officinalis	Callus	*Bacillus cereus*	[17]
Barleria lupulina	Leaf callus	*Staphylococcus aureus* *Bacillus pumilus*	[18]
Ricinus communis	Cell suspension	*Sarcina lutea,* *Staphylococcus aureus,* *Bacillus megaterium,* *Bacillus subtilis,* *Bacillus halodurans.* Shigella sonnei, Klebsiella species, Proteus species, Escherichia coli, Pseudomonas aeruginosa, Salmonella typhi.	[19]
Holarrhena antidsenterica	Callus	*Staphylococcus aureus* **Gram Negative** Salmonella, Escherchia coli	[20]

Elicitation

In many plants, the presence of secondary metabolites was observed from their *in vitro* cultures. Few studies showed better antimicrobial efficacies of *in vitro* plants over *in vivo* plants. In general, the plants growing in nature have shown more antimicrobial activities than their *in vitro* cultures [7, 10, 21, 22]. This difference is directly related to their growing conditions. Micropropagated plants are being grown under a controlled condition and lack plant-microbe interactions and environmental fluctuations. But, the tissue culture of medicinal plants provides efficient propagation methods for their mass multiplication, and the availability of plant materials is possible throughout the year. For making it cost-effective and commercially feasible, treating micropropagules by elicitors is highly successful in getting enhanced production of these compounds [23]. In some plants, the novel compound formation was also observed, thus showing the wide application of tissue culture. The presence of secondary metabolites was observed in micropropagules of different plants. There is evidence that the induction of secondary metabolite production from primary compounds is more effective in the stationary growth phase. For this reason, a good strategy for a plant cell factory is to establish a two-stage culture, in which the cells are first maintained in a proliferation medium for biomass formation and are then transferred to an optimal production medium, which induces the synthesis of secondary compounds. The elicitation creates artificial stress, which stimulates the cells to produce more secondary metabolites [24]. The elicitation can be divided into two types- abiotic and biotic. Biotic elicitation can be sub-divided into two types: physical and chemical. Physical elicitation to *in vitro* cultures can be done by altering the pH of the medium, altering growth conditions of the culture (such as temperature, humidity, light) and by their irradiation for a short period [25]. Chemical elicitation can be achieved by altering media composition, and treatment with plant growth regulators such as Abscisic acid and other chemicals such as Salicyclic acid. Inorganic chemicals like salts or metal ions are being used to increase the production of bioactive compounds by their modification of plant secondary metabolism. The receptors of the cell membrane recognize most of the biotic elicitors, and in response, the cell produces phytoalexins. In nature, plants face constant attack due to microbes and their immune response helps in combating such attacks. Therefore, plant cells are capable to recognize conserved microbe specific molecules, also termed as microbe or pathogen associated molecular patterns (MAMPs or PAMPs). Receptors of plant membranes are capable to recognize elicitors like microbial cell wall products, extracts of dead pathogens, *etc.* Therefore, this strategy has been adopted by many researcher for the enhanced production of compounds showing antimicrobial potential (Table **2**).

Table 2. Enhanced production of phytochemicals from *in vitro* cultures of some plants after elicitation.

Name of Plant	Type of Cultures	Elicitation	Type of Metabolites Induced/Stimulated Synthesis	References
Solanum malacoxylon	Cell Cultures	Benzothiadozole	B- sitosterol, campestoron, stigmasterol & vitamines	[26]
Petroselinum crispum	Cell suspensions	2,6- dichloroisonicotinic, 4,5- or 5- chlorosalicyclic acid & 3,5- dichlorosalicyclic acid	Phenylpropanol derivatives	[27]
Vitis vinifera	Calli	Extract of yeast *Aureobasidium pullans*	Stilbene	[28]

(Table 2) cont.....

Name of Plant	Type of Cultures	Elicitation	Type of Metabolites Induced/Stimulated Synthesis	References
Pinus ginseng	Cell suspensions & hairy root culture	Yeast extract	Saponin and other metabolites	[29, 30]
H. perforatum	Cell Suspension	Fungal extract	Naphtodianthrones, total phenolics, flavonoids & anthocyanins	[31]
Fagopyrum tataricum	Hairy root cultures	Yeast polysachharides	Flavonoids	[32]
Psoralea corylifolia	Cell cultures	*Aspergillus niger & Penicillium notatum* extract	Psoralen	[33]
Coleus forskohlii	Suspension culture	Fungal elicitors	forskolin	[34]
Euphorbia pekinensis	Cell suspension	Endophytic fungal elicitor	Terpenoid & polyphenol	[35]
Andrographis paniculata	Suspension cultures	*Aspergillus niger* extract	Flavonoid	[36]
Linum sp.	Cell suspension	Several fungal extract	Lignan production	[37, 38]
Linum album	Cell suspension	Commercial yeast extract	Podophyllotoxin	[39]
Cayratia trifolia	Cell suspension	Yeast extract	Stilbenes	[40]
Silybum marianum	Cell Suspension	Yeast extract	Silymarin	[41]
Artemesia annua	Hairy root	Yeast extract	Artemesin	[42]
Taxus	Cell Cultures	Fungal extract alone or in combination with other elicitors	Paclitaxel and other taxanes	[43 - 45]

Metabolic Engineering

There are different metabolic pathways for the biosynthesis of different metabolites: shikimate, polyketide and terpenoid. Terpenoid biosynthesis in plants occur by two pathways; mevalonic acid pathway (MVA) and methyl-D-erythrito (MEP) pathway. Now it is possible to manipulate these endogenous pathways: by overexpression or downregulation of these pathways by precursors, enzymes, and regulatory proteins with the help of recombinant DNA technology. Phenylalanine acts as the substrate in the first reaction of the phenylpropanoid biosynthetic pathway and is used as a precursor for the production of flavonoids, phenolic acids, lignans, and coumarins [46]. Identification of biosynthetic pathways of metabolites has great applications. Precursors of these pathways can enhance the production of metabolites, when supplied exogenously to *in vitro* cultures. Some researchers have used precursors for enhancing antimicrobial efficacy of plants (Table **3**).

Table 3. Some examples of antimicrobial activities of *in vitro* cultures after precursor feeding.

Name of Plant	Types of Micropropagules	Precursor Used	Effective Against	References
Nasturtium officinale	Microshoots	L-phenylalanine	*Propionibacterium* spp	[47]
Daucas carota	Callus	tryptophan	*Bacillus subtilis, Staphylococcus aureus, Pseudomonas floureceans, Escherichia coli, Bacillus thuringiensis, Saccharomyces cervisiae, Candida albicans*	[48]
Dionaea muscipula	Micropropagated plants	l-phenylalanine	*Enterococcus faecalis, Staphylococcus aureus, Klebsiella pneumoniae, Pseudomonas aeruginosa*	[49]

Therefore, a holistic approach is required for the production of antimicrobial compounds from the plants. There are different mechanisms of antimicrobials' action against microbes: antimicrobials perform as inhibitors for microbial biosynthetic pathway, act as chelating agents which reduce the availability of micronutrients needed for bacterial growth, they permeabilize or destabilize the cell membrane, cause higher ion leakage and proton influx in the damaged bacterial cell, inhibition of supercoiling activity of DNA gyrase thus impairing DNA or RNA synthesis and cause the death of bacterial cell [23]. Thus, phytochemicals provide an efficient option for the treatment of microbial infections [50]. Plant phenolics can act synergistically with antibiotics and will be an effective solution for the treatment against multidrug-resistant (MDR) bacteria. Researchers have identified their activities as antibiotic potentiators and virulence attenuators.

CONCLUSION

Therefore, there is a great need to explore plants with antimicrobial efficacy and *in vitro* technology must be applied for their enhanced production to make the medicines cost-effective. Phytochemicals will provide better substitute of antibiotics. They will help in dealing deleted with antibiotic resistance and multi drug resistance problems.

REFERENCES

[1]   Bandow JE, Brötz H, Leichert LIO, Labischinski H, Hecker M. Proteomic approach to understanding antibiotic action. Antimicrob Agents Chemother 2003; 47(3): 948-55.
[http://dx.doi.org/10.1128/AAC.47.3.948-955.2003] [PMID: 12604526]

[2]   Parekh J, Chanda S. Antibacterial activity of aqueous and alcoholic extracts of 34 indian medicinal plants against some *staphylococcus* Species. Turk J Biol 2008; 32: 63-71.

[3]   Othman L, Sleiman A, Abdel-Massih RM. Antimicrobial activity of polyphenols and alkaloid in middle eastern plants. Front Microbiol 2019; 10: 911.
[http://dx.doi.org/10.3389/fmicb.2019.00911] [PMID: 31156565]

[4]   Marchev AS, Yordanova ZP, Georgiev MI. Green (cell) factories for advanced production of plant secondary metabolites. Crit Rev Biotechnol 2020; 40(4): 443-58.
[http://dx.doi.org/10.1080/07388551.2020.1731414] [PMID: 32178548]

[5]   Gutierrez- Valdes N, hakkinen ST, lemasson C, *et al.* Hairy root cultures: A versatile tool with multiple applications. Front Plant Sci 2020; 11.
[http://dx.doi.org/10.3389/fpls.2020,00033]

[6]   De souza Barboza TJ, Ferreira AF, de Paula rosa Ignacio AC, Albarello N. Antimicrobial activity of annona mucosa (jacq.) grown *in vivo* and obtained by *in vitro* culture. Brazilian J Microbiol 2015; 46(3): 785-9.

[7]   Haque SM, Chakraborty A, Dey D, Mukherjee S, Nayak S, Ghosh B. Improved micropropagation of *Bacopa monnieri* (L.) Wettst. (Plantaginaceae) and antimicrobial activity of *in vitro* and *ex vitro* raised plants against multidrug-resistant clinical isolates of urinary tract infecting (UTI) and respiratory tract infecting (RTI) bacteria. Clinical Phytoscience 2017; 3(1): 17.
[http://dx.doi.org/10.1186/s40816-017-0055-6]

[8]   Ozdemir FA, Kilic O, Atalan E. *In vitro* callus propagation and antibacterial activities of callus an edible endemic and medicinal plant *Scutellaria orientalis* L. subsp. bicolor. Prog Nutr 2016; 18(1): 81-6.

[9]   Mahmoud Al O. Evaluation of antimicrobial activity of *ex vitro* and callus extracts from *Commiphora gileadensis*. Pak J Biol Sci 2019; 22(2): 73-82.
[http://dx.doi.org/10.3923/pjbs.2019.73.82] [PMID: 30972989]

[10] Chipeva VA, Petrova DC, Geneva ME, Dimitrova MA, Moncheva PA, Kapchina-Toteva VM. Antimicrobial activity of extracts from *in vivo* and *in vitro* propagated *Lamium album* l. plants. Afr J Tradit Complement Altern Med 2013; 10(6): 559-62.
[http://dx.doi.org/10.4314/ajtcam.v10i6.30] [PMID: 24311888]

[11] Kumari A, Baskaran P, Van Staden J. *In vitro* propagation and antibacterial activity in *Cotyledon orbiculata*: A valuable medicinal plant. Plant Cell Tissue Organ Cult 2016; 124(1): 97-104.
[http://dx.doi.org/10.1007/s11240-015-0878-0]

[12] Fraternale D, Giamperi L, Ricci D. Chemical composition and antifungal activity of essential oil obtained from *in vitro* plants of Thymus mastichina L. J Essential Oil Research 2003; 15(4): 278-81.

[13] Simoes-Gurgel C, Rocha AS, Cordeiro LS, *et al.* Antibacterial activity of field-grown plants, *in vitro* propagated plants, callus and cell suspension cultures of cleome rosea vahl. JPR 2012; 5: 3304-8.

[14] Arumugam M, Panneerselvam R. *In vitro* propagation and antibacterial activity of *Clitoria ternatea* Linn. Asian Pac J Trop Biomed 2012; 2(2): S870-5.
[http://dx.doi.org/10.1016/S2221-1691(12)60326-8]

[15] Noor J, Razia K, Anwar S, Mohammad S, Siraj A. Comparison of antibacterial activity of parent plant of *Tylophora indica* Merr. with its *in vitro* raised plant and leaf callus. Afr J Biotechnol 2013; 12(31): 4891-6.
[http://dx.doi.org/10.5897/AJB2013.12488]

[16]   Thenmozhi M, Sivaraj R. *In Vitro* evaluation of the antibacterial activity of *Petunia* leaf and callus extracts. Agric Tech 2011; 7: 321-30.

[17]   Khorasani A, Sani W, Philip K, Taha RM, Rafat A. Antioxidant and antibacterial activities of ethanolic extracts of *Asparagus officinalis* cv. Mary Washington: Comparison of *in vivo* and *in vitro* grown plant bioactivities. Afr J Biotechnol 2010; 9(49): 8460-6.

[18]   Moin S, Babu SS, Mahalakshmipriya A. *In vitro* callus production and antibacterial activity of *Barleria lupulina* Lindl. Asia Pac J Mol Biol Biotechnol 2012; 20(2): 59-64.

[19]   Rahman M, Bari MA. Antibacterial activity of cell suspension cultures of Castor (*Ricinus communis* L. cv. Roktima). European J Med Plants 2013; 3(1): 65-77.
[http://dx.doi.org/10.9734/EJMP/2013/1722]

[20]   Mahato S, Mehta A, Roy S. Studies on antibacterial effects of bark, seed and callus extracts of *Holarrhena antidysenterica* Wall. Bioscan 2013; 8(2): 717-21.

[21]   Shokrian T, Noori SAS, Nematzadeh GA, Alavi SM. Evaluating antibacterial activity of *in vitro* culture of Ajwain (*Trachyspermum copticum*) extract and comparison with seed extract and essential oils. Journal of Plant Molecular Breeding 2016; 4(2): 41-6.
[http://dx.doi.org/10.22058/jpmb.2016.25528]

[22]   Mahendran G, Bai VN. An efficient *in vitro* propagation, antioxidant and antimicrobial activities of *Aphyllorchis montana* Rchb.f. Plant Biosyst 2016; 150(5): 1087-95.
[http://dx.doi.org/10.1080/11263504.2015.1008597]

[23]   Christopher A, Sarkar D, Shetty K.) Elicitation of Stress- Induced Phenolic Metabolites for Antimicrobial Applications against Foodborne Human Bacterial Pathogens. Antibiotics 2021; 10(109).

[24]   Ramirez-Estrada K, Vidal-Limon H, Hidalgo D, *et al.* Elicitation, an effective strategy for the biotechnological production of bioactive high-added value compounds in plant cell factories. Molecules 2016; 21(2): 182.
[http://dx.doi.org/10.3390/molecules21020182] [PMID: 26848649]

[25]   Cusido RM, Onrubia M, Sabater-Jara AB, *et al.* A rational approach to improving the biotechnological production of taxanes in plant cell cultures of Taxus spp. Biotechnol Adv 2014; 32(6): 1157-67.
[http://dx.doi.org/10.1016/j.biotechadv.2014.03.002] [PMID: 24681092]

[26]   Burlini N, Iriti M, Daghetti A, Faoro F, Ruggiero A, Bernasconi S. Benzothiadiazole (BTH) activates sterol pathway and affects vitamin D3 metabolism in *Solanum malacoxylon* cell cultures. Plant Cell Rep 2011; 30(11): 2131-41.
[http://dx.doi.org/10.1007/s00299-011-1119-6] [PMID: 21779826]

[27]   Kauss H, Franke R, Krause K, *et al.* Conditioning of parsley (petroselinum crispum l.) suspension cells increases elicitor- induced incorporation of cell wall phenolics. Plant Physiol 1993; 102(2): 459-66.
[http://dx.doi.org/10.1104/pp.102.2.459] [PMID: 12231833]

[28]   Rühmann S, Pfeiffer J, Brunner P, *et al.* Induction of stilbene phytoalexins in grapevine *(Vitis vinifera)* and transgenic stilbene synthase-apple plants (*Malus domestica*) by a culture filtrate of *Aureobasidium pullulans.* Plant Physiol Biochem 2013; 72: 62-71.
[http://dx.doi.org/10.1016/j.plaphy.2013.03.011] [PMID: 23578977]

[29]   Kim CY, Im HW, Kim HK, Huh H. Accumulation of 2,5-dimethoxy-1,4-benzoquinone in suspension cultures of *Panax ginseng* by a fungal elicitor preparation and a yeast elicitor preparation. Appl Microbiol Biotechnol 2001; 56(1-2): 239-42.
[http://dx.doi.org/10.1007/s002530000557] [PMID: 11499937]

[30]   Jeong GT, Park DH, Ryu HW, *et al.* Production of antioxidant compounds by culture of *Panax ginseng* C.A. Meyer hairy roots: I. Enhanced production of secondary metabolite in hairy root cultures by elicitation. Appl Biochem Biotechnol 2005; 124(1-3): 1147-58.
[http://dx.doi.org/10.1385/ABAB:124:1-3:1147] [PMID: 15930588]

[31] Gadzovska Simic S, Tusevski O, Maury S, *et al.* Fungal elicitor-mediated enhancement in phenylpropanoid and naphtodianthrone contents of *Hypericum perforatum* L. cell cultures. Plant Cell Tissue Organ Cult 2015; 122(1): 213-26.
[http://dx.doi.org/10.1007/s11240-015-0762-y]

[32] Zhao JL, Zou L, Zhang CQ, *et al.* Efficient production of flavonoids in *Fagopyrum tataricum* hairy root cultures with yeast polysaccharide elicitation and medium renewal process. Pharmacogn Mag 2014; 10(39): 234-40.
[http://dx.doi.org/10.4103/0973-1296.137362] [PMID: 25210309]

[33] Ahmed SA, Baig MMV. Biotic elicitor enhanced production of psoralen in suspension cultures of *Psoralea corylifolia* L. Saudi J Biol Sci 2014; 21(5): 499-504.
[http://dx.doi.org/10.1016/j.sjbs.2013.12.008] [PMID: 25313287]

[34] Swaroopa G, Anuradha M, Pullaiah T. Elicitation of forskolin in suspension cultures of *Coleus forskohlii* (willd.) Briq. using elicitors of fungal origin. Curr Trends Biotechnol Pharm 2013; 7: 755-62.

[35] Gao F, Yong Y, Dai C. Effects of endophytic fungal elicitor on two kinds of terpenoids production and physiological indexes in *Euphorbia pekinensis* suspension cells. Faslnamah-i Giyahan-i Daruyi 2011; 5: 4418-25.

[36] Mendhulkar VD, Vakil MMA. Chitosan and Aspergillus Niger mediated elicitation of total flavonoids in suspension culture of *Andrographis paniculata* (Burm. f.) Nees. Int J Pharma Bio Sci 2013; 4: 731-40.

[37] Baldi A, Srivastava AK, Bisaria VS. Fungal elicitors for enhanced production of secondary metabolites in plant cell suspension cultures. In: Varma A, Kharkwal AC, Eds. Symbiotic Fungi, Soil Biology. Berlin/Heidelberg, Germany: Springer-Verlag 2009; Vol. 18: pp. 373-80.
[http://dx.doi.org/10.1007/978-3-540-95894-9_23]

[38] Tahsili J, Sharifi M, Safaie N, Esmaeilzadeh-Bahabadi S, Behmanesh M. Induction of lignans and phenolic compounds in cell culture of *Linum album* by culture filtrate of *Fusarium graminearum*. J Plant Interact 2014; 9(1): 412-7.
[http://dx.doi.org/10.1080/17429145.2013.846419]

[39] van Fürden B, Humburg A, Fuss E. Influence of methyl jasmonate on podophyllotoxin and 6-methoxypodophyllotoxin accumulation in *Linum album* cell suspension cultures. Plant Cell Rep 2005; 24(5): 312-7.
[http://dx.doi.org/10.1007/s00299-005-0954-8] [PMID: 15818489]

[40] Roat C, Ramawat KG. Elicitor-induced accumulation of stilbenes in cell suspension cultures of Cayratia trifolia (L.) Domin. Plant Biotechnol Rep 2009; 3(2): 135-8.
[http://dx.doi.org/10.1007/s11816-009-0082-y]

[41] Sánchez-Sampedro MA, Fernández-Tárrago J, Corchete P. Yeast extract and methyl jasmonate-induced silymarin production in cell cultures of *Silybum marianum* (L.) Gaertn. J Biotechnol 2005; 119(1): 60-9.
[http://dx.doi.org/10.1016/j.jbiotec.2005.06.012] [PMID: 16054261]

[42] Putalun W, Luealon W, De-Eknamkul W, Tanaka H, Shoyama Y. Improvement of artemisinin production by chitosan in hairy root cultures of *Artemisia annua* L. Biotechnol Lett 2007; 29(7): 1143-6.
[http://dx.doi.org/10.1007/s10529-007-9368-8] [PMID: 17426924]

[43] Yuan YJ, Li C, Hu ZD, Wu JC, Zeng AP. Fungal elicitor-induced cell apoptosis in suspension cultures of Taxus chinensis var. mairei for taxol production. Process Biochem 2002; 38(2): 193-8.
[http://dx.doi.org/10.1016/S0032-9592(02)00071-7]

[44] Zhang JF, Gong S, Guo ZG. Effects of different elicitors on 10-deacetylbaccatin III-10-O-acetyltransferase activity and cytochrome P450 monooxygenase content in suspension cultures of

Taxus cuspidata cells. Cell Biol Int Rep 2010; 18(1): e00009.
[PMID: 23119144]

[45]   Badi H, Abdoosi V, Farzin N. New approach to improve taxol biosynthetic. Trakia J Sci Ser Biomed Sci 2015; 13(2): 115-24.
[http://dx.doi.org/10.15547/tjs.2015.02.002]

[46]   Smetanska I. Production of secondary metabolites using plant cell cultures. Adv Biochem Eng Biotechnol 2008; 111: 187-228.
[http://dx.doi.org/10.1007/10_2008_103] [PMID: 18594786]

[47]   Klimek-Szczykutowicz M, Dziurka M, Blažević I, *et al.* Precursor boosted production of metabolites in *Nasturtium officinale* microshoots grown in plant form bioreactors, and antioxidant and antimicrobial activities of biomass extracts. Molecules 2021; 26(15): 4660.
[http://dx.doi.org/10.3390/molecules26154660] [PMID: 34361814]

[48]   Arafa NM, Mohamed SS, Aly US. *In vitro* antimicrobial activity of carrot callus extracts as affected by tyrosine and tryptophan precursor. Int J Pharm Tech Res 2016; 9(9): 121-9.

[49]   Krolicka A, Szpitter A, Gilgenast E, Romanik G, Kaminski M, Lojkowska E. Stimulation of antibacterial naphthoquinones and flavonoids accumulation in carnivorous plants grown *in vitro* by addition of elicitors. Enzyme Microb Technol 2008; 42(3): 216-21.
[http://dx.doi.org/10.1016/j.enzmictec.2007.09.011]

[50]   Vaishnav P, Demain AL. Unexpected applications of secondary metabolites. Biotechnol Adv 2011; 29(2): 223-9.
[http://dx.doi.org/10.1016/j.biotechadv.2010.11.006] [PMID: 21130862]

CHAPTER 11

The Contemporary Facts Towards *In Vitro* Production of the Plant-derived Medicinal Metabolites

Boregowda Nandini[1], Kiran S. Mawale[1] and Parvatam Giridhar[1,*]

[1] *Plant Cell Biotechnology Department, CSIR-Central Food Technological Research Institute (CFTRI), Mysuru-570 020, Karnataka, India*

Abstract: Plants are active biochemical factories of a vast group of secondary metabolites (SMs) and these SMs are indeed a basic source of various commercial pharmaceutical drugs. From the prehistoric time, plants have been used for therapeutic resolutions. Medicinal and aromatic plants are the biogenic pond of diverse forms of SMs, which results in their overexploitation. There is an increasing need for the natural phytochemicals from plants for sustainable and economical value forces their mass production through *in vitro* plant tissue culture (PTC) methods. A vast quantity of medicinal plants and their metabolites have been developed by *in vitro* culture techniques in a small time period related to conventional methods. *In vitro* plant cell cultures assist in a potential role in the commercial production of SMs. The novel prime practices of *in vitro* techniques facilitate transgenic cultures and enlighten the understanding lane of regulation and expression of biosynthetic pathways. SMs have composite chemical alignment and are created in response to different forms of stress to accomplish various physiological tasks in the plant host system. They are immensely utilized in pharmaceutical industries, dietary supplements, cosmetics, fragrances, dyes, flavors, *etc.* SMs are also termed specialised metabolites, secondary products, toxins or natural products; these are basically organic compounds produced by plants and are not directly involved in the growth and development of the plant. Instead, they usually intervene with ecological interactions and conceivably produce selective support for the plant host by increasing its survivability or productivity. Few SMs are specific for a narrow set of plant species within a phylogenetic group. SMs habitually play a vital role in the defense systems of plants against herbivory and other interspecies defences. Human beings uses SMs mainly for medicines, pigments, flavourings and recreational drugs. Prolonged use of these SMs in several industrial areas still needs to be focused to enhance the fabrication by using *in vitro* PTC practices and optimizing their large-scale fabrication using bioreactors. The present book chapter intends to highlight the rationale of the *in vitro* production of SMs from medicinal plants and their progress in the modern epoch for the mass production facts toward the step of commercial and economical forte.

* **Corresponding author Parvatam Giridhar:** Plant Cell Biotechnology Department, CSIR-Central Food Technological Research Institute (CFTRI), Mysuru- 70 020, Karnataka, India; Tel: +91-821-2516510, Fax: +91-821-2517332; E-mail: giridharp@cftri.res.in

Keywords: Bioreactor,   Micropropagation,   Phytochemicals,   Secondary metabolites.

INTRODUCTION

Secondary metabolites (SMs) of plant species are the chemical building blocks for their therapeutically beneficial effects. They are also important indicators for determining the quality of pharmaceutical materials [1]. Plant SMs are naturally occurring sources of biologically active compounds that are used in a healthy diet, traditional medicine, and a variety of industrial applications [2]. In response to various forms of stress, plants produce SMs with a complex chemical composition. These metabolites are used to perform various physiological tasks. There is a wide range of applications for these chemicals in the pharmaceutical and cosmetic industries, cosmetics, dietary supplements, fragrances, flavors, dyes, *etc.* It has become necessary to focus research efforts on increasing the production of these metabolites by employing plant tissue culture (PTC) techniques and optimizing their large-scale production using bioreactors [3]. When it comes to health benefits, medicinal plants are superior to synthetic drugs in terms of safety and cost [4 - 6]. The herbal medicine industry has recently emerged as one of the fastest-growing in the world. It is estimated that the global trade in medicinal plants and their metabolites will reach US$ 5 trillion by 2050, with an average annual growth rate of 7% [7]. It takes a long time for the plant to grow to the point where it can produce the amount of metabolites desired. To overcome this situation, one alternative method is to use PTC techniques for the rapid production of SMs for commercial use [8].

Because of the wide variety of SMs, most of the plants have medicinal properties that can be attributed to a diverse group of naturally occurring metabolic products. Although these metabolites are not essential for the growth and development of plants [9, 10], they play an important role as signaling molecules and defense agents. They're viewed as economically significant products as insecticides, dyes, flavors, and fragrances are just a few of the many things they're used [11]. When developing SMs for the market, consistency and high yield are critical factors [12, 13]. Secondary metabolite production has been improved using traditional and metabolic engineering methods [14]. Elicitor-mediated augmentation of SMs in plants *ex vitro* and *in vitro* is reported to be a very effective and highly reproducible strategy [15 - 18]. Microbes, considered biotic elicitors, activate a wide range of secondary metabolic pathways (fungi, bacteria, viruses, yeast, *etc.*). Bacterial, fungal, and yeast extracts are increasingly being used to induce SMs because of their better yield and quality [18 - 20]. Fungal elicitors are the best way to increase the production of SMs in PTC [21]. It activates secondary metabolic pathways and phytoalexins in plant disease resistance physiological progressions [3]. Alkaloids, terpenoids, steroids, saponins, phenolics, flavanoids and amino acids are just a few examples of the many SMs that are used in pharmaceutical preparations. Bioreactor design, nutrient optimization, selection of highly productive lines, elicitation, two-phase cultivation, and metabolic engineering have all been employed in PTC to augment the SMs production in a large scale [22 - 24].

There are approximately 100,000 SMs in the plant kingdom, all of which are restricted to specific taxonomic groups. The three major groups of SMs in plants are nitrogen-containing compounds (cyanogenic glycosides, alkaloids, and glucosinolates), phenolic compounds (flavonoids and phenylpropanoids), and terpenes (isoprenoids) based on their biosynthetic pathways [25]. In the current book chapter, a few selected botanicals are overviewed for their SMs under *in vitro* conditions, like a callus, suspension cells, and root cultures. The Table **1** provides an overview of the growth and development of a few selected plants' secondary metabolites under *in vitro* conditions. A new solution for the production and conservation of natural products is to use PTC of higher plants as a renewable and environmentally friendly raw material source.

Table 1. List of selected plants and elicitors used to induce secondary metabolites under *in vitro* culture conditions.

S. No	Plant Species	Elicitors	Secondary Metabolites	Type of Culture	References
1.	*Artemisia absinthium*	MeJA, JA and GA	Total phenolic and Total flavonoid content	Suspension	[378]
2.	*Artemisia absinthium*	silver and copper nanoparticles	Secondary metabolites and antioxidants	Callus cultures	[379]
3.	*Artemisia vulgaris*	Farnesyl Diphosphate	ß-Caryophyllene	Callus and Hairy Root Cultures	[380]
4.	*Codonopsis pilosula*	Methyl Jasmonate	Atractylenolide, lobetyolinin and polysaccharide	Adventitious roots and multiple shoots	[381]
5.	*Achillea gypsicola*	MeJA and SA	Camphor and phenolic content	Cell suspension	[382]
6.	*Thevetia peruviana*	MeJA and SA	Phenolic content	cell suspension	[383]
7.	*Catharanthus roseus*	cyclodextrins and MeJA	Terpenoid indole alkaloid	Cell cultures	[128]
8.	*Catharanthus roseus*	artemisinic acid	Vindoline and vinblastine	Cell suspension	[384]
9.	*Catharanthus roseus*	Sodium Nitroprusside	Terpenoid Indole Alkaloid	Hairy Root Cultures	[385]

(Table 1) cont.....

S. No	Plant Species	Elicitors	Secondary Metabolites	Type of Culture	References
10.	*Catharanthus roseus*	JA	Fatty Acid and Terpenoid Indole Alkaloid	Cell suspension	[126]
11.	*Hypericum perforatum*	light	Secondary metabolites	Adventitious root	[386]
12.	*Hypericum perforatum*	perlite nanoparticles and TiO2/perlite	Secondary metabolites	Callus cultures	[387]
13.	*Hypericum Perforatum*	Fungal mycelia	Secondary metabolite	Cell suspensions	[388]
14.	*Hypericum Perforatum*	Polysaccharide	Secondary Metabolite and Antioxidant	Shoot culture	[389]
15.	*Portulaca oleracea*	MeJaA and SA	Dopamine	Hairy root	[390]
16.	*Taxus baccata*	MeJA and Squalestatin	Phenolic content	Cell suspension	[391]
17.	*Taxus* spp.	MeJA and Cyclodextrins	Taxane	Cell	[392]
18.	*Nothapodytes foetida*	Gamma Irradiation	Camptothecin	Callus Cultures	[393]
19.	*Chlorophytum borivilianum*	JA and SA	Diosgenin	Cell cultures	[394]
20.	*Lavandula angustifolia*	JA and SA	Biochemical	Cell culture	[395]
21.	*Aloe arborescens*	Meta-topolin (mT), (mTR), (MemT) and (BAR),	Secondary metabolite and antioxidant	Adventitious shoot	[33]
22.	*Cupressus sempervirens*	-	Secondary metabolite	Callus cultures	[175]
23.	*Arnebia euchroma*	-	Shikonin	Suspension culture	[47]
24.	*Arnebia spp.*	-	Napthoquinone metabolite (shikonin)	Cell suspension	[396]
25.	*Lychnis fos-cuculi*	-	Ecdysteroids, triterpenoid saponins, flavonoids, and phenolic acids	Shoot cultures, fast-growing roots, and callus	[266]
26.	*Podophyllum Hexandrum*	MeJA	Podophylloxin (ptox)	Cell	[397]
27.	*Ajuga bracteosa*	MeJA	Phytoecydysteroids	Hairy root	[398]

(Table 1) cont.....

S. No	Plant Species	Elicitors	Secondary Metabolites	Type of Culture	References
28.	*Satureja khuzistanica*	MeJA	Rosmarinic acid	Cell suspension	[399]
29.	*Silybum marianum*	MeJA and Cyclodextrin	Silymarin	Cell	[400]
30.	*Salvia miltiorrhiza*	MeJA	Tashinones	Hairy root	[401]
31.	*Bacopa monnieri*	MeJA	Bacoside	Shoot	[278]
32.	*Centella asiatica*	MeJA	Centelloside	Cell suspension	[402]
33.	*Gymnema sylvestre*	MeJA	Gymnemic acid	Cell suspension	[403]
34.	*Panax gingseng*	MeJA	Ginsenosides	Hairy root lines	[404]
35.	*Panax gingseng*	Cerium	Ginsenosides	Hairy root lines	[405]
36.	*Panax gingseng*	MeJA	Gingsenosides (Rg 3)	-	[406]
37.	*Hypericum perforatum*	SA	Hypericin and pseudo hypericin	Cell suspension	[407]
38.	*Plumbago indica*	JA	Plumbagin	Hairy root	[408]
39.	*Stephania venosa*	SA and Chitosan	Dicentrine	Cell suspension	[356]
40.	*Withania somnifera*	MeJA and SA	Withanolide A, Witholide, Withaferin A	Hairy root	[409]

Aloe arborescens Mill

Aloe arborescens (Asphodelaceae), also known as krantz aloe, is harvested in the wild in South Africa and exported to Japan, where it is used in traditional Japanese medicine [26]. Several *Aloe* species have been micropropagated for topolins production under *in vitro* conditions by various researchers [27 - 30]. With the exception of *A. vera*, all Aloe species are protected as a conservation measure by the Convention on International Trade in Endangered Species [26]. The use of topolins in micropropagation studies of Aloe species has only been reported in a few studies [31, 32]. A study found that the type and concentration of cytokinins used exogenously during tissue culture have a significant impact on not only shoot proliferation but also the *in vitro* production of bioactive SMs [33 - 35].

Aralia elata (Miq.) Seem

Araliaceae has 50 genera and 1412 species [36]. The Araliaceae family has 71 species, many of which are used as food and medicine in Eurasian countries [37 - 39]. *A. elata* is a well-known traditional medicine and wild vegetable due to its high flavonoid and saponin content. Heavy shoot hunting has nearly depleted this species' natural reserve, but its traditional culture regime is heavily reliant on land use [40]. Explants and Plant growth regulators (PGRs) have been used to establish a somatic embryogenesis micropropagation system for *A. elata* [41]. and induced somatic embryogenic callus from winter buds of 10-year-old trees nurtured on MS medium basal salts [42]. Plantlets from somatic embryo germination emerged after a five-month culture period [43]. Kang *et al* . [44] grew embryogenic callus from hairy roots in the same conditions. When leaflet petioles were grown on MS medium containing 1.0 mg/l, 2,4-D and 0.5 mg/l, 6-benzyladenine (BA) for one month in early spring, they produced somatic embryogenic callus. After co-cultivation with *A. rhizogenes* ATCC 15834, transgenic hairy roots were induced from petiole and root segments of the *in vitro* plant *A. elata*. Putative hairy root induction from root segments was higher (26.7%) in contrast to 10% of petiole explants.

Arnebia euchroma (Royle) J onst.

Arnebia is a genus of about 25 species in the Boraginaceae family. *Arnebia euchroma* is a perennial Alpine grass that can be found in the Pamirs, Tien Shan, western Tibet, and the Himalayas [45]. Rabinovich and Davydenkov initiated *A. euchroma* tissue culture in Russia in 1987 [46]. In suspension culture, the composition of the naphthoquinone fraction differed from that of the intact plant. In contrast to the intact plant, benzoquinones were found to accumulate in cultured cells. It was found that in suspension culture, cell aggregate cloning was effective in increasing shikonin production [47]. Kumar *et al* . [48] found that stimulation of shikonin biosynthesis was mutual with a reduction in cell growth, and adding 102 μM ethyl jasmonate and 10 μM 12-oxophytodienoic acid to suspension culture for 5-6 days increases the level of shikonin by 12- and 8-fold, respectively. Kozlovtseva *et al* . [49] reported that the shikonin extraction *in situ* with paraffin oil and hexadecane did not result in increased shikonin production during the second step of cultivation. To increase shikonin production, Sokha [50] optimised the macroelement composition of the medium and selected procedures (mainly transferring tissue in the stationary growth phase). Also, the accumulation of triterpene saponin and coumarin in tissue culture was reported. An elicitor from *Rhizoctonia solani* increases shikalkin production in *A. euchroma* callus. The effects of Cu^{2+}, MeJA, and SA on shikalkin production in *A. euchroma* callus were compared. At 25°C, indole acetic acid (IAA) (1M) and kinetin (10M) induced pigment production on White medium. *R. solani* increased pigment production by 7 fold over White medium. Cu^{2+} doubled shikalkin output. MeJA and SA had similar enhancement effects as Cu^{2+} [51].

Artemisia annua L.

The Chinese aromatic annual herb *A. annua* (Sweet wormwood) belongs to the Asteraceae family and produces the most potent antimalarial drug 'artemisinin,' a sesquiterpene lactone that is efficacious against chloroquine and quinine-resistant *Plasmodium falciparum* and many other malaria-causing parasites [52]. Several *in vitro* studies have shown that artemisinin accumulates in callus [53, 54], suspension cells [55], shoots [56 - 58], and hairy root cultures [57, 59]. In terms of artemisinin production, *A. annua* callus and cell suspension cultures are disappointing. Artemisinin biosynthesis appears to necessitate some degree of differentiation of shoot cultures [60]. Previous studies have documented the effect of medium composition on the growth and production of phytochemicals in a variety of plant cell cultures [58, 61]. PTC *in vitro* could be a viable alternative to traditional methods of producing artemisinin. *A. annua* shoot cultures were established on MS basal medium containing 30 g sucrose, 0.5 mg 6-benzyladenine, and 0.05 mg naphthaleneacetic acid per litre. With enhanced artemisinin production of 26.7 mg/l under *in vitro* conditions [58]. However, numerous attempts have been made to improve artemisinin production, including genetic transformations through the over-expression of artemisinin biosynthetic pathway genes in plants [62], microorganisms [63], and other expression systems such as hairy roots [64] and cell cultures [65], but little success has been reported due to the high cost of production and difficulties posed. As a result, simpler, less expensive, and more effective approaches are required for the drug's rapid commercialization. A short-term application of UV-B to *in vitro* grown plantlets of *A. annua* may be a safe method of ensuring a steady supply of artemisinin-producing plantlets and also simultaneously regulating the plant's stress response genes [66].

Chamomile spp.

Matricaria chamomilla (synonym: *Matricaria recutita*), more commonly referred to as chamomile (also spelled camomile), German chamomile, Hungarian chamomile (kamilla), wild chamomile, blue chamomile, or scented mayweed, is an annual plant in the Asteraceae family [67, 68]. Most herbal teas are made from chamomile (*Matricaria chamomilla*), which has anti-inflammatory, analgesic, antibiotic, antispasmodic, An antispasmodic (synonym: spasmolytic) is a pharmaceutical drug or other agent that suppresses muscle spasms and sedative properties [69]. The therapeutic use of chamomile is due to its high phenolic, terpenoids, essential oil, and flavonoid content [70, 71]. Inflammatory and bacterial diseases of the skin and internal organs have traditionally been treated with chamomile (*C. recutita*) [72, 73]. Čellárová *et al* . [74, 75] cultured chamomile callus from young receptacles in LS medium [76]. Reichling &

Becker [77] used stem- and leaf explants to induce callus cultures from two chamomile varieties ('E40' and 'BK2') on a modified MS medium supplemented with 2.4 µM NAA. Riechling *et al* . [78] established callus cultures and a successful micropropagation system from seeds of five chamomile varieties cultured on MS medium supplemented with NAA (27.7 µM) and Kinetin (11.9 µM). Passamonti *et al* . [79] established callus cultures and a successful micropropagation system from seeds of five chamomile varieties cultured on MS medium supplemented with 0.05 µM NAA and 11.6 µM kinetin. Chamomile hairy root culture was used to increase the essential oil content and pharmacologically bioactive compounds α - bisabolol and ß - eudesmol in large quantities [80]. On MS proliferating like, medium enriched with NAA, chamomile callus tissue grows into a large mass [81]. The steroidal hormone 17-estradiol will be helpful in optimising the growth of German chamomile cells *in vitro* [82].

Cannabis sativa L.

Cannabis sativa, or marijuana, is an annual dioecious herb from eastern Asia in the Cannabaceae family [83]. *Cannabis sativa* has been used medicinally since 1000 B.C [84]. The Cannabis plant contains over 560 natural product components [85 - 87]. Cannabinoids, terpenes, phenolics, carotenoids, alkaloids, and amino acids are all found in cannabis [88, 89]. Many traditions have used cannabis for centuries to treat pain, spasms, asthma, insomnia, depression, and appetite loss [90]. Cannabinoids are significant chemical compounds including 9-tetrahydrocannabinol, cannabidiol, cannabinol, cannabigerol, and cannabichromene [89]. Callus cultures was initially used to produce cannabinoids, resulting in the conversion of olivetol and cannabidiol to cannabielsoin [91 - 93]. However, cannabinoid production was found to be unstable and insufficient. The primary application of *in vitro* culture in cannabis is micropropagation [94 - 97]. Several reports describe aseptically propagating cannabis stem, cotyledon, and flower explants [98 - 102]. Δ9 -tetrahydrocannabinolic acid synthase (THCAS) was isolated and cloned from cannabis leaves [103]. In cannabis cell suspension cultures [104], used biotic (*Pythium aphanidermatum* and *Botrytis cinerea*) and abiotic (methyl jasmonate, salicylic acid, jasmonic acid, UV-B, $AgNO_3$, $NiSO_4H_2O$, and $CoCl_2H_2O$) elicitors, but no improved cannabinoid production was obtained. In *C. sativa*, meta-topolin (2.0 M) is used in a one-step protocol to promote adventitious shoot formation and root induction under *in vitro* conditions [100]. Recently, a study was published that addressed the issues mentioned above in conventional cannabis micropropagation [105] by employing a two-step *in vitro* photoautotrophic method for cannabis micropropagation. Traditional (photomixotrophic) cannabis micropropagation methods are time-consuming, exhibit high hyperhydricity, and have low shoot proliferation, rooting and acclimation success rates [99, 106]. *In vitr C. sativa* flowering explants responded best to 12.0- and 13.2-hour photoperiod treatments [107]. Explant rooting was evaluated using a photoautotrophic micropropagation system that uses passive ventilation to reduce costs and labour, as well as a number of factors that influence rooting success [108].

Catharanthus roseus (L.) G. Don

Catharanthus roseus is a medicinal plant from Madagascar that belongs to the Apocynaceae family, which is a medicinal plant rich in monoterpene and terpenoid indole alkaloids [109]. *C. roseus* produces a total of 120 alkaloids, with 70 of them having pharmacological activity. Traditional medicine uses it to treat cancer, diabetes, hypertension, and infections. The highest alkaloid content was found during flowering [110]. All Kin/IAA growth hormone combinations produced the highest concentration of vincristine. Only the growth hormone combinations Kin/IAA, IAA/Gb, BAP/Gb, and NAA/Gb showed vinblastine potentiation [111]. Nitrogen (N) and Phosphorus (P) both promote growth while inhibiting alkaloid production [112]. Plant and leaf-organ cultures of *C. roseus* were established by Krueger *et al* . [113] from aseptically germinated seeds on MS Revised Tobacco medium supplemented with benzyladenine (BA). Hirata et al. [114] patented a method for growing *C. roseus* plant organ cultures that yield significant amounts of indole alkaloids like vinblastine, vincristine, vindoline, catharanthine, and ajmalicine. Hirata & Miyamoto [114] made root and shoot cultures from *C. roseus* seedlings. Root cultures and cell suspension cultures showed alkaloid spectra similar to intact plant roots. In multiple-shoot cultures of *C. roseus*, near UV light with a 370 nm peak stimulated the production of leurosine, one of the major dimeric indole alkaloids. Miura *et al* . [115] isolated vinblastine from a callus initiated from young leaf segments of *C. roseus* in MS medium with NAA at 1.0 mg/l and kinetin at 0.1 mg/l. Yokoyama [116] patented a method for extracting arbutin from *C. roseus* callus cultures using Linsmaier-Skoog (LS) medium supplemented with hydroquinone with a yield as high as 306 mg of the compound from 2 g of callus [76]. *C. roseus* hairy root cultures and growth kinetics for indole alkaloid production. Indole alkaloid production in *C. roseus* cell cultures has been extensively studied for the last 20 years [117, 118]. The alkaloid composition of callus tissue was extracted from the roots, stems, leaves, and flowers of *Catharanthus roseus*, encompassing both white and pink-purple varieties. [119]. *In vitro* studies by Pietrosiuk & Furmanowa [120] examined the production of indole alkaloids in different *C. roseus* roots, in which B5/2 liquid medium supplemented with 0.5 mg/l and 0.25 mg/l NAA produced the best results in untransformed root culture. The C. roseus calli culturing procedure proved effective and promising with increasing anthocyanin production with the highest levels of total anthocyanins (78.73 g/gm) in MS medium with 3 and 0.5 M L-phenylalanine and calcium chloride ($CaCl_2$) [121]. MeJA elicited the accumulation of alkaloids (ajmalicine, serpentine, ajmaline, and catharanthine) in *C. roseus* hairy root cultures [122]. In the presence of flavin mononucleotide and manganese ions, non-enzymatic coupling of catharanthine and vindoline occurs under *in vitro* conditions [123]. *Agrobacterium rhizogenes* transformed hairy root cultures of *C. roseus* and effectively produced catharanthine, tabersonine, lochnericine, and horhammericine indole alkaloids [124]. Many *in vitro* cultures have been reported as superior to conventional breeding methods for producing therapeutically important alkaloids [125, 126]. The alkaloid, Alstonine from calli; antirhine and cathindine from cell suspensions; acuamicine and lochnericine from calli and suspensions; horhammericine and vindoline from suspensions and sprouts; tabersonine from calli and suspensions; 3,4-anhydrovinblastine and catharine from suspensions and sprouts; vinblastine from calli, sprouts, and somatic embryos are studied in this plant [109, 127 - 129] used artemisinic acid as an elicitor to increase vindoline and vinblastine production in *C. roseus* cell suspension. Since plants contain only a small amount of these compounds, *in vitro* methods are being used to improve phytochemical production [130].

Chlorophytum borivilianum SANT. Et. FERN

The Liliaceae family's *C. borivilianum* is a small perennial herb. The plant is native to Rajasthan, western M. P., and north Gujarat forests. The adaptogenic and aphrodisiac properties of this plant's tubers are well-known [131, 132]. *C. borivilianum* tubers are the main constituents of over a hundred ayurvedic preparations due to their high therapeutic value [133]. It is known that *C. borivilianum* can be propagated using tissue culture [134 - 136]. Steroidal and tri-terpenoidal saponins, alkaloids, vitamins, minerals, proteins, polysaccharides, and steroids are all abundant in tubers. Fructans, simple sugars like glucose and fructose, phenolics, triterpenoids, gallo-tannins, and mucilage are also present [137]. Because of its medicinal properties, demand for *C. borivilianum* tubers has increased all over the world, with India being a major market [138]. *In vitro* regenerated plantlets produce more SMs, notably saponins, than wild plants, proving that micropropagation can open up new avenues for the study of phytopharmaceuticals and bioprospecting of rare and important medicinal plants [139].

Coleus spp.

In Indian Ayurvedic Medicine, the medicinal plant *Coleus forskohlii* (Lamiaceae/Labiatae) is commonly used. SMs, labdane diterpenoid forskolin, is reported to have numerous biological and pharmacological properties [140]. As an adenylate cyclase activator, forskolin has been found [141]. The roots of *C.*

forskohlii plants are the only source of forskolin, but the concentration of the metabolite from wild plants in natural habitats is extremely low [142]. Forskolin was found in callus derived from young leaves of *C. forskohlii* plants. The micropropagation and *in vitro* culture of different Coleus species, as well as the production of forskolin and rosmarinic acid, is known [143]. There have also been reports of large-scale production of rosmarinic acid (RA) and forskolin from cell cultures of *C. blumei* and *C. forskohlii*, respectively. In transformed cultures of *C. blumei* and *C. forskohlii*, genetic transformation using *Agrobacterium* has been shown to increase RA and forskolin production [143]. Forskolin production was observed in untransformed suspension cultures of *C. forskohlii* [144]. Nodal segments to achieve *in vitro* clonal multiplication of C. forskolii and discovered that the forskolin content (0.1%) in tubers of micropropagated plants was the same as that found in wild plants [145]. Forskolin production in different *C. forskohlii in vitro* culture systems [145]. On MS and White's basal medium, shoot tips, callus, and root tip cultures were established with and without plant growth regulators (PGRs). The root callus cells of *C. forskohlii* produce coleonol (forskolin) [146]. The effect of 35 differently substituted phenoxyacetic acids (10-5 M) was investigated on the production of RA and discovered that 2,4-D had the greatest effect, increasing RA production by 40% [147]. The amount of RA accumulated by *C. blumei* suspension cultures is strongly influenced by the amount of carbohydrates added to the culture media [147 - 149]. Cell suspension cultures of *C. blumei* are among the highest-producing plant cell cultures in terms of secondary product formation, according to Inomata *et al* . [150], who reported an accumulation of RA up to 21% of the cell dry weight in *C. blumei* cell cultures. Martinez & Park [151] investigated the effects of sucrose concentration on cell viability, cell growth, RA production, sugar consumption, product yield, and cell yield in suspension cultures of preconditioned and non-preconditioned *C. blumei.*

Coptis japonica (Thunb.) Makino

Coptis japonica, also known as Japanese goldthread, is a flowering plant in the Ranunculaceae family that is native to central and southern Japan. Berberine, the main alkaloid, is grown for medicinal purposes in Asia. Berberine is an antibacterial, stomachic, and anti-inflammatory alkaloid. In the source plant's roots, Yamada and Sato established Coptis cell cultures and selected highly productive cell lines using a small cell aggregate selection method. Few publications report that berberine production in cell cultures is higher than in plants [152, 153]. The addition of gibberellic acid (GA$_3$) to the culture medium increased the production of berberine by *Coptis japonica* cell cultures [154]. The high-density culture method improved berberine yield from highly productive *Coptis japonica* cells [155].

Curcuma longa L.

Curcuma longa (Zingiberaceae), often known as turmeric and recognized as the "golden spice" and "spice of life," is widely utilised in Ayurvedic, Unani, and Siddha medicine as well as a home cure for a variety of ailments [156]. Concerning *C. longa* and other curcuma species, micropropagation and plant regeneration from callus, as well as *in-vitro* culture investigations, have been described [157 - 161]. Microrhizomes were grown in liquid media *in vitro*. Sucrose levels increased in correlation with rhizome size, and larger microrhizomes were capable of field survival without acclimation [157, 162]. Large microrhizomes of turmeric can be produced in bigger culture vessels with mild agitation [163]. Regardless of the unpredictability associated with international exporting of seasonal agricultural products, *in vitro* prepared rhizomes are a readily available source of fresh turmeric tissue [164]. Cousins *et al* . [165] investigated secondary metabolism-inducing treatments on turmeric rhizomes *in vitro*. Micropropagation of a disease-free elite clone of turmeric *in vitro* has been established using clonal multiplication [166], organogenesis [167], somatic embryogenesis [161], and bioreactor [168]. Curcumin, demethoxycurcumin, and bis-demethoxycurcumin were studied in several systems. Studies has also been performed to directly quantify curcuminoids in turmeric shoots and microrhizomes used in nutritional supplements [169]. Depending on the nutritional media, phytohormones, concentration, and cell line, the callus culture of fresh lateral buds of C. longa can produce significant amounts of polyphenols and curcumin [170]. Curcumin has been shown in previous in silico studies to inhibit the binding of the spike (S) glycoprotein of SARS-CoV-2 to the angiotensin-converting enzyme 2 (ACE-2) receptor [171, 172]. When curcumin was added to cell culture supernatants, the amount of SARS-CoV-2 RNA was considerably reduced. SARS-CoV-2 was successfully eliminated in Vero E6 and human Calu3 cells by turmeric root extract, dissolved turmeric capsule content, and pure curcumin [173]. Turmeric PB009 and ST018 were acclimated *in vitro* to greenhouse settings using 6%t sucrose and 4% glucose, which resulted in a higher percentage of survival, physiological adaption, and overall growth performance [174].

Cupressus sempervirens L.

Cupressus sempervirens (Cupressaceae) is commonly referred to as the Mediterranean cypress and is primarily grown as an ornamental. *C. sempervirens* has recognized therapeutic qualities due to the presence of a range of SMs that are the subject of pharmacological patents. and/or cosmetics currently on the market. The plant's aerial parts are used as an astringent in folk medicine to treat haemorrhoids, varicose veins, and venous circulation disorders. *In vitro* studies have shown that *C. sempervirens* callus can produce rutin, quercetin, and other metabolites for commercial use at appropriate quantities. [175]. There was little or no information on the production of SMs from the *C. sempervirens* plant using the *in vitro* callus culture technique.

Dioscorea spp.

Chinese traditional medicine uses *Dioscorea* species (Dioscoreaceae) as a tonic. *Dioscorea deltoidea* is an endangered medicinal plant widely used in traditional medicine and pharmaceutical industries. *D. deltoidea* is a tropical and subtropical plant that grows in India's northwestern Himalayas [176]. It has a long history in both traditional and modern medicine. The effect of elicitors MeJA and SA, and precursors (squalene, sitosterol, and cholesterol) on diosgenin production from *D. deltoidea* shoot cultures [177] and in *D. galesttiana* cells was studied [178]. Endophytic fungus *F. oxysporum* Dzf17 significantly enhanced diosgenin accumulation in *D. zingiberensis* cell cultures. Oligosaccharides from the endophytic fungus *F. oxysporum* Dzf17 show to increase diosgenin production in *D. zingiberensis* cell cultures [179].

Echinacea spp.

Echinacea is a perennial plant genus in the Asteraceae family native to North America. Native Americans used *Echinacea purpurea*, *Echinacea angustifolia*, and *Echinacea pallida* to treat a variety of inflammatory and allergic conditions, including swollen gums, inflamed skin, sore throats, and gastrointestinal disorders [180]. Most studies on caffeic acid derivatives, alkamides, and anthocyanins used *in vitro* grown *Echinacea* species [181]. Also, cinnamic acid and caffeic acid were isolated from Echinacea callus cultures [182]. According to the literature, the reproductive stems of *Echinacea purpurea* contained significantly more alkamides than the leaves [183]. The main difference was in *E. angustifolia in vitro* alkamide content. The amount of alkamide in cultured tissues was higher than in greenhouse leaves [184, 185]. Many such studies focused on establishing an effective regeneration system with callus and/or shoot cultures [186 - 189], providing mass production with micropropagation [190] and obtaining secondary metabolites of standard quality and efficiency [121, 191]. The presence of echinacoside, caffeic acid derivatives, and polysaccharides was merely found in cell suspension cultures from *E. angustifolia* seedling tissues [192]. However, after the first subcultures, *E. angustifolia* shoots showed high hyperhydricity, abundant callus, and *de novo* shoot formations on the veins of intact leaves, as observed by [193]. Cell, callus, and hairy root cultures were used to investigate the biosynthetic pathways of significant phytochemicals in Echinacea [194]. Echinacea cell cultures have been successfully used to produce polysaccharides on a small and large scale [195, 196]. Transgenic Echinaceae hairy roots demonstrated significant differences in root growth and caffeic acid derivatives production [197 - 201]. SOD and APX are upregulated in *Echinacea purpurea* AR cultures by 100M sodium nitroprusside, promoting phenolic, flavonoid, and caffeic acid derivative accumulation [202]. *E. purpurea* hairy root cultures accumulate dicaffeoyl tartaric, caffeoylquinic, and caffeoyl tartaric acid derivatives when exposed to light [199]. *In vitro* plants treated with gibberellic acid (GA3), paclobutrazol, uniconazole, or both increased the concentration of caftaric acid in the roots but had little effect on the concentration in the shoots of *E. purpurea* [203]. The active shoot organogenesis from flower stalks of *E. angustifolia* adult plants was established, as well as the first report on caffeic acid derivative and alkamide production from *E. angustifolia* adult plant *in vitro* regenerated shoots [204]. *Agrobacterium rhizogenes* strain A4 and *Agrobacterium tumefaciens* strain GV3101, containing only the rolABC genes, were used to transform hairy root cultures of three *Echinacea* species (*E. angustifolia, E. purpurea, and E. pallida*). The effects of sucrose, media composition, jasmonic acid, and indolebutyric acid on transformed cultures were studied [205]. Caffeic acid derivatives, phenolics, and flavonoids have been successfully produced in bioreactors using Echinacea ARs from several species, including *E. pallida, E. purpurea, and E. angustifolia* [206 - 208]. Experimenting with different plant extract compositions and their potential therapeutic effects may help to better understand the potential therapeutic effects of different Echinacea preparations [209]. Caffeic acid production *in vitro* and RAPD analysis of some *E. purpurea* plant varieties are being studied [210]. Active compounds and biological activity of some *Echinacea purpurea* cultivars cultured *in vitro*. The Echinacea extracts investigated (*in vitro* and *in vivo* plants and calli of the two varieties) demonstrated a moderate level of activity against the microbial strains tested [211]. It was found 5.63 mg/g cichoric acid in the callus of *E. purpurea* root explants cultured in 2.0 mg/l 2.4-D + 1.0 mg/l modified 1/2 MS medium containing KIN [212]. ARs from *E. pallida* and *E. purpurea* co-cultured can reduce pro-inflammatory mediator production in mouse peritoneal macrophages by regulating MAPK signalling pathways [213]. New lines of *E. purpurea* micropropagated*via* somatic embryogenesis have been studied for secondary metabolites and genetic stability [214]. Compared to l-phenylalanine, 24-epibrassinolide can successfully increase secondary metabolite production in transgenic hairy roots of *E. purpurea* [215]. Physical and biochemical differences between transgenic hairy root lines of *E. purpurea* mediated by *Agrobacterium rhizogenes* [216]. On co-cultured Echinacea adventitious roots showed that antioxidant enzyme activity increased with 25 μM MeJA, indicating that antioxidant enzyme activity increases with secondary metabolite synthesis [217].

Eryngium alpinum L.

Eryngium alpinum L. (*Alpine eryngo*), a member of the Apiaceae subfamily Saniculoideae, is listed in Annex II of the Habitats Directive and Appendix I of the Bern Convention on the Conservation of European Wildlife and Natural Habitats (The Bern Convention), and is protected by the European Habitats Directive—Natura 2000 as well as national red lists in some European countries [218]. The International Union for Conservation of Nature (IUCN) classifies the species as vulnerable [219]. Shoots cultured on media supplemented with different phytohormones were able to produce the desired phenolics—phenolic acids and flavonoids [220]. Even though there are approximately 230–250, *Eryngium* species in the world, still a few have been invented into *in vitro* cultures, such as *E. foetidum* [220 - 223], *E. planum* [224 - 226], *E. maritimum* [227], *E. campestre* [228], and *E. viviparum* [229]. Some Eryngium species have their phenolic acid content measured qualitatively and quantitatively in *in vitro* biomass [224, 225, 227, 228]. The *E. planum* callus and cell suspension were high in rosmarinic, chlorogenic, and caffeic acids. Shoots cultured on solid MS medium had 3.5 times the RA and 24.33 times the caffeic acid content of intact plant basal leaves [224]. The presence of rosmarinic, chlorogenic, and caffeic acids was confirmed in *E. planum* shoots agitated in the liquid MS media [225]. Two phenolic acids, RA and chlorogenic acid, were found in *E. maritimum* shoots and roots. The levels of RA and chlorogenic acid (CA) in cultured shoots are 4.96 and 8.02 times higher, respectively, than in whole plant basal leaves. [227]. Kikowska *et al* . [230] illustrated the effect of different culture systems on phenolic compound production in *E. alpinum in vitro* shoots culture.

Ginkgo biloba L.

Ginkgophyta (Ginkgoaceae) is only known from the Ginkgo or maidenhair tree. It is a 'living fossil' because it is one of the oldest plants capable of living over 1,000 years [231]. It is also known for its unique properties that contribute to its longevity and disease resistance. It has been around for 200 million years [232]. Tulecke [233] established the first *G. biloba* cell culture, using pollen grains as explants in a modified White medium supplemented with 0.25% yeast extract and 1 mg/l a-naphthalene acetic acid (NAA). Nakanishi *et al* . [234] were the first to cultivate *G. biloba* cultures in order to decipher the ginkgolide biosynthetic pathway. Park *et al* . [235] investigated the effect of various media on the production of ginkgolides and bilobalides. The results indicated that MS medium produced significantly more ginkgolides and bilobalides than Gamborg B5, SH, or WPM. Using cell culture, Kang *et al* . [236] investigated the impact of precursor feeding on the synthesis of bilobalides and ginkgolides. After treatment with the bacteria *Staphylococcus aureus* and the yeast *Candida albicans*. Kang *et al* . [237] observed an increase in ginkgolides and bilobalides. Treatment of 800 mM KCl increased the concentration of GA, GB, and bilobalide in both cells and culture medium in ginkgo [238].

Hypericum perforatum L.

Hypericum perforatum (Hypericaceae) is an herb that is widely used in both traditional and modern medicine. Clinical studies *in vitro* and *in vivo* demonstrate antiviral, antifungal, antibacterial, wound-healing, antidepressant, and antioxidant properties [239, 240]. The medicinal properties of the plant are attributed to the presence of SMs such as phloroglucinols (hyperfoliatin, hyperforin, adhyperforin), naphtodianthrones (pseudohypericin, hypericin), tannins (cathechin and epicatechin), flavonoids (rutin, quercetin, isoquercitrin, quercitrin, amentoflavone and hyperoside), proanthocyanidins (procyanidin B_2) and bioflavonoids (biapigenin and amentoflavone) and minor quantities of essential oil [241 - 244]. *In vitro* culture systems have been reported to be a viable alternative to large-scale production of pharmaceutically active metabolites [245, 246]. Using phytohormones and various elicitors, the overproduction of naphtodianthrones from *H. perforatum* cell suspension cultures has been adapted [244, 247, 248].

Hypericum spp.

Regarding naphthodianthrone hypericin isolation, several *Hypericum* spp. grown *in vitro* produce this economically important metabolite [249 - 251]. *In vitro* hypericin extraction from *H. canariense* shoots and plantlets was described by [251]. Several authors also reported that 6-benzylaminopurine did not affect the hypericin content of *in vitro* regenerated *H. perforatum* plants [249, 252].

Lavandula spp.

Lavenders (*Lavandula* spp., Lamiaceae) are fragrant ornamental plants that are extensively used in the food, fragrance, and pharmaceutical industries. Lavenders are mint-family flowering plants that are endemic to the Mediterranean region, the Arabian Peninsula, the Canary Islands, and India. There are 39 species, numerous hybrids, and nearly 400 registered cultivars [253], many of which have highly valued aromatic and medicinal properties in the fragrance, pharmaceutical, food, and flavour industries. Additionally, lavenders are popular as ornamental and decorative plants [254]. Calvo *et al* . [255] found that increasing the osmolarity of the medium or supplementing it with 25–50 mM ABA increased monoterpene yield while keeping the profile qualitatively similar to the parent plants. Banthorpe *et al* . [256] used terpenoids-accumulating callus lines to boost alkaloid biosynthesis in other species. The effect of elicitors on RA production by *L. vera* cells is well documented, and its accumulation can be induced by modifying nutrient supply like, cis and trans p-coumaric acids and ß-sitostero l [257 - 259]. The cultivation mode influences the volatile metabolite profile of *L. vera* cell suspension cultures, resulting in differences between two-phase systems with resin and stirred tank bioreactors [260]. SMs have been found in *L. angustifolia* Mill. *angustifolia* suspension cell cultures.

Lithospermum erythrorhizon Sieb. et Zucc.

L. erythrorhizon (Boraginaceae) is a Japanese, Korean, and Chinese perennial herbaceous plant. Because this plant's root bark (cork layers) contains a high concentration of red naphthoquinone pigments (shikonin derivatives), the roots of *L. erythrorhizon* are red-purple in colour and have been used as a dye since ancient times. Shikonin, an SM of *L. erythrorhizon*, was first produced industrially in the 1980s. In the 1970s and 1980s, Mitsui Chemicals (formerly Mitsui Petrochemical Industries) began producing shikonin from *Lithospermum erythrorhizon* cell cultures. *L. erythrorhizon* cells couldn't produce enough shikonin due to the high concentration of ammonium ions in the medium [261]. Stable transformation methods for non-model plants like *L. erythrorhizon* are difficult to establish, but they can improve secondary metabolite productivity and by genetic engineering. This plant has been used traditionally to treat wounds, burns, frostbite, haemorrhoids and tumours [262]. The roots of this plant are medicinal, producing large amounts of shikonin derivatives, which are red naphthoquinone derivatives. In M9 medium, *L. erythrorhizon* cells produce large amounts of lithospermic acid B [263]. Shikonin-producing plant species *L. erythrorhizon* has been the most studied because shikonin-producing cultured cells were established in the 1970s and used in the 1980s for industrial production. One of the most striking features of this cell culture system is that shikonin production is negatively regulated by light irradiation [264].

Lychnis flos-cuculi L.

Lychnis flos-cuculi is an herbaceous plant of the caryophyllaceae family, growing on wet meadows and flood plains throughout Europe and Northern Asia. Plant populations are dwindling due to changes in traditional meadow cultivation and exploitation, as well as in the drainage of those meadows to create arable land. Many studies have shown that *L. flos-cuculi* contains phenolic acids, flavonoids and ecdysteroids, and a significant amount of complex triterpenoid saponins [265 - 268]. Additionally, *L. flos-cuculi* has the highest antioxidant activity of any plant whose inflorescences have been studied. *L. flos-cuculi* plants grown *in vitro*, including their roots, were studied for the first time for their total polyphenol content and antioxidant activity. Such *in vitro* raised biomass is suitable for further investigations on phytochemical composition and biological activities [267].

Morinda citrifolia L.

Morinda citrifolia (Rubiaceae) has been used for food and medicine in Polynesia for over 2,000 years. This plant's leaf, fruit, bark, and root all contain medicinally active components with antibacterial, antiviral, and anticancer properties [269]. Baque *et al* . [270] investigated the ability of a wide range of auxins to induce anthraquinone (AQ) production in *M. citrifolia* cells. AQs in *M. citrifolia* cell suspensions was illustrated *via* a model system for analyzing secondary and primary metabolism interactions. AQ levels ranged from 0.2-43.4 mmol (100-200 mg) g^{-1} dry weight during growth and stationary phases [271]. AQs from *M. citrifolia* suspension cultures have been widely reported [272 - 274], but commercialization has been hampered may be due to fluctuations in AQs content and excessive foaming in *M. citrifolia* callus cell cultures [275]. Large-scale production of AQs from *M. citrifolia* is difficult due to low AQ content and continuous bioreactor foaming during suspension cultures [275, 276]. This plant has around 160 phytochemicals, mainly polyphenols, organic acids, and alkaloids are reported [277]. Conversely, *in vitro*-induced adventitious roots showed rapid proliferation and metabolic activity [278]. Controlled feeding of the carbon source in the growth medium and elicitor treatment increased AQ accumulation in *M. citrifolia* suspension cultures [279]. Using a balloon-type bubble bioreactor, the effects of aeration rate, inoculum density, and MS medium salt strengths were investigated to improve root growth and production of bioactive compounds such as AQs, phenolics, and flavonoids [280]. AQ s are the most commonly reported phenolic compounds. Chitosan shells of shrimps (*Penaeus monodon*) were used as an elicitation method to increase AQ compounds on the callus leaf of *M. citrifolia* [281].

Nicotiana tabacum L.

Nicotiana is a member of the Solanaceae family and consists of 21 species, of which *N. tabacum* and *N. rustica* are well-known sources of smoking tobacco [282]. Early studies on nicotine biosynthesis using tissue cultures produced inconclusive findings. According to [283], nicotine content in explanted tobacco tissues (*N. glutinosa*) decreased rapidly at the start of the culture and was undetectable once the callus was fully established. Similarly, suspension cultures of tobacco cells derived from *N. tabacum* var. Bright Yellow and stem callus of *N. tabacum* var. P-19 [284] produced similar results [285, 286]. The optimal sucrose and available nitrogen concentrations in the culture medium for nicotine production in tobacco tissue culture were 3% and 840 mg N/l, respectively [282].

The lysine decarboxylase (ldc) bacterial gene increases cadaverine and anabasine alkaloids production in hairy roots of *N. tabacum* [287]. Exogenous hyoscyamine increases tropane alkaloids secretion in *N. tabacum* hairy roots [288]. *In vitro* studies on the elicitation of biomass and SMs, as well as the establishment of stable Nicotiana hairy root cultures *via Agrobacterium rhizogenes* transformation, were documented [289]. By decreasing NUP1 (nicotine uptake permease) gene expression in N. tabacum hairy roots, it increased nicotine release in the culture medium [290, 291]. The Geraniol synthase gene isolated from *Valeriana officinalis* was used to produce geraniol in the hairy root culture of *N. tabacum* [292]. *N. tabacum* is a versatile model system for PTC and genetic engineering research [293]. The relationship between tobacco leaf structures (trichomes) and SMs with antimicrobial activity was studied *in vitro* and in silico approaches [294]. The expression of the ß-cryptogein gene in tobacco hairy roots (*N. tabacum*) suggests a possible channelling of the carbon pool toward phenylpropanoid/benzenoid pathways, lipoxygenase pathways and nicotine biosynthesis [295].

Nothapodytes foetida (Wight)

Nothapodytes foetida is an endangered species found in India's Western Ghats that has gained international attention due to its pharmacological and therapeutic properties. It produces camptothecin, a monoterpenoid indole alkaloid used in the formulation of anticancer drugs [296]. *Camptotheca acuminata, Ophiorrhiza* species, *Ervatamia he yneana, Meriilliodendron megacarpum*, and *N. nimmoniana* are among the plants that produce it [297, 298]. Camptothecin is produced in a variable amount in several parts of *N. foetida* [299], and the alkaloid content rises with the plant's age [300].

Ocimum spp.

Ocimum species are among the world's most vital therapeutic plants [301]. It belongs to the Lamiaceae family, subfamily Ocimoideae, and has over 150 species and varieties [302] in tropical Africa, Asia, and South and Central America [303]. RA was the major phenolic compound in *O. basilicum* hairy root cultures, according to [304]. Monoterpene derivatives (linalool, camphor, 1,8-cineole, geraniol, limonene, and citral), phenyl propanoid derivatives (methyleugenol, eugenol, methylchavicol, chavicol, methylcinnamate), and sesquiterpenoids (bergamotene, bisabolene, and caryophyllene) were the most common constituents in Ocimum species [305 - 307]. Six triterpene acids as oleanolic, betulinic, ursolic, euscaphic, 3-epimaslinic and alphitolic acids were isolated from *O. basilicum* hairy roots cultures by [308] by using *Agrobacterium rhizogenes*. *O. americanum* plantlets grown in MS medium with 1.0 mg/l BA and

0.25 mg/l IAA accumulated a significant amount of RA [309]. Red basil cell line from *O. basilicum* shows improved RA and AC accumulation in cell suspension cultures and identified RA-related molecules such as caffeic acid, coumaric acid, and flavones [310]. Explants and leaf-derived suspension cultures of *O. basilicum* were grown for three weeks in airlift bioreactors, and the fresh weight of the suspension was increased by a factor of 2.5, with an increase in RA accumulation of 29 µg/g DW. It was found that immobilising sweet basil (*O. basilicum*) cells in a high density gel matrix increased RA accumulation (1400 times) [311], also found immobilised *O. basilicum* cells accumulated 5g/l RA) [312]. Cell suspension cultures of *O. basilicum, O. sanctum,* and *O. gratissimum* allow for the industrial production of major SMs of Ocimum species such as phenols, flavanoids, alkaloids, terpenoids, and essential oils [313]. According to El-Kadafy *et al* . [314], shoot and callus cultures of *O. basilicum* grown on a medium containing 5mg/l BA and 1mg/l NAA accumulated higher levels of RA (9.42 to 38.25g/mg DW) than the control. To select elite (high RA producing) cultivars of *O. basilicum*, an *in vitro* growth system followed by *A. rhizogenes*-mediated transformation to select three transformed root lines. *R. irregularis* has greater potential as a biotic elicitor for the production of RA, caffeic acid, and antioxidants under *in vitro* conditions [315, 316]. Chicoric acid levels in callus cultures of *O. bascilicum* ranged from the highest (43.89 mg/g DW) in 5 mg/L TDZ to the lowest (9.17 mg/g DW) in 0.1 mg/L NAA [315]. SMs such as phenols, alkaloids, and terpenoids were measured in *O. basilicum, O. sanctum* and *O. gratissimum* cell cultures elicited with MeJA and chitosan (treatments alone and in combination) [317]. *In vitro* callus cultures of *O. basilicum* produce enhanced phenylpropanoid metabolites like hydroxycinnamic acid derivatives (caffeic acid, chicoric acid, RA) and anthocyanins (cyanidin and peonidin) [318]. *In vitro* cultures of *O. tenuiflorum* and *O. basilicum* were measured and compared for eugenol (leaf), total phenolic content (stem), somatic embryos (leaf, stem), and inflorescence callus (inflorescence callus) [319].

Oenothera biennis L.

Oenothera, commonly referred to as evening primrose, is a genus of Onagraceae family herbaceous flowering plants that contains roughly 145 species. This genus is widely known for its therapeutic characteristics, which include antioxidant, anti-inflammatory, antibacterial, anticancer, and anti-obesity effects. *O. biennis* transformed tissues had increased cytokinin levels and developed as teratomas, creating clumps of short, branching shoots with modified leaves [320]. The 2D TLC method (fingerprinting) was used to analyse flavonoid chemicals and phenolic acids in microshoots and leaves of soil plants grown *in vitro* [321]. Evening primrose seed oil is beneficial for rheumatoid arthritis, breast pain, eczema, and alcoholism [322]. Evening primrose *in vitro* production research has been done on single genotypes and/or explants [320, 323, 324]. Evening primrose is a valuable oil-rich wild flower. Indeterminate inflorescence and diverse germination impede the commercial production of this plant. The hypocotyl tissue of evening primrose is ideal for callus development and somatic embryogenesis [325]. The best medium for *Oenothera biennis* cluster bud induction was MS+6-BA, 2 mg. +NAA, 0.4 mg 30 g L^{-1} sucrose The optimum rooting media for *O. biennis* was 1/2MS+NAA 0.5 mg [326]. For growth and roots, the solid medium of 1/2 MS medium supplemented with 0.1 mg NAA/litre was optimal. Using 0.75 mg L^{-1} BAP for direct regeneration, 0.5 mg L^{-1} 2, 4-D, and 1.25 mg L^{-1} BAP for indirect regeneration, increased *in vitro* synthesis of evening primrose [327].

Panax ginseng C.A. Meyer

Ginseng, or *Panax ginseng* C. A. Meyer (Araliaceae), is a medicinal plant widely used in Asia as a tonic and adaptogenic agent. It is also popular in North America and Europe as a nutraceutical or functional food. *Panax ginseng* produces glycosylated triterpenes called ginsenosides (ginseng). Elicitation strategies have been developed to increase the production of ginsenosides due to the low productivity of metabolite in ginseng cell culture. Many studies have shown that the most commonly known oxylipin compounds, JA and MeJA, can increase ginsenosides production in ginseng adventitious root cultures when used in combination [328 - 332]. Various types of airlift bioreactors for adventitious root growth and ginsenoside accumulation, and they reported that bulb type bubble bioreactors were suitable for biomass accumulation (41.92 g DW) because the oxygen transfer capacity (K L a) was optimum with bulb-type reactors, whereas biomass accumulation was less in cylinder type bioreactors (38.55 g DW) [235]. Various polyunsaturated fatty acids (PUFAs) were used as elicitors to boost biomass accumulation and ginsenoside production in Panax ginseng adventitious root cultures [333]. An investigation was also made into ginsenoside production in liquid media and a pilot-scale culture system using bioreactors [328, 334]. Globally, ginseng products are sold in 35 countries, with an estimated 80,000 tonnes produced annually [335]. Numerous ginsenosides have been shown to have physiological and pharmacological activity in the treatment of heart disease, antifatigue, hepato-protective and anti-tumor and cancer [332, 336, 337]. In the absence of NH^{4+} ions, it was found the highest ginsenoside content of 10.96 mg g^{-1} DW [334]. Elicitation by organic and inorganic elicitors and other additives of *in vitro* grown *P. ginseng* adventitious roots increased ginsenosides production [338]. Nitrogen and phosphorus affect ginsenoside production in *Panax quinquefolium* hairy root cultures grown in shake flasks and nutrient sprinkle bioreactors [339]. Tissue-specific phytohormone distribution correlated with hormone biosynthesis genes that influenced ginsenoside synthesis and distribution [340].

Solanum spp.

There are approximately 1,500 species of Solanum (Solanaceae) in tropical and subtropical regions of the world and South America. The Solanum genus contains many bioactive metabolites, including steroidal alkaloids, pyridines, withanolides, sesquiterpenes and diterpenes, glycoalkaloids, and flavonoids, among others. Numerous compounds with anti-tumor, anti-fungal, and cytotoxic properties can be derived from this species [341, 342]. Solasodine and its glycosides, solasonine and ß-solamardine, have been isolated from various Solanaceae plant cell and tissue cultures [343 - 345]. Solasodine, a pharmaceutically important compound, was yielded at 2% dry weight from 4-month-old callus tissue with rhizogenesis in a medium with 2 mg/l NAA [346]. *In vitro* grown *S. nigrium* shows 150mM NaCl had the best effect on solasodine and proline accumulations. Even at 200mM, NaCl reduced solasodine production [347]. In *S. khasianum*, hairy root cultures had higher levels of solasodine production than cultures without shoot regeneration [348]. Secondary metabolite production and accumulation of Solanum spp. were higher in the dark condition, regardless of kinetin doses, implying that hormones may reduce the cost of *in vitro* metabolite production [341]. Biotechnologically useful metabolites such as chlorogenic and ferulic acids, orientin, quercetin, and, in higher concentrations, quercetin, were detected in *S. aculeatissimum* cell cultures [349].

Stephania spp.

About 10,000 plant alkaloids have been identified in Stephania (Menispermaceae), many of which are involved in pathogen, insect, and herbivore defense. Due to its toxicity, alkaloids are "privileged" drug structures [350]. *S. venosa* is a red sap climbing plant [351]. The plant is used in Thai traditional medicine for neuronal function, as an appetizer, and to treat diabetes. *S. venosa* tubers contain many bioactive alkaloids, including dicentrine, an aporphine isoquinoline. Dicentrine has been shown to have antiarrhythmic [352], antitumor [353], antiplatelet [354], and acetylcholinesterase inhibitory activities [355]. The highest dicentrine content (19.5 mg/g dry weight) was obtained from *Stephania venosa* callus cultured on MS medium with 0.5 mg/L TDZ and 1.0 mg/L NAA [356]. It was found that the Chinese medicinal herb "Fan fang ji," also known as *S. tetrandra* can be effectively induced to form calluses *in vitro* using a combination of auxins (2,4D, IAA, and NAA), as well as other cytokinins and cytokines (BA, kinetin, TDZ, and zeatin) at various concentrations (0.5 to 2.0 mg/L) [357]. Stepharine can be produced in large quantities by using morphogenic cell cultures of *S. glabra* [358]. *S. glabra* young leaf callus cultures produce high levels of stepharine (over 0.9% dry weight) [359].

Taxus baccata L.

Taxus baccata (Taxaceae) is a deciduous conifer that grows in abundance throughout central and southern Europe [3] reported that taxol (plaxitaxol), a diterpene alkaloid isolated from the bark of the Taxus tree, is one of the most potent anticancer agents due to its mechanism of action on microtubules. Christen *et al* . were the first to report *in vitro* taxol production [360]. *In vitro* cultures have been shown to be a highly effective and sustainable method of producing paclitaxel from *Taxus baccata, Taxus yunnanensis, Taxus cuspidate, Taxus chinensis, Taxus canadensis,* and *Taxus globosa* [361]. Effective methods for increasing paclitaxel yields have been reported to include the use of high-yielding cell lines, two-stage culture systems, carbohydrate optimization, pre-feeding strategies, and fungal inducers such as fungal extracts in combination with elicitors such as salicylic acid, chitosan, squalene, MeJA *etc* [362], and described high taxane production in deep brown cell cultures with a low growth index.

Tripterygium wilfordii Hook. f.

Since the 1960s, *T. wilfordii,* an annual vine belonging to the Celastraceae family, has been used as an allopathic medicine in China to treat rheumatoid arthritis and inflammation [363]. For kidney disease, cancer, and systemic lupus erythematosus *T. wilfordii* roots have been used [364 - 366]. In *T. wilfordi*, aggregate cell size had no effect on wilforgine or wilforine content [367]. The inclusion of 50 mM of MeJA resulted in a substantial increase in the synthesis of triptolide and wilforine, whereas 50mM SA had no effect on hairy root growth but slightly increased the production of both SMs under *in vitro* conditions [368]. *T. wilfordii* adventitious root fragment liquid cultures produced more SMs in a shake flask and a modified bubble column bioreactor [368]. Cambial meristematic cells (CMCs) isolated from *T. wilfordii* were grown, characterised and applied for the first time. The significant enrichment in terpenoids found in *T. wilfordii* CMCs suggests that these cells could serve as a more efficient and controllable platform for long-term terpene production than dedifferentiated cells (DDCs) [369]. Sesquiterpene alkaloids, diterpenoids, triterpenoids, and other SMs have been found in the Tripterygium genus [370]. Nine compounds were found in *T. wilfordii* hairy root cultures. The ratio of NH^{4+}/NO^{3-} and phosphate concentration in *T. wilfordii* hairy root cultures were modified to enhance wilforgine and wilforine production [371]. It illustrated the effects of various MeJA and SA concentrations on root growth and celastrol production [371].

Vaccinium spp.

Vaccinium berry crops (Ericaceae), including blueberry, cranberry and lingonberry, are well-known for their commercial and nutritive values with high antioxidant metabolite contents, which have high potential to prevent several degenerative diseases. Blueberry and lingonberry leaves contain substantially higher levels of polyphenolics, flavonoids and proanthocyanidins than those in the fruits [372]. Both biotic (purified 13-glucan and chitosan) and abiotic (sodium ferric ethylenediamine di-(o-hydroxyphenylacetate) FeEDDHA, and $CuSO_4$) elicitors significantly increased anthocyanin accumulation in *V. pahalae* [373]. The phenolic compounds in tissue culture leaves are higher than in naturally growing leaves [374]. Despite the fact that both plants were grown in the same greenhouse environment, micropropagated lowbush blueberry clones had higher phenolics, flavonoids, and antioxidant activity than blueberries grown from conventional SCs [375]. The phenolic and flavonoid content of micropropagated bilberry and lingonberry berries is similar [376]. It was found that phytochemical differences between donor and somatic embryogenesis (SE) regenerated blueberry plants [377]. They found that in partially blueberry cultivars, SE-regenerated plants had higher total phenolic and flavonoid contents than SC donor plants.

CONCLUSION

Plant tissue culture (PTC) is a promising avenue for investigating the limitless potential of a wide range of medicinal plants. Plants produce a variety of compounds (SMs) as a result of the metabolic activities that occur within them. Most ethnopharmacology resources were available in the form of comprehensive medical manuals in the last decade. The Indian Ayurvedic Pharmacopoeia is one of them. The problem of multidrug-resistant pathogens is a global health threat that is continually challenging the scientific community in the current scenario. Researchers in the pharmaceutical industry use phytochemicals as a source of new molecules that can be used to create innovative new drugs. For drug discovery scientists, comprehending the critical molecular mechanisms involved in the screening of bioactive small molecule compounds has become a significant challenge. Unfortunately, pandemics are likely to recur on a smaller or larger scale in the future, owing to the diversity of known and unknown pathogens. Plant biotechnology tools and methods, such as *in vitro* culture, enable us to exploit the diversity of secondary metabolites produced by various plants. *In vitro* culture technologies have the potential to grow any plant in any location and provide added value through increased production of secondary metabolites and the generation of novel medicinal compounds. In the future, it is critical to continue developing research models to support the development of botanicals that are resistant to antibiotics, as well as regulatory reforms of clinical development programmes.

REFERENCES

[1]   Li Y, Kong D, Fu Y, Sussman MR, Wu H. The effect of developmental and environmental factors on secondary metabolites in medicinal plants. Plant Physiol Biochem 2020; 148: 80-9.
[http://dx.doi.org/10.1016/j.plaphy.2020.01.006] [PMID: 31951944]

[2]   Calabrò S, Rana CS. Plant secondary metabolites: A review. Int J Eng Res Gen Sci 2015; 3: 153-9.
[http://dx.doi.org/10.1007/978-81-322-2401-3_11]

[3]   Chandran H, Meena M, Barupal T, Sharma K. Plant tissue culture as a perpetual source for production of industrially important bioactive compounds. Biotechnol Rep 2020; 26: e00450.
[http://dx.doi.org/10.1016/j.btre.2020.e00450] [PMID: 32373483]

[4]   Ekor M. The growing use of herbal medicines: Issues relating to adverse reactions and challenges in monitoring safety. Front Pharmacol 2014; 4(JAN): 177.
[http://dx.doi.org/10.3389/fphar.2013.00177] [PMID: 24454289]

[5]   Thomford N, Senthebane D, Rowe A, *et al.* Natural products for drug discovery in the 21st century: Innovations for novel drug discovery. Int J Mol Sci 2018; 19(6): 1578.
[http://dx.doi.org/10.3390/ijms19061578] [PMID: 29799486]

[6]   Anand U, Jacobo-Herrera N, Altemimi A, Lakhssassi N. A comprehensive review on medicinal plants as antimicrobial therapeutics: Potential avenues of biocompatible drug discovery. Metabolites 2019; 9(11): 258.
[http://dx.doi.org/10.3390/metabo9110258] [PMID: 31683833]

[7]   GOI. National population policy 2020 Gvernment of India. 2002; 2-15.

[8]   Kolewe ME, Gaurav V, Roberts SC. Pharmaceutically active natural product synthesis and supply *via* plant cell culture technology. Mol Pharm 2008; 5(2): 243-56.
[http://dx.doi.org/10.1021/mp7001494] [PMID: 18393488]

[9]   Yang L, Wen KS, Ruan X, Zhao YX, Wei F, Wang Q. Response of plant secondary metabolites to environmental factors. Molecules 2018; 23(4): 762.
[http://dx.doi.org/10.3390/molecules23040762] [PMID: 29584636]

[10]   Rehab A. Hussein, Amira A. El-Anssary. Plants secondary metabolites: The key drivers of the pharmacological actions of medicinal plants. Herb Med. intechopen 2019; p. 76139.
[http://dx.doi.org/10.5772/intechopen.76139]

[11]   Guerriero G, Berni R, Muñoz-Sanchez J, *et al.* Production of plant secondary metabolites: Examples, tips and suggestions for biotechnologists. Genes 2018; 9(6): 309.
[http://dx.doi.org/10.3390/genes9060309] [PMID: 29925808]

[12]   Vijaya SN. Advancements in the production of secondary metabolites. J Nat Prod 2010; 3: 112-23.

[13]   Gonçalves S, Romano A. Production of plant secondary metabolites by using biotechnological tools. Second Metab - Sources Appl. intechopen 2018; p. 76414.
[http://dx.doi.org/10.5772/intechopen.76414]

[14]   Isah T, Umar S, Mujib A, *et al.* Secondary metabolism of pharmaceuticals in the plant *in vitro* cultures: Strategies, approaches, and limitations to achieving higher yield. Plant Cell Tissue Organ Cult 2018; 132(2): 239-65.
[http://dx.doi.org/10.1007/s11240-017-1332-2]

[15]   Giridhar P, Parimalan R. A biotechnological perspective towards improvement of annatto color production for value addition :The influence of biotic elicitors. Asia Pac J Mol Biol Biotechnol 2010; 18: 75-7.

[16]   Mahendranath G, Venugopalan A, Giridhar P, Ravishanakar GA. Improvement of annatto pigment yield in achiote through laminarin Spray: An ecofriendly approach. Int J Agric Environ Biotechnol 2011; 4: 163-6.

[17] Parimalan R, Mahendranath G, Giridhar P. Abiotic elicitor mediated augmentation of annatto pigment production in standing Crop of *Bixa orellana* L . 1:229–236 Ind J Fund App Life Sci 2011; 1(4): 229-36.

[18] Gururaj HB, Giridhar P, Ravishankar GA. Laminarin as a potential non-conventional elicitor for enhancement of capsaicinoid metabolites. Asian J Plant Sci Res 2012; 2: 490-5.

[19] Burman U, Saini M, Kumar P. Effect of zinc oxide nanoparticles on growth and antioxidant system of chickpea seedlings. Toxicol Environ Chem 2013; 95(4): 605-12.
[http://dx.doi.org/10.1080/02772248.2013.803796]

[20] Saini RK, Harish Prashanth KV, Shetty NP, Giridhar P. Elicitors, SA and MJ enhance carotenoids and tocopherol biosynthesis and expression of antioxidant related genes in *Moringa oleifera* Lam. leaves. Acta Physiol Plant 2014; 36(10): 2695-704.
[http://dx.doi.org/10.1007/s11738-014-1640-7]

[21] Thakur M, Bhattacharya S, Khosla PK, Puri S. Improving production of plant secondary metabolites through biotic and abiotic elicitation. J Appl Res Med Aromat Plants 2019; 12: 1-12.
[http://dx.doi.org/10.1016/j.jarmap.2018.11.004]

[22] Weathers PJ, Towler MJ, Xu J. Bench to batch: Advances in plant cell culture for producing useful products. Appl Microbiol Biotechnol 2010; 85(5): 1339-51.
[http://dx.doi.org/10.1007/s00253-009-2354-4] [PMID: 19956945]

[23] Hussain MS, Fareed S, Ansari S, Rahman MA, Ahmad IZ, Saeed M. Current approaches toward production of secondary plant metabolites. J Pharm Bioallied Sci 2012; 4(1): 10-20.
[http://dx.doi.org/10.4103/0975-7406.92725] [PMID: 22368394]

[24] Marchev AS, Yordanova ZP, Georgiev MI. Green (cell) factories for advanced production of plant secondary metabolites. Crit Rev Biotechnol 2020; 40(4): 443-58.
[http://dx.doi.org/10.1080/07388551.2020.1731414] [PMID: 32178548]

[25] Fang X, Yang C-Q, Wei Y. Genomics grand for diversified plants secondary metabolites. Plant Divers Resour 2011; 33: 53-64.

[26] Smith GF, Klopper RR, Figueiredo E, Crouch NR. Aspects of the taxonomy of *Aloe arborescens* Mill. (Asphodelaceae: Alooideae). Bradleya 2012; 30(30): 127-37.
[http://dx.doi.org/10.25223/brad.n30.2012.a15]

[27] Chukwujekwu JC, Fennell CW, van Staden J. Optimisation of the tissue culture protocol for the endangered *Aloe polyphylla*. S Afr J Bot 2002; 68(4): 424-9.
[http://dx.doi.org/10.1016/S0254-6299(15)30368-9]

[28] Bedini C, Caccia R, Triggiani D, Mazzucato A, Soressi GP, Tiezzi A. Micropropagation of *Aloe arborescens* Mill: A step towards efficient production of its valuable leaf extracts showing antiproliferative activity on murine myeloma cells. Plant Biosyst 2009; 143(2): 233-40.
[http://dx.doi.org/10.1080/11263500902722402]

[29] Kumar V, Van Staden J. A review of *Swertia chirayita* (Gentianaceae) as a traditional medicinal plant. Front Pharmacol 2016; 6: 308.
[http://dx.doi.org/10.3389/fphar.2015.00308] [PMID: 26793105]

[30] Niguse M, Sbhatu DB, Abraha HB. *In Vitro* Micropropagation of *Aloe adigratana* Reynolds Using Offshoot Cuttings. ScientificWorldJournal 2020; 2020: 1-7.
[http://dx.doi.org/10.1155/2020/9645316]

[31] Bairu MW, Stirk WA, Dolezal K, Van Staden J. Optimizing the micropropagation protocol for the endangered *Aloe polyphylla*: can meta-topolin and its derivatives serve as replacement for benzyladenine and zeatin? Plant Cell Tissue Organ Cult 2007; 90(1): 15-23.
[http://dx.doi.org/10.1007/s11240-007-9233-4]

[32] van der Westhuizen A. The use of meta-topolin as an alternative cytokinin in the tissue culture of

Eucalyptus species. Acta Hortic 2014; (1055): 25-8.
[http://dx.doi.org/10.17660/ActaHortic.2014.1055.4]

[33] Amoo SO, Aremu AO, Van Staden J. *In vitro* plant regeneration, secondary metabolite production and antioxidant activity of micropropagated *Aloe arborescens* Mill. Plant Cell Tissue Organ Cult 2012; 111(3): 345-58.
[http://dx.doi.org/10.1007/s11240-012-0200-3]

[34] Hlatshwayo NA, Amoo SO, Olowoyo JO, Doležal K. Efficient micropropagation protocol for the conservation of the endangered *Aloe peglerae*, an ornamental and medicinal species. Plants 2020; 9(4): 506.
[http://dx.doi.org/10.3390/plants9040506] [PMID: 32295312]

[35] Kodad S, Melhaoui R, Hano C, *et al.* Effect of culture media and plant growth regulators on shoot proliferation and rooting of internode explants from moroccan native almond (*Prunus dulcis* Mill.) Genotypes. Int J Agron 2021; 2021: 1-10.
[http://dx.doi.org/10.1155/2021/9931574]

[36] Guo S, Wei H, Li J, *et al.* Geographical distribution and environmental correlates of eleutherosides and isofraxidin in eleutherococcus senticosus from natural populations in forests at northeast China. Forests 2019; 10(10): 872.
[http://dx.doi.org/10.3390/f10100872]

[37] Shikov AN, Pozharitskaya ON, Makarov VG. Aralia elata var. mandshurica (Rupr. & Maxim.) J.Wen: An overview of pharmacological studies. Phytomedicine 2016; 23(12): 1409-21.
[http://dx.doi.org/10.1016/j.phymed.2016.07.011] [PMID: 27765361]

[38] Sun Y, Li B, Lin X, *et al.* Simultaneous Determination of Four Triterpenoid saponins in *Aralia elata* Leaves by HPLC-ELSD Combined with Hierarchical Clustering Analysis. Phytochem Anal 2017; 28(3): 202-9.
[http://dx.doi.org/10.1002/pca.2662] [PMID: 28071864]

[39] Wei H, Chen X, Chen G, Zhao H. Foliar nutrient and carbohydrate in Aralia elata can be modified by understory light quality in forests with different structures at Northeast China. Ann For Res 2019; 62(2): 125-37.
[http://dx.doi.org/10.15287/afr.2019.1395]

[40] Wei H, Chen G, Chen X, Zhao H. Growth and nutrient uptake in aralia elata seedlings exposed to exponential fertilization under different illumination spectra. Int J Agric Biol 2020; 23: 644-52.
[http://dx.doi.org/10.17957/IJAB/15.1336]

[41] Moon H k, Youn Y, Yi JS. Somatic embryogenesis, plant regeneration, and field establishment from tissue culture of winter buds of 10-year-old Aralia elata.pdf. J korean Soc For Sci 1998; 87: 57-61.

[42] Murashige T, Skoog F. A revised medium for rapid growth and bio assay with tobacco tissue culture. Physiol Plant 1962; 15(3): 473-97.
[http://dx.doi.org/10.1111/j.1399-3054.1962.tb08052.x]

[43] Amemiya K, Mochizuki T. Somatic Embryo Formation and Plant Regeneration in 'Zaoh' line No.2 of Japanese Angelica Tree (*Aralia elata* seem.). Plant Biotechnol (Tsukuba) 2002; 19(5): 383-7.
[http://dx.doi.org/10.5511/plantbiotechnology.19.383]

[44] Kang HJ, Anbazhagan VR, You XL, Moon HK, Yi JS, Choi YE. Production of transgenic Aralia elata regenerated from Agrobacterium rhizogenes-mediated transformed roots. Plant Cell Tissue Organ Cult 2006; 85(2): 187-96.
[http://dx.doi.org/10.1007/s11240-005-9070-2]

[45] Chukavina A. Flora of Tajik SSR. Nauk Leningr 7: 1984.

[46] Davydenkov V. Cell culture of *Arnebia euchroma* (Royle) Jonst. : Novel source of shikonin production. Him Farm Zh 1991; 1: 53-5.

[47] Zakhlenjuk OV, Kunakh VA. *Arnebia euchroma: In Vitro* culture and the production of shikonin and

other secondary metabolites. In: Biotechnology in Agriculture and Foresty. Med Aromat Plants 1998; 41: 28-44.

[48] Kumar P, Sharma P, Kumar V. Plant resources: *In vitro* production, challenges and prospects of secondary Metabolites from medicinal plants. In: Industrial Biotechnology 2019; 89-104.

[49] Kozlovtseva L. Suspension culturing of macrotomia Arnebia euchroma cells. Optimization of conditions for shikonin production. Biotechnologia 1994; 3: 24-6.

[50] Sokha V. Shikonin sources in tissue culture.PhD Thesis. Russian: Chemical Pharmaceutical Institute of St. Petersburg 1996.

[51] Arghavani P, Haghbeen K, Mousavi A. Enhancement of shikalkin production in arnebia euchroma callus by a fungal elicitor, *Rhizoctonia solani.* Iran J Biotechnol 2015; 13(4): 10-6.
[http://dx.doi.org/10.15171/ijb.1058] [PMID: 28959304]

[52] Klayman DL. Qinghaosu (artemisinin): An antimalarial drug from China. Science 1985; 228: 1049-55.
[http://dx.doi.org/10.1126/science.3887571]

[53] Martinez BC, Staba EJ. The Production of Artemisinin in *Artemisia annua* L. Tissue Cultures. ACADEMIC PRESS, INC. 1988.

[54] Nair MSR, Basile DV. Bioconversion of arteannuin B to artemisinin. J Nat Prod 1993; 56(9): 1559-66.
[http://dx.doi.org/10.1021/np50099a015] [PMID: 8254350]

[55] Tawfiq NK, Anderson LA, Roberts MF, Phillipson JD, Bray DH, Warhurst DC. Antiplasmodial activity of *Artemisia annua* plant cell cultures. Plant Cell Rep 1989; 8(7): 425-8.
[http://dx.doi.org/10.1007/BF00270085] [PMID: 24233369]

[56] Woerdenbag HJ, Bos R, Salomons MC, Hendriks H, Pras N, Malingré TM. Volatile constituents of *Artemisia annua* L. (Asteraceae). Flavour Fragrance J 1993; 8(3): 131-7.
[http://dx.doi.org/10.1002/ffj.2730080303]

[57] Paniego NB, Giulietti AM. Artemisinin production by *Artemisia annua* L.-transformed organ cultures. Enzyme Microb Technol 1996; 18(7): 526-30.
[http://dx.doi.org/10.1016/0141-0229(95)00216-2]

[58] Liu CZ, Guo C, Wang Y, Ouyang F. Factors influencing artemisinin production from shoot cultures of *Artemisia annua* L. World J Microbiol Biotechnol 2003; 19(5): 535-8.
[http://dx.doi.org/10.1023/A:1025158416832]

[59] Liu CZ, Wang YC, Ouyang F, Ye HC, Li GF. Production of artemisinin by hairy root cultures of *Artemisia annua* L. Biotechnol Lett 1997; 19(9): 927-9.
[http://dx.doi.org/10.1023/A:1018362309677]

[60] Paniego NB, Giulietti AM. *Artemisia annua* L.: dedifferentiated and differentiated cultures. Plant Cell Tissue Organ Cult 1994; 36(2): 163-8.
[http://dx.doi.org/10.1007/BF00037715]

[61] Akalezi CO, Liu S, Li QS, Yu JT, Zhong JJ. Combined effects of initial sucrose concentration and inoculum size on cell growth and ginseng saponin production by suspension cultures of *Panax ginseng.* Process Biochem 1999; 34(6-7): 639-42.
[http://dx.doi.org/10.1016/S0032-9592(98)00132-0]

[62] Chen DH, Ye HC, Li GF. Expression of a chimeric farnesyl diphosphate synthase gene in *Artemisia annua* L. transgenic plants *via Agrobacterium tumefaciens*-mediated transformation. Plant Sci 2000; 155(2): 179-85.
[http://dx.doi.org/10.1016/S0168-9452(00)00217-X] [PMID: 10814821]

[63] Ro DK, Paradise EM, Ouellet M, *et al.* Production of the antimalarial drug precursor artemisinic acid in engineered yeast. Nature 2006; 440(7086): 940-3.
[http://dx.doi.org/10.1038/nature04640] [PMID: 16612385]

[64] Xie D, Ye H, Li G, Guo Z, Zou Z, Guo Z. Selection of hairy root clones of *Artemisia annua* L. for

artemisinin production. Isr J Plant Sci 2001; 49(2): 129-34.
[http://dx.doi.org/10.1560/N11N-6BLG-ER7C-XKCT]

[65]   Durante M, Caretto S, Quarta A, De Paolis A, Nisi R, Mita G. β-Cyclodextrins enhance artemisinin production in *Artemisia annua* suspension cell cultures. Appl Microbiol Biotechnol 2011; 90(6): 1905-13.
[http://dx.doi.org/10.1007/s00253-011-3232-4] [PMID: 21468706]

[66]   Pandey N, Pandey-Rai S. Short term UV-B radiation-mediated transcriptional responses and altered secondary metabolism of *in vitro* propagated plantlets of *Artemisia annua L*. Plant Cell Tissue Organ Cult 2014; 116(3): 371-85.
[http://dx.doi.org/10.1007/s11240-013-0413-0]

[67]   Fitter R, Fitter A, Blamey M. The wild flowers of Britain and Northern Europe. Viking Pr 1989.

[68]   Stace C. The new flora of the british isles. Cambridge Univ Press 1991.

[69]   Singh O, Khanam Z, Misra N, Srivastava M. Chamomile (*Matricaria chamomilla* L.): An overview. Pharmacogn Rev 2011; 5(9): 82-95.
[http://dx.doi.org/10.4103/0973-7847.79103] [PMID: 22096322]

[70]   Raal A, Orav A, Püssa T, Valner C, Malmiste B, Arak E. Content of essential oil, terpenoids and polyphenols in commercial chamomile (*Chamomilla recutita* L. Rauschert) teas from different countries. Food Chem 2012; 131(2): 632-8.
[http://dx.doi.org/10.1016/j.foodchem.2011.09.042]

[71]   Sotiropoulou NS, Megremi SF, Tarantilis P. Evaluation of antioxidant activity, toxicity, and phenolic profile of aqueous extracts of chamomile (*Matricaria chamomilla* L.) and sage (*Salvia ocinalis* L.) prepared at different temperatures. Appl Sci 2020; 10(7): 2270.
[http://dx.doi.org/10.3390/app10072270]

[72]   Schilcher H. the chamomile. Handbook for doctors, pharmacists and other natural scientists scientific publishing company. mbH struttgart 1987.

[73]   Podlech D. Herbs and medicinal plants of britain and europe. London: Harper Collins Publ 1996.

[74]   Čellárová E, Greláková K, Repčák M, Hončariv R. Morphogenesis in callus tissue cultures of some *Matricaria* and *Achillea species*. Biol Plant 1982; 24(6): 430-3.
[http://dx.doi.org/10.1007/BF02880439]

[75]   Čellárová E, Repčáková K, Hončariv R. Salt tolerance of *Chamomilla recutita* (L.) Rauschert tissue cultures. Biol Plant 1986; 28(4): 275-9.
[http://dx.doi.org/10.1007/BF02902293]

[76]   Linsmaier EM, Skoog F. Organic growth factor requirements of tobacco tissue cultures. Physiol Plant 1965; 18(1): 100-27.
[http://dx.doi.org/10.1111/j.1399-3054.1965.tb06874.x]

[77]   Reichling J, Becker H. Tissue culture of *Matricaria chamomilla* L. I. Communication: Isolations and maintainance of the tissue culture. Preliminary phytochemical investigations (author's transl). Planta Med 1976; 30(3): 258-68.
[http://dx.doi.org/10.1055/s-0028-1097727] [PMID: 1005528]

[78]   Reichling J, Bisson W, Becker H. Vergleichende untersuchungen zur bildung und akkumulation von etherischem öl in der intakten pflanze und in der calluskultur von *Matricaria chamomilla*. Planta Med 1984; 50(4): 334-7.
[http://dx.doi.org/10.1055/s-2007-969724]

[79]   Passamonti F, Piccioni E, Standardi A, Veronesi F. Micropropagation of *Chamomilla recutita* L. Rauschert. Acta Hortic 1998; 457.

[80]   Éva Szőke, Lemberkovics Éva, Standardi A. Comparative investigation of sesquiterpene components of essential oils originating from intact plants and hairy root chamomile cultures. GSC Advanced

Research and Reviews 2021; 6(2): 28-49.
[http://dx.doi.org/10.30574/gscarr.2021.6.2.0016]

[81] Mazur P. The effect of NAA and BAP on the multiplication of chamomile (*Matricaria chamomilla* L.) callus tissue *in vitro*. World Sci News 2019; 125: 245-51.

[82] Nozari E, Asghari-zakaria R, Zare N. Effect of 17β -estradiol on seedling and callus growth of German chamomile (*Matricaria chamomilla* L .). J Plant Physiol Breed 2020; 10: 77-87.

[83] Russo EB. History of cannabis and its preparations in saga, science, and sobriquet. Chem Biodivers 2007; 4(8): 1614-48.
[http://dx.doi.org/10.1002/cbdv.200790144] [PMID: 17712811]

[84] Mechoulam R. The pharmacohistory of *Cannabis sativa*. Chapman and Hall/CRC 2019.
[http://dx.doi.org/10.1201/9780429260667-1]

[85] ElSohly MA, Slade D. Chemical constituents of marijuana: The complex mixture of natural cannabinoids. Life Sci 2005; 78(5): 539-48.
[http://dx.doi.org/10.1016/j.lfs.2005.09.011] [PMID: 16199061]

[86] Kovalchuk I, Pellino M, Rigault P, *et al.* The genomics of *Cannabis* and its close relatives. Annu Rev Plant Biol 2020; 71(1): 713-39.
[http://dx.doi.org/10.1146/annurev-arplant-081519-040203] [PMID: 32155342]

[87] Hesami M, Pepe M, Alizadeh M, Rakei A, Baiton A, Phineas Jones AM. Recent advances in cannabis biotechnology. Ind Crops Prod 2020; 158: 113026.
[http://dx.doi.org/10.1016/j.indcrop.2020.113026]

[88] Andre CM, Hausman JF, Guerriero G. *Cannabis sativa*: The plant of the thousand and one molecules. Front Plant Sci 2016; 7: 19.
[http://dx.doi.org/10.3389/fpls.2016.00019] [PMID: 26870049]

[89] Elsohly MA. Marijuana and the Cannabinoids. NJ: Humana Totowa Publishers 2007.
[http://dx.doi.org/10.1007/978-1-59259-947-9]

[90] Fattore L. cannabinoids in neurologic and mental disease. Acad Press 2015; pp. 1-452.

[91] Turner JC, Hemphill JK, Mahlberg PG. Quantitative determination of cannabinoids in individual glandular trichomes of *Cannabis sativa* L. (Cannabaceae). Am J Bot 1978; 65(10): 1103-6.
[http://dx.doi.org/10.1002/j.1537-2197.1978.tb06177.x]

[92] Loh WHT, Hartsel SC, Robertson LW. Tissue culture of *cannabis sativa* L. and *in vitro* biotransformation of phenolics. Z Pflanzenphysiol 1983; 111(5): 395-400.
[http://dx.doi.org/10.1016/S0044-328X(83)80003-8]

[93] Braemer R, Paris M. Biotransformation of cannabinoids by a cell suspension culture of *Cannabis sativa* L. Plant Cell Rep 1987; 6(2): 150-2.
[http://dx.doi.org/10.1007/BF00276675] [PMID: 24248499]

[94] Schachtsiek J, Hussain T, Azzouhri K, Kayser O, Stehle F. Virus-induced gene silencing (VIGS) in *Cannabis sativa* L. Plant Methods 2019; 15(1): 157.
[http://dx.doi.org/10.1186/s13007-019-0542-5] [PMID: 31889981]

[95] Wróbel T, Dreger M, Wielgus K, Słomski R. Modified nodal cuttings and shoot tips protocol for rapid regeneration of *Cannabis sativa* L. J Nat Fibers 2020; 00: 1-10.
[http://dx.doi.org/10.1080/15440478.2020.1748160]

[96] Monthony AS, Page SR, Hesami M, Jones AMP. The past, present and future of *Cannabis sativa* tissue culture. Plants 2021; 10(1): 185.
[http://dx.doi.org/10.3390/plants10010185] [PMID: 33478171]

[97] Adhikary D, Kulkarni M, El-Mezawy A, *et al.* Medical cannabis and industrial hemp tissue culture: Present status and future potential. Front Plant Sci 2021; 12: 627240.
[http://dx.doi.org/10.3389/fpls.2021.627240] [PMID: 33747008]

[98]   Wang GS, Le Lait MC, Deakyne SJ, Bronstein AC, Bajaj L, Roosevelt G. Unintentional pediatric exposures to marijuana in Colorado, 2009-2015. JAMA Pediatr 2016; 170(9): e160971.
[http://dx.doi.org/10.1001/jamapediatrics.2016.0971] [PMID: 27454910]

[99]   Chandra S, Lata H, ElSohly MA. *Cannabis sativa* L. - botany and biotechnology. *Cannabis sativa* L. Bot Biotechnol 2009; 1-474.
[http://dx.doi.org/10.1007/978-3-319-54564-6]

[100] Lata H, Chandra S, Techen N, Khan IA, ElSohly MA. *In vitro* mass propagation of *Cannabis sativa* L.: A protocol refinement using novel aromatic cytokinin meta-topolin and the assessment of eco-physiological, biochemical and genetic fidelity of micropropagated plants. J Appl Res Med Aromat Plants 2016; 3(1): 18-26.
[http://dx.doi.org/10.1016/j.jarmap.2015.12.001]

[101] Chaohua C, Gonggu Z, Lining Z, *et al.* A rapid shoot regeneration protocol from the cotyledons of hemp (*Cannabis sativa* L.). Ind Crops Prod 2016; 83: 61-5.
[http://dx.doi.org/10.1016/j.indcrop.2015.12.035]

[102] Piunno KF, Golenia G, Boudko EA. Regeneration of shoots from immature and mature inflorescences of *Cannabis sativa.* Can J Plant Sci 2019; 1-11.

[103] Sirikantaramas S, Morimoto S, Shoyama Y, *et al.* The gene controlling marijuana psychoactivity: molecular cloning and heterologous expression of Δ1-tetrahydrocannabinolic acid synthase from *Cannabis sativa* L. J Biol Chem 2004; 279(38): 39767-74.
[http://dx.doi.org/10.1074/jbc.M403693200] [PMID: 15190053]

[104] Flores-Sanchez IJ, Peč J, Fei J, Choi YH, Dušek J, Verpoorte R. Elicitation studies in cell suspension cultures of *Cannabis sativa* L. J Biotechnol 2009; 143(2): 157-68.
[http://dx.doi.org/10.1016/j.jbiotec.2009.05.006] [PMID: 19500620]

[105] Kodym A, Leeb CJ. Back to the roots: Protocol for the photoautotrophic micropropagation of medicinal *Cannabis.* Plant Cell Tissue Organ Cult 2019; 138(2): 399-402.
[http://dx.doi.org/10.1007/s11240-019-01635-1] [PMID: 31404230]

[106] Page RL II, Allen LA, Kloner RA, *et al.* Medical marijuana, recreational cannabis, and cardiovascular health: A scientific statement from the american heart association. Circulation 2020; 142(10): e131-52.
[http://dx.doi.org/10.1161/CIR.0000000000000883] [PMID: 32752884]

[107] Moher M, Jones M, Zheng Y. Photoperiodic response of *in vitro Cannabis sativa* plants. HortScience 2021; 56(1): 108-13.
[http://dx.doi.org/10.21273/HORTSCI15452-20]

[108] Zarei A, Behdarvandi B, Tavakouli Dinani E, Maccarone J. *Cannabis sativa* L. photoautotrophic micropropagation: A powerful tool for industrial scale *in vitro* propagation. Vitr Cell Dev Biol - Plant 2021.
[http://dx.doi.org/10.1007/s11627-021-10167-3]

[109] Heijden R, Jacobs D, Snoeijer W, Hallard D, Verpoorte R. The Catharanthus alkaloids: Pharmacognosy and biotechnology. Curr Med Chem 2004; 11(5): 607-28.
[http://dx.doi.org/10.2174/0929867043455846] [PMID: 15032608]

[110] Schmelzer GH, Gurib-Fakim A, Arroo R, *et al.* Plant resources of tropical africa. Medicinal plants 2008; 11(1): 1.

[111] Mekky H, Al-Sabahi J, Abdel-Kreem MFM. Potentiating biosynthesis of the anticancer alkaloids vincristine and vinblastine in callus cultures of *Catharanthus roseus.* S Afr J Bot 2018; 114: 29-31.
[http://dx.doi.org/10.1016/j.sajb.2017.10.008]

[112] Mishra MRM, Srivastava RK, Akhtar N. Effect of nitrogen, phosphorus and medium ph to enhance alkaloid production from *Catharanthus roseus* cell suspension culture. Int J Second Metab 2019; 137-53.
[http://dx.doi.org/10.21448/ijsm.559679]

[113] Krueger RJ, Carew DP. Production of vindoline in root regeneration of *Catharanthus roseus.* Planta Med 1982; 45: 56-6.
[http://dx.doi.org/10.1055/s-2007-971245] [PMID: 17396784]

[114] Hirata K, Miyamoto K. *Catharanthus roseus* L. (Periwinkle): Production of vindoline and catharanthine. In: Bajaj YPS, Ed. Medicinal and Aromatic Plants VI Biotechnology in Agriculture and Forestry. Berlin, Heidelberg.: Springer 1994; 26: pp. 46-55.

[115] Miura Y, Hirata K, Kurano N. Isolation of vinblastine in callus culture with differentiated roots of *Catharanthus roseus* (L).G.Don. Agric Biol Chem 1987; 51(2): 611-4.
[http://dx.doi.org/10.1271/bbb1961.51.611]

[116] Yokoyama M. Plant cell culture secondary metabolism: Toward industrial application. In: By DiCosmo F, Misawa M, Eds. Boca Raton, New York, London, Tokyo: CRC Press 1996; pp. 79-121.

[117] Toivonen L, Ojala M, Kauppinen V. Indole alkaloid production by hairy root cultures of *Catharanthus roseus*: Growth kinetics and fermentation. Biotechnol Lett 1990; 12.

[118] Lounasmaa M, Galambos J. Indole alkaloid production in *Catharanthus roseus* cell suspension cultures. In: Fortschritte der Chemie Organischer Naturstoffe 1989; 89-115.

[119] EC M, AA A. Alkaloid yield variation incallus cultures derived from different plant parts ofthe white and rosy purple periwinkle, *Catharanthus roseus* (L). Don. Philipp J Biotechnol 1993; 4: 1-8.

[120] Pietrosiuk A, Furmanowa M. Preliminary results of indole alkaloids production in different roots of *Catharanthus roseus* cultured *in vitro*. Acta Soc Bot Pol 2014; 70(4): 261-5.
[http://dx.doi.org/10.5586/asbp.2001.033]

[121] Taha HS, Lashin II, Sharaf AM. *In vitro* studies and RAPD analysis of *Echinacea angustifolia*. J Am Sci 2010; 6: 781-90.

[122] Ruiz-May E, Galaz-Ávalos RM, Loyola-Vargas VM. Differential secretion and accumulation of terpene indole alkaloids in hairy roots of *Catharanthus roseus* treated with methyl jasmonate. Mol Biotechnol 2009; 41(3): 278-85.
[http://dx.doi.org/10.1007/s12033-008-9111-2] [PMID: 18841500]

[123] Asano M, Harada K, Yoshikawa T, Bamba T, Hirata K. Synthesis of anti-tumor dimeric indole alkaloids in *catharanthus roseus* was promoted by irradiation with near-ultraviolet light at low temperature. Biosci Biotechnol Biochem 2010; 74(2): 386-9.
[http://dx.doi.org/10.1271/bbb.90545] [PMID: 20139608]

[124] Neha Verma, Abhishek Sharma. Agrobacterium rhizogenes mediated transformation studies in *Catharanthus roseus* : A status update. Jigyasa - 2014At: CSIR-CIMAP, Lucknow.

[125] Moreno PRH, Van der Heijden R, Verpoorte R. Cell and tissue cultures of *Catharanthus roseus*: A literature survey. Plant Cell Tissue Organ Cult 1995; 42(1): 1-25.
[http://dx.doi.org/10.1007/BF00037677]

[126] Goldhaber-Pasillas G, Mustafa N, Verpoorte R. Jasmonic acid effect on the fatty acid and terpenoid indole alkaloid accumulation in cell suspension cultures of *Catharanthus roseus*. Molecules 2014; 19(7): 10242-60.
[http://dx.doi.org/10.3390/molecules190710242] [PMID: 25029072]

[127] El-Sayed M, Verpoorte R. Catharanthus terpenoid indole alkaloids: Biosynthesis and regulation. Phytochem Rev 2007; 6(2-3): 277-305.
[http://dx.doi.org/10.1007/s11101-006-9047-8]

[128] Almagro L, Gutierrez J, Pedreño MA, Sottomayor M. Synergistic and additive influence of cyclodextrins and methyl jasmonate on the expression of the terpenoid indole alkaloid pathway genes and metabolites in *Catharanthus roseus* cell cultures. Plant Cell Tissue Organ Cult 2014; 119(3): 543-51.
[http://dx.doi.org/10.1007/s11240-014-0554-9]

[129] Liu J, Zhu J, Tang L, Wen W, Lv S, Yu R. Enhancement of vindoline and vinblastine production in suspension-cultured cells of *Catharanthus roseus* by artemisinic acid elicitation. World J Microbiol Biotechnol 2014; 30(1): 175-80.
[http://dx.doi.org/10.1007/s11274-013-1432-z] [PMID: 23864440]

[130] Naeem M, Aftab T, Khan MMA. *Catharanthus roseus*: Current research and future prospects. springer 2017.

[131] Singh M, Singh A, Singh S, Tripathi RS, Patra DD. Production potential and economics of safed musli (*Chlorophytum borivilianum*) under intercropping system. Arch Agron Soil Sci 2011; 57(6): 669-78.
[http://dx.doi.org/10.1080/03650341003785768]

[132] Kothari SK, Reddy PS. Response of safed musli (*Chlorophytum borivilianum* Santapau and Fernandes) to methods of planting, spacing, harvesting age and cropping system. Curr Res Med Aromat Plants 2016.

[133] Misra A, Shasany AK, Shukla AK, *et al.* AFLP-based detection of adulterants in crude drug preparations of the "Safed Musli" complex. Nat Prod Commun 2007; 2(1): 1934578X0700200.
[http://dx.doi.org/10.1177/1934578X0700200119]

[134] Weathers PJ, DeJesus-Gonzalez L, Kim YJ, Souret FF, Towler MJ. Alteration of biomass and artemisinin production in *Artemisia annua* hairy roots by media sterilization method and sugars. Plant Cell Rep 2004; 23(6): 414-8.
[http://dx.doi.org/10.1007/s00299-004-0837-4] [PMID: 15551137]

[135] Rizvi MZ, Kukreja AK, Khanuja SPS. *In vitro* culture of *Chlorophytum borivilianum* Sant. et Fernand. in liquid culture medium as a cost-effective measure. Curr Sci 2007; 92: 87-90.

[136] Ashraf MF, Aziz MA, Kemat N, Ismail I. Effect of cytokinin types, concentrations and their interactions on *in vitro* shoot regeneration of *Chlorophytum borivilianum* Sant. & Fernandez. Electron J Biotechnol 2014; 17(6): 275-9.
[http://dx.doi.org/10.1016/j.ejbt.2014.08.004]

[137] Thakur M, Dixit VK. A review on some important medicinal plants of *Chlorophytum* spp. Pharmacognosy Res 2008; 2: 168-72.

[138] Kemat N, Kadir MA, Abdullah NAP, Ashraf F. Rapid multiplication of safed musli (*Chlorophytum borivilianum*) through shoot proliferation. Afr J Biotechnol 2010; 9: 4595-600.
[http://dx.doi.org/10.4314/ajb.v9i29]

[139] A J, K BY. Estimation of some secondary metabolites from the *in vitro* cultures of *chlorophytum borivilianum* sant. et. fern. Int J Pharm Pharm Sci 2018; 10(1): 36-45.
[http://dx.doi.org/10.22159/ijpps.2018v10i1.20757]

[140] Kanne H, Prasanna V, Burte NP, Gujjula R. Extraction and elemental analysis of *Coleus forskohlii* extract. Pharmacognosy Res 2015; 7(3): 237-41.
[http://dx.doi.org/10.4103/0974-8490.157966] [PMID: 26130934]

[141] Mastan A, Rane D, Dastager SG, Vivek Babu CS. Development of low-cost plant probiotic formulations of functional endophytes for sustainable cultivation of *Coleus forskohlii*. Microbiol Res 2019; 227: 126310.
[http://dx.doi.org/10.1016/j.micres.2019.126310] [PMID: 31421714]

[142] Bhowal M, Mehta DM. *Coleus forskholii*: Phytochemical and pharmacological profile. Int J Pharm Sci Res 2017; 8(9): 3599-618.
[http://dx.doi.org/10.13040/IJPSR.0975-8232.8(9).3599-18]

[143] Nagpal A, Balwinder Singh B, Sanjeev Sharma B. Coleus spp.: Micropropagation and *in vitro* production of secondary metabolites. In: Medicinal and Aromatic Plant Science and Biotechnology. 2008.

[144] Mersinger R, Dornauer H, Reinhard E. Formation of forskolin by suspension cultures of *Coleus*

forskohlii. Planta Med 1988; 54(3): 200-4.
[http://dx.doi.org/10.1055/s-2006-962403] [PMID: 3174855]

[145] Sen J, Sharma A, Sahu N, Mahato S. Production of forskolin in *in vitro* cultures of *Coleus forskohlii.* Planta Med 1992; 58(4): 324-7.
[http://dx.doi.org/10.1055/s-2006-961477] [PMID: 17226481]

[146] Tripathi CKM, Basu SK, Jain S, Tandon JS. Production of coleonol (forskolin) by root callus cells of plant Coleus forskohlii. Biotechnol Lett 1995; 17(4): 423-6.
[http://dx.doi.org/10.1007/BF00130801]

[147] Zenk MH, El-Shagi H, Ulbrich B. Production of rosmarinic acid by cell-suspension cultures of *Coleus blumei.* Naturwissenschaften 1977; 64(11): 585-6.
[http://dx.doi.org/10.1007/BF00450645]

[148] Ulbrich B, Wiesner W, Arens H. Large-scale production of rosmarinic acid from plant cell cultures of coleus blumei benth. In: Primary and Secondary Metabolism of Plant Cell Cultures. springer 1985; pp. 293-303.

[149] Petersen M, Alfermann AW. Two new enzymes of rosmarinic acid biosynthesis from cell cultures of coleus blumei: Hydroxyphenylpyruvate reductase and rosmarinic acid synthase. Z Naturforsch C J Biosci 1988; 43(7-8): 501-4.
[http://dx.doi.org/10.1515/znc-1988-7-804]

[150] Inomata S, Yokoyama M, Seto S, Yanagi M. High-level production of arbutin from hydroquinone in suspension cultures of *Catharanthus roseus* plant cells. Appl Microbiol Biotechnol 1991; 36(3): 315-9.
[http://dx.doi.org/10.1007/BF00208148]

[151] Martinez BC, Park CH. Characteristics of batch suspension cultures of preconditioned *Coleus blumei* cells: Sucrose effect. Biotechnol Prog 1993; 9(1): 97-100.
[http://dx.doi.org/10.1021/bp00019a014]

[152] Yamada Y, Sato F. Production of berberine in cultured cells of *Coptis japonica.* Phytochemistry 1981; 20(3): 545-7.
[http://dx.doi.org/10.1016/S0031-9422(00)84193-X]

[153] Sato F, Yamada Y. High berberine-producing cultures of *coptis japonica* cells. Phytochemistry 1984; 23(2): 281-5.
[http://dx.doi.org/10.1016/S0031-9422(00)80318-0]

[154] Hara Y, Yoshioka T, Morimoto T, Fujita Y, Yamada Y. Enhancement of berberine production in suspension cultures of *coptis japonica* by gibberellic acid treatment. J Plant Physiol 1988; 133(1): 12-5.
[http://dx.doi.org/10.1016/S0176-1617(88)80077-4]

[155] Matsubara K, Kitani S, Yoshioka T, Morimoto T, Fujita Y, Yamada Y. High density culture of *Coptis japonica* cells increases berberine production. J Chem Technol Biotechnol 1989; 46(1): 61-9.
[http://dx.doi.org/10.1002/jctb.280460107]

[156] Ammon H, Wahl M. Pharmacology of *Curcuma longa.* Planta Med 1991; 57(1): 1-7.
[http://dx.doi.org/10.1055/s-2006-960004] [PMID: 2062949]

[157] Ashkanani J, Sudhersan C, Jibimanuel S. Micropropagation and field evaluation of micropropagated plants of *Ziziphus spinachristi.* Acta Hortic 2013; (993): 77-83.
[http://dx.doi.org/10.17660/ActaHortic.2013.993.11]

[158] Salvi ND, George L, Eapen S. Plant regeneration from leaf base callus of turmeric and random amplified polymorphic DNA analysis of regenerated plants. Plant Cell Tissue Organ Cult 2001; 66(2): 113-9.
[http://dx.doi.org/10.1023/A:1010638209377]

[159] Babu NK, Divakaran M, Raj RP. Biotechnological approaches in improvement of spices. A review. In: Bahadur B, Venkat Rajam M, Sahijram L, Krishnamurthy K, Eds. Plant Biology and Biotechnology.

New Delhi: Springer 2015; pp. 487-516.

[160]   Kou Y, Ma G, Teixeira da Silva JA, Liu N. Callus induction and shoot organogenesis from anther cultures of *Curcuma attenuata* Wall. Plant Cell Tissue Organ Cult 2013; 112(1): 1-7.
[http://dx.doi.org/10.1007/s11240-012-0205-y]

[161]   Soundar Raju C, Aslam A, Shajahan A. High-efficiency direct somatic embryogenesis and plant regeneration from leaf base explants of turmeric (*Curcuma longa* L.). Plant Cell Tissue Organ Cult 2015; 122(1): 79-87.
[http://dx.doi.org/10.1007/s11240-015-0751-1]

[162]   Zaremba LS, Smoleński WH, Nadgauda RS. Factors affecting *in vitro* microrhizome production in turmeric. Ann Oper Res 2000; 97(1/4): 131-41.
[http://dx.doi.org/10.1023/A:1018996712442]

[163]   Adelberg JW, Cousins MM. Development of micro- and minirhizomes of turmeric, *Curcuma longa* L.,*in vitro*. Acta Hortic 2007; (756): 103-8.
[http://dx.doi.org/10.17660/ActaHortic.2007.756.11]

[164]   Cousins M, Adelberg J, Chen F, Rieck J. Antioxidant capacity of fresh and dried rhizomes from four clones of turmeric (*Curcuma longa* L.) grown *in vitro* . Ind Crops Prod 2007; 25(2): 129-35.
[http://dx.doi.org/10.1016/j.indcrop.2006.08.004]

[165]   Cousins MM, Adelberg J, Chen F, Rieck J. Secondary metabolism-inducing treatments during *in vitro* development of turmeric (*Curcuma longa* L.) rhizomes. J Herbs Spices Med Plants 2010; 15(4): 303-17.
[http://dx.doi.org/10.1080/10496470903507841]

[166]   Naz S, Ilyas S, Javad S, Ali A. *In vitro* clonal multiplication and acclimatization of different varieties of turmeric (*Curcuma longa* L.). Pak J Bot 2009; 41: 2807-16.

[167]   Roopadarshini V. High frequency shoot multiplication and callus regeneration of turmeric. Plant Biotechnol 2010; 6: 723-33.

[168]   El-Hawaz RF, Bridges WC, Adelberg JW. *In vitro* growth of *Curcuma longa* L. in response to five mineral elements and plant density in fed-batch culture systems. PLoS One 2015; 10(4): e0118912.
[http://dx.doi.org/10.1371/journal.pone.0118912] [PMID: 25830292]

[169]   Pistelli L, Bertoli A, Gelli F, Bedini L, Ruffoni B, Pistelli L. Production of Curcuminoids in different *in vitro* organs of *Curcuma longa.* Nat Prod Commun 2012; 7(8): 1934578X1200700.
[http://dx.doi.org/10.1177/1934578X1200700819] [PMID: 22978224]

[170]   Gurav SS, Gurav NS, Patil AT, Duragkar NJ. Effect of explant source, culture media, and growth regulators on callogenesis and expression of secondary metabolites of *Curcuma Longa*. J Herbs Spices Med Plants 2020; 26(2): 172-90.
[http://dx.doi.org/10.1080/10496475.2019.1689542]

[171]   Shanmugarajan D, P P, Kumar BRP, Suresh B. Curcumin to inhibit binding of spike glycoprotein to ACE2 receptors: computational modelling, simulations, and ADMET studies to explore curcuminoids against novel SARS-CoV-2 targets. RSC Advances 2020; 10(52): 31385-99.
[http://dx.doi.org/10.1039/D0RA03167D] [PMID: 35520671]

[172]   Jena AB, Kanungo N, Nayak V, Chainy GBN, Dandapat J. Catechin and curcumin interact with S protein of SARS-CoV2 and ACE2 of human cell membrane: insights from computational studies. Sci Rep 2021; 11(1): 2043.
[http://dx.doi.org/10.1038/s41598-021-81462-7] [PMID: 33479401]

[173]   Bormann M, Alt M, Schipper L, *et al.* Turmeric root and its bioactive ingredient curcumin effectively neutralize SARS-CoV-2 *In Vitro* . Viruses 2021; 13(10): 1914.
[http://dx.doi.org/10.3390/v13101914] [PMID: 34696344]

[174]   Chintakovid N, Tisarum R, Samphumphuang T, Sotesaritkul T, Cha-um S. *In vitro* acclimatization of *Curcuma longa* under controlled *iso*-osmotic conditions. Plant Biotechnol 2021; 38(1): 37-46.

[http://dx.doi.org/10.5511/plantbiotechnology.20.1021a] [PMID: 34177323]

[175] Abd Alhady M, Abo El-Fadl R, Hegazi G, Desoukey S. *In vitro* production of some secondary metabolites from cupressus sempervirens. J Adv Biomed Pharm Sci 2020.
[http://dx.doi.org/10.21608/jabps.2020.24700.1074]

[176] Prakash N, Ansari MA, Punitha P, Sharma PK. indigenous traditional knowledge and usage of folk bio-medicines among rongmei tribe of tamenglong district of manipur, India. Afr J Tradit Complement Altern Med 2014; 11(3): 239-47.
[http://dx.doi.org/10.4314/ajtcam.v11i3.34] [PMID: 25371589]

[177] Nazir R, Gupta S, Kumar V. Enhanced *in vitro* production of diosgenin in shoot cultures of *Dioscorea deltoidea* by elicitation and precursor feeding. 2020; 1-16.
[http://dx.doi.org/10.21203/rs.3.rs-41829/v1]

[178] Rojas R, Alba J, Magaña-Plaza I, Cruz F, Ramos-Valdivia AC. Stimulated production of diosgenin in *Dioscorea galeottiana* cell suspension cultures by abiotic and biotic factors. Biotechnol Lett 1999; 21(10): 907-11.
[http://dx.doi.org/10.1023/A:1005598623728]

[179] Li P, Mao Z, Lou J, *et al.* Enhancement of diosgenin production in Dioscorea zingiberensis cell cultures by oligosaccharides from its endophytic fungus *Fusarium oxysporum* Dzf17. Molecules 2011; 16(12): 10631-44.
[http://dx.doi.org/10.3390/molecules161210631] [PMID: 22183887]

[180] Kindscher K. Ethnobotany of purple coneflower (*Echinacea angustifolia*, Asteraceae) and OtherEchinacea Species. Econ Bot 1989; 43(4): 498-507.
[http://dx.doi.org/10.1007/BF02935924]

[181] Schöllhorn C, Schecklies E, Wagner H. Immunochemical investigations of polysaccharides from *Echinacea purpurea* Cell Suspension Cultures. Planta Med 1993; 59(S 1): A662-3.
[http://dx.doi.org/10.1055/s-2006-959930]

[182] JH S, H B, J D. Callus cultures of the genus Echinacea II. Effect of phenylalanineon the growth of cultures and production of cinnamic acids. Pharmazie 1991; 46: 363-4.

[183] Perry N, van Klink J, Burgess E, Parmenter G. Alkamide levels in echinacea purpurea: A rapid analytical method revealing differences among roots, rhizomes, stems, leaves and flowers. Planta Med 1997; 63(1): 58-62.
[http://dx.doi.org/10.1055/s-2006-957605] [PMID: 17252329]

[184] Bauer R, Wagner H. Echinacea species as potential immunostimulatory drugs. Econ Med Plant Res 1997; 5: 253-321.

[185] Bauer R. Chemistry, analysis and immunological investigations of Echinacea phytopharmaceuticals.Immunomodulatory Agents from Plants In: Progress in Inflammation Research. 1999.
[http://dx.doi.org/10.1007/978-3-0348-8763-2_2]

[186] Choffe KL, Victor JMR, Murch SJ, Saxena PK. *In vitro* regeneration of *Echinacea purpurea* L.: Direct somatic embryogenesis and indirect shoot organogenesis in petiole culture. Vitr Cell Dev Biol - Plant 2000; 36: 30-6.
[http://dx.doi.org/10.1007/s11627-000-0008-4]

[187] Coker PS, Camper ND. *In vitro* culture of *Echinacea purpurea* L. J Herbs Spices Med Plants 2000; 7(4): 1-7.
[http://dx.doi.org/10.1300/J044v07n04_01]

[188] Koroch A, Kapteyn J, Juliani HR, Simon JE. *In Vitro* regeneration and agrobacterium transformation of *Echinacea purpurea* Leaf Explants *. Plant Biol 2002; 522-6.

[189] Zebarjadi A, Motamedi J, Ismaili A. Indirect shoot regeneration of iranian purple coneflower (*Echinacea purpurea* L.) from cotyledon and hypocotyl explants. Acta Agron Hung 2011; 59(1): 65-

72.
[http://dx.doi.org/10.1556/AAgr.59.2011.1.7]

[190] Jones MPA, Cao J, O'Brien R, Murch SJ, Saxena PK. The mode of action of thidiazuron: Auxins, indoleamines, and ion channels in the regeneration of *Echinacea purpurea* L. Plant Cell Rep 2007; 26(9): 1481-90.
[http://dx.doi.org/10.1007/s00299-007-0357-0] [PMID: 17483954]

[191] Butiuc-Keul AL, Vlase L, Crăciunaş C. Clonal propagation and production of cichoric acid in three species of echinaceae. *In Vitro* Cell Dev Biol Plant 2012; 48: 249-58.
[http://dx.doi.org/10.1007/s11627-012-9435-2]

[192] Smith MAL, Kobayashi H, Gawienowski M, Briskin DP. An *in vitro* approach to investigate medicinal chemical synthesis by three herbal plants. Plant Cell Tissue Organ Cult 2002; 70(1): 105-11.
[http://dx.doi.org/10.1023/A:1016081913719]

[193] Lakshmanan P, Danesh M, Taji A. Production of four commercially cultivated *Echinacea* species by different methods of *in vitro* regeneration. J Hortic Sci Biotechnol 2002; 77(2): 158-63.
[http://dx.doi.org/10.1080/14620316.2002.11511473]

[194] Billah MM, Hosen MB, Khan F, Niaz K. Echinacea. Nonvitamin and nonmineral nutritional supplements. Cambridge: Academic Press 2018.

[195] Li WW, Barz W. Structure and accumulation of phenolics in elicited *Echinacea purpurea* cell cultures. Planta Med 2006; 72(3): 248-54.
[http://dx.doi.org/10.1055/s-2005-873201] [PMID: 16534730]

[196] Misawa M. An alternative for production of useful metabolites. Biotechnol Adv 1994; 13(3): 425-53.

[197] Liu CZ, Abbasi BH, Gao M, Murch SJ, Saxena PK. Caffeic acid derivatives production by hairy root cultures of *Echinacea purpurea*. J Agric Food Chem 2006; 54(22): 8456-60.
[http://dx.doi.org/10.1021/jf061940r] [PMID: 17061821]

[198] Liu R, Li W, Sun LY, Liu CZ. Improving root growth and cichoric acid derivatives production in hairy root culture of *Echinacea purpurea* by ultrasound treatment. Biochem Eng J 2012; 60: 62-6.
[http://dx.doi.org/10.1016/j.bej.2011.10.001]

[199] Abbasi BH, Saxena PK, Murch SJ, Liu CZ. Echinacea biotechnology: Challenges and opportunities. Vitr Cell Dev Biol - Plant 2007; 43: 481-92.
[http://dx.doi.org/10.1007/s11627-007-9057-2]

[200] Abbasi BH, Stiles AR, Saxena PK, Liu CZ. Gibberellic acid increases secondary metabolite production in *Echinacea purpurea* hairy roots. Appl Biochem Biotechnol 2012; 168(7): 2057-66.
[http://dx.doi.org/10.1007/s12010-012-9917-z] [PMID: 23076568]

[201] Abdoli M, Moieni A, Naghdi Badi H. Morphological, physiological, cytological and phytochemical studies in diploid and colchicine-induced tetraploid plants of *Echinacea purpurea* (L.). Acta Physiol Plant 2013; 35(7): 2075-83.
[http://dx.doi.org/10.1007/s11738-013-1242-9]

[202] Wu CH, Murthy HN, Hahn EJ, Paek KY. Large-scale cultivation of adventitious roots of *Echinacea purpurea* in airlift bioreactors for the production of chichoric acid, chlorogenic acid and caftaric acid. Biotechnol Lett 2007; 29(8): 1179-82.
[http://dx.doi.org/10.1007/s10529-007-9399-1] [PMID: 17589811]

[203] Jones AMP, Saxena PK, Murch SJ. Elicitation of secondary metabolism in *Echinacea purpurea* L. by gibberellic acid and triazoles. Eng Life Sci 2009; 9(3): 205-10.
[http://dx.doi.org/10.1002/elsc.200800104]

[204] Lucchesini M, Bertoli A, Mensuali-Sodi A, Pistelli L. Establishment of *in vitro* tissue cultures from *Echinacea angustifolia* D.C. adult plants for the production of phytochemical compounds. Sci Hortic 2009; 122(3): 484-90.
[http://dx.doi.org/10.1016/j.scienta.2009.06.011]

[205] Romero FR, Delate K, Kraus GA. Alkamide production from hairy root cultures of Echinacea. Vitr Cell Dev Biol - Plant 2009; 45: 599-609.
[http://dx.doi.org/10.1007/s11627-008-9187-1]

[206] Jeong JA, Wu CH, Murthy HN, Hahn E-J, Paek K-Y. Application of an airlift bioreactor system for the production of adventitious root biomass and caffeic acid derivatives of *Echinacea purpurea*. Biotechnol Bioprocess Eng 2009; 14(1): 91-8.
[http://dx.doi.org/10.1007/s12257-007-0142-5]

[207] Cui HY, Abdullahil Baque M, Lee EJ, Paek KY. Scale-up of adventitious root cultures of *Echinacea angustifolia* in a pilot-scale bioreactor for the production of biomass and caffeic acid derivatives. Plant Biotechnol Rep 2013; 7(3): 297-308.
[http://dx.doi.org/10.1007/s11816-012-0263-y]

[208] Chen XL, Zhang JJ, Chen R, Li QL, Yang YS, Wu H. An uncommon plant growth regulator, diethyl aminoethyl hexanoate, is highly effective in tissue cultures of the important medicinal plant purple coneflower (*Echinacea purpurea* L.). BioMed Res Int 2013; 2013: 1-12.
[http://dx.doi.org/10.1155/2013/540316] [PMID: 24455702]

[209] Guarnerio CF, Fraccaroli M, Gonzo I, *et al.* Metabolomic analysis reveals that the accumulation of specific secondary metabolites in *Echinacea angustifolia* cells cultured *in vitro* can be controlled by light. Plant Cell Rep 2012; 31(2): 361-7.
[http://dx.doi.org/10.1007/s00299-011-1171-2] [PMID: 22009052]

[210] Aboul-Enein AM, Afify AE-MM, Rady MR. *In vitro* Clonal Propagation, Caffeic Acid Production and RAPD Analysis of Some Varieties of *Echinacea purpurea* Plant. J Appl Sci Res 2013.

[211] Rady MR, Aboul-Enein AM, Ibrahim MM. Active compounds and biological activity of *in vitro* cultures of some *Echinacea purpurea* varieties. Bull Natl Res Cent 2018; 42(1): 20.
[http://dx.doi.org/10.1186/s42269-018-0018-1]

[212] Ramezannezhad R, Aghdasi M, Fatemi M. Enhanced production of cichoric acid in cell suspension culture of *Echinacea purpurea* by silver nanoparticle elicitation. Plant Cell Tissue Organ Cult 2019; 139(2): 261-73.
[http://dx.doi.org/10.1007/s11240-019-01678-4]

[213] Fan M zhi, Wu X han, Li X feng. Co-cultured adventitious roots of echinacea pallida and *echinacea purpurea* inhibit lipopolysaccharide-induced inflammation *via* mapk pathway in mouse peritoneal macrophages. Chinese Herb Med 2021; 13(2): 228-34.
[http://dx.doi.org/10.1016/j.chmed.2021.01.001]

[214] Lema-Rumińska J, Kulus D, Tymoszuk A, Varejão JMTB, Bahcevandziev K. Profile of secondary metabolites and genetic stability analysis in new lines of *Echinacea purpurea* (L.) Moench micropropagated *via* somatic embryogenesis. Ind Crops Prod 2019; 142: 111851.
[http://dx.doi.org/10.1016/j.indcrop.2019.111851]

[215] Demirci T, Çelikkol Akçay U, Göktürk Baydar N. Effects of 24-epibrassinolide and l-phenylalanine on growth and caffeic acid derivative production in hairy root culture of *Echinacea purpurea* L. Moench. Acta Physiol Plant 2020; 42(4): 66.
[http://dx.doi.org/10.1007/s11738-020-03055-7]

[216] Demirci T, Akçay UÇ, Göktürk Baydar N. Physical and biochemical differences in Agrobacterium rhizogenes-mediated transgenic hairy root lines of *Echinacea purpurea*. Vitr Cell Dev Biol - Plant 2020; 56: 875-81.
[http://dx.doi.org/10.1007/s11627-020-10090-z]

[217] An D, Wu CH, Wang M. Methyl jasmonate elicits enhancement of bioactive compound synthesis in adventitious root co-culture of *Echinacea purpurea* and *Echinacea pallida*. Vitr Cell Dev Biol - Plant 2021; 58(1): 181-7.
[http://dx.doi.org/10.1007/s11627-021-10195-z]

[218] Gygax A. *Eryngium alpinum*. In: The IUCN Red List of Threatened species. Version 2014 2013.

[219] Gillot P, Garraud L. *Eryngium alpinum* (L.) In: red book of threatened flora,. natl museum of history nat conserv bot natl porquerolles. Paris, Fr: Ministry of the Environment 1995.

[220] Kikowska M, Thiem B, Szopa A, *et al*. Comparative analysis of phenolic acids and flavonoids in shoot cultures of *Eryngium alpinum* L.: an endangered and protected species with medicinal value. Plant Cell Tissue Organ Cult 2019; 139(1): 167-75.
[http://dx.doi.org/10.1007/s11240-019-01674-8]

[221] Arockiasamy S, Prakash S, Ignacimuthu S. Direct organogenesis from mature leaf and petiole explants of Eryngium.L. Biol Plant 2002; 45(1): 129-32.
[http://dx.doi.org/10.1023/A:1015177330589]

[222] Martin KP. Efficacy of different growth regulators at different stages of somatic embryogenesis in *Eryngium foetidum* L. - A rare medicinal plant. Vitr Cell Dev Biol - Plant 2004; 40: 459-63.
[http://dx.doi.org/10.1079/IVP2004543]

[223] Chandrika UG, Prasad Kumara PAAS. Gotu kola (*centella asiatica*). Adv Food Nutr Res 2015; 76: 125-57.
[http://dx.doi.org/10.1016/bs.afnr.2015.08.001] [PMID: 26602573]

[224] Kikowska M, Budzianowski J, Krawczyk A, Thiem B. Accumulation of rosmarinic, chlorogenic and caffeic acids in *in vitro* cultures of *Eryngium planum* L. Acta Physiol Plant 2012; 34(6): 2425-33.
[http://dx.doi.org/10.1007/s11738-012-1011-1]

[225] Kikowska M, Kędziora I, Krawczyk A, Thiem B. Methyl jasmonate, yeast extract and sucrose stimulate phenolic acids accumulation in *Eryngium planum* L. shoot cultures. Acta Biochim Pol 2015; 62(2): 197-200.
[http://dx.doi.org/10.18388/abp.2014_880] [PMID: 25856557]

[226] Thiem A, Duşa A. QCA: A package for qualitative comparative analysis. R J 2013; 5(1): 87-97.
[http://dx.doi.org/10.32614/RJ-2013-009]

[227] Kikowska M, Thiem B, Sliwinska E, *et al*. The effect of nutritional factors and plant growth regulators on micropropagation and production of phenolic acids and saponins from plantlets and adventitious root cultures of *Eryngium maritimum* L. J Plant Growth Regul 2014; 33(4): 809-19.
[http://dx.doi.org/10.1007/s00344-014-9428-y]

[228] Kikowska M, Thiem B, Sliwinska E, *et al*. Micropropagation of *eryngium campestre* l. *via* shoot culture provides valuable uniform plant material with enhanced content of phenolic acids and antimicrobial activity. Acta Biol Cracov Ser; Bot 2016; 58(1): 43-56.
[http://dx.doi.org/10.1515/abcsb-2016-0009]

[229] Ayuso M, Pinela J, Dias MI, *et al*. Phenolic composition and biological activities of the *in vitro* cultured endangered *Eryngium viviparum* J. Gay. Ind Crops Prod 2020; 148: 112325.
[http://dx.doi.org/10.1016/j.indcrop.2020.112325]

[230] Kikowska M, Thiem B, Szopa A, Ekiert H. Accumulation of valuable secondary metabolites: phenolic acids and flavonoids in different *in vitro* systems of shoot cultures of the endangered plant species—*Eryngium alpinum* L. Plant Cell Tissue Organ Cult 2020; 141(2): 381-91.
[http://dx.doi.org/10.1007/s11240-020-01795-5]

[231] Jacobs BP, Browner WS. *Ginkgo biloba*: A living fossil. Am J Med 2000; 108(4): 341-2.
[http://dx.doi.org/10.1016/S0002-9343(00)00290-4] [PMID: 11014729]

[232] Singh B, Kaur P, Gopichand , Singh RD, Ahuja PS. Biology and chemistry of *Ginkgo biloba*. Fitoterapia 2008; 79(6): 401-18.
[http://dx.doi.org/10.1016/j.fitote.2008.05.007] [PMID: 18639617]

[233] Tulecke W. The pollen of ginkgo biloba: *In Vitro* culture and tissue formation. Am J Bot 1957; 44(7): 602-8.

[http://dx.doi.org/10.1002/j.1537-2197.1957.tb10583.x]

[234] Nakanishi K, Habaguchi K, Nakadaira Y. Structure of bilobalide, a rare tert-butyl containing sesquiterpenoid related to the cla-ginkgolide. J fhe Am Chem Soc 1971; 4491: 3544-6.

[235] Park YG, Kim SJ, Jung HY, *et al.* Variation of ginkgolides and bilobalide contents in leaves and cell cultures of *Ginkgo biloba* L. Biotechnol Bioprocess Eng 2004; 9(1): 35-40.
[http://dx.doi.org/10.1007/BF02949319]

[236] Kang SM, Min JY, Kim YD, *et al.* Effect of supplementing terpenoid biosynthetic precursors on the accumulation of bilobalide and ginkgolides in *Ginkgo biloba* cell cultures. J Biotechnol 2006; 123(1): 85-92.
[http://dx.doi.org/10.1016/j.jbiotec.2005.10.021] [PMID: 16364482]

[237] Kang SM, Min JY, Kim YD, *et al.* Effect of biotic elicitors on the accumulation of bilobalide and ginkgolides in *Ginkgo biloba* cell cultures. J Biotechnol 2009; 139(1): 84-8.
[http://dx.doi.org/10.1016/j.jbiotec.2008.09.007] [PMID: 18983879]

[238] Kang SM, Min JY, Park DJ, *et al.* Potassium chloride elicits enhancement of bilobalide and Ginkgolides production by *Ginkgo biloba* cell cultures. Forest Sci Technol 2010; 6(2): 49-54.
[http://dx.doi.org/10.1080/21580103.2010.9671972]

[239] Kladar N, Srđenović B, Grujić N, *et al.* Ecologically and ontogenetically induced variations in phenolic compounds and biological activities of *Hypericum maculatum* subsp. *maculatum*, Hypericaceae. Rev Bras Bot 2015; 38(4): 703-15.
[http://dx.doi.org/10.1007/s40415-015-0177-3]

[240] You M, Kim DW, Jeong KS, *et al.* St. John's Wort (*Hypericum perforatum*) stimulates human osteoblastic MG-63 cell proliferation and attenuates trabecular bone loss induced by ovariectomy. Nutr Res Pract 2015; 9(5): 459-65.
[http://dx.doi.org/10.4162/nrp.2015.9.5.459] [PMID: 26425274]

[241] Nahrstedt A, Butterweck V. Biologically active and other chemical constituents of the herb of *Hypericum perforatum* L. Pharmacopsychiatry 1997; 30(S 2) (2): 129-34.
[http://dx.doi.org/10.1055/s-2007-979533] [PMID: 9342774]

[242] Greeson JM, Sanford B, Monti DA. St. John's wort (*Hypericum perforatum*): a review of the current pharmacological, toxicological, and clinical literature. Psychopharmacology 2001; 153(4): 402-14.
[http://dx.doi.org/10.1007/s002130000625] [PMID: 11243487]

[243] Bagdonaitė E, Mártonfi P, Repčák M, Labokas J. Variation in concentrations of major bioactive compounds in *Hypericum perforatum* L. from Lithuania. Ind Crops Prod 2012; 35(1): 302-8.
[http://dx.doi.org/10.1016/j.indcrop.2011.07.018]

[244] Shakya P, Marslin G, Siram K, Beerhues L, Franklin G. Elicitation as a tool to improve the profiles of high-value secondary metabolites and pharmacological properties of *Hypericum perforatum*. J Pharm Pharmacol 2018; 71(1): 70-82.
[http://dx.doi.org/10.1111/jphp.12743] [PMID: 28523644]

[245] Zhou T, Chen B, Fan G, Chai Y, Wu Y. Application of high-speed counter-current chromatography coupled with high-performance liquid chromatography–diode array detection for the preparative isolation and purification of hyperoside from *Hypericum perforatum* with online purity monitoring. J Chromatogr A 2006; 1116(1-2): 97-101.
[http://dx.doi.org/10.1016/j.chroma.2006.03.041] [PMID: 16620843]

[246] Karuppusamy S. A review on trends in production of secondary metabolites from higher plants by *in vitro* tissue, organ and cell cultures. J Med Plants Res 2009; 3: 1222-39.

[247] Zhao J, Davis LC, Verpoorte R. Elicitor signal transduction leading to production of plant secondary metabolites. Biotechnol Adv 2005; 23(4): 283-333.
[http://dx.doi.org/10.1016/j.biotechadv.2005.01.003] [PMID: 15848039]

[248] Gadzovska-Simic S, Tusevski O, Antevski S, *et al.* Secondary metabolite production in *Hypericum*

perforatum L. cell suspensions upon elicitation with fungal mycelia from *Aspergillus flavus*. Arch Biol Sci 2012; 64(1): 113-21.
[http://dx.doi.org/10.2298/ABS1201113G]

[249]   Čellárová E, Brutovská R, Bruňáková K, Daxnerová Z, Weigel RC. Correlation between hypericin content and the ploidy of somaclones of *Hypericum perforatum* L. Acta Biotechnol 1997; 17(1): 83-90.
[http://dx.doi.org/10.1002/abio.370170111]

[250]   Zaremba LS, Smoleński WH. RFLP analysis of *Hypericum perforatum* L. somaclones and their progenies. Ann Oper Res 2000; 97(1/4): 131-41.
[http://dx.doi.org/10.1023/A:1018996712442]

[251]   Mederos-Molina S. Micropropagation of Hypericum canariense L. for the Production of Hypericin.In: Medicinal and Aromatic Plants XII. Biotechnology in Agriculture and Forestry 2002.
[http://dx.doi.org/10.1007/978-3-662-08616-2_6]

[252]   Umek A, Kreft S, Kartnig T, Heydel B. Quantitative phytochemical analyses of six *Hypericum* species growing in slovenia. Planta Med 1999; 65(4): 388-90.
[http://dx.doi.org/10.1055/s-2006-960798] [PMID: 17260265]

[253]   Upson T, Andrews S. The genus Lavandula. Portl Timber Press 2004.

[254]   Touati B, Chograni H, Hassen I, Boussaïd M, Toumi L, Brahim NB. Chemical composition of the leaf and flower essential oils of Tunisian *Lavandula dentata* L. (Lamiaceae). Chem Biodivers 2011; 8(8): 1560-9.
[http://dx.doi.org/10.1002/cbdv.201000357]

[255]   Del Carmen Calvo M, Sánchez-Gras MC. Accumulation of monoterpenes in shoot-proliferation cultures of *Lavandula latifolia* Med. Plant Sci 1993; 91(2): 207-12.
[http://dx.doi.org/10.1016/0168-9452(93)90143-N]

[256]   Banthorpe DV, Bates MJ, Ireland MJ. Stimulation of accumulation of terpenoids by cell. Phytochemistry 1995; 40.

[257]   Park SU, Uddin MR, Xu H, *et al.* Biotechnological applications for rosmarinic acid production in plant. Afr J Biotechnol 2008; 7: 4959-65.

[258]   Pavlov AI, Ilieva MP, Panchev IN. Nutrient medium optimization for rosmarinic acid production by *Lavandula vera* MM cell suspension. Biotechnol Prog 2000; 16(4): 668-70.
[http://dx.doi.org/10.1021/bp000041z] [PMID: 10933844]

[259]   TopÇu G, Herrmann G, Kolak U, Gören C, Porzel A, Kutchan TM. Isolation of fatty acids and aromatics from cell suspension cultures of *Lavandula angustifolia*. Nat Prod Res 2007; 21(2): 100-5.
[http://dx.doi.org/10.1080/14786410500462884] [PMID: 17365695]

[260]   Georgiev M, Georgiev V, Penchev P, *et al.* Volatile metabolic profiles of cell suspension cultures of *Lavandula vera*, *Nicotiana tabacum* and *Helianthus annuus*, cultivated under different regimes. Eng Life Sci 2010; 10: NA.
[http://dx.doi.org/10.1002/elsc.200900090]

[261]   Fujita Y, Hara Y, Suga C, Morimoto T. Production of shikonin derivatives by cell suspension cultures of Lithospermum erythrorhizon. Plant Cell Rep 1981; 1(2): 61-3.
[http://dx.doi.org/10.1007/BF00269273] [PMID: 24258860]

[262]   Yazaki K. *Lithospermum erythrorhizon* cell cultures: Present and future aspects. Plant Biotechnol 2017; 34(3): 131-42.
[http://dx.doi.org/10.5511/plantbiotechnology.17.0823a] [PMID: 31275019]

[263]   Yamamoto H, Yazaki K, Inoue K. Simultaneous analysis of shikimate-derived secondary metabolites in *Lithospermum erythrorhizon* cell suspension cultures by high-performance liquid chromatography. J Chromatogr, Biomed Appl 2000; 738(1): 3-15.
[http://dx.doi.org/10.1016/S0378-4347(99)00473-9] [PMID: 10778921]

[264] Takanashi K, Nakagawa Y, Aburaya S, *et al.* Comparative proteomic analysis of *Lithospermum erythrorhizon* reveals regulation of a variety of metabolic enzymes leading to comprehensive understanding of the shikonin biosynthetic pathway. Plant Cell Physiol 2019; 60(1): 19-28.
[http://dx.doi.org/10.1093/pcp/pcy183] [PMID: 30169873]

[265] Maliński MP, Michalska AD, Tomczykowa M, Tomczyk M, Thiem B. Ragged Robin *(Lychnis flos-cuculi)* - a plant with potential medicinal value. Rev Bras Farmacogn 2014; 24(6): 722-30.
[http://dx.doi.org/10.1016/j.bjp.2014.11.004]

[266] Maliński MP, Kikowska M, Kruszka D, *et al.* Various *in vitro* systems of Ragged Robin *(Lychnis flos-cuculi* L.): A new potential source of phytoecdysteroids? Plant Cell Tissue Organ Cult 2019; 139(1): 39-52.
[http://dx.doi.org/10.1007/s11240-019-01660-0]

[267] Maliński MP, Budzianowski J, Kikowska M, *et al.* Two ecdysteroids isolated from micropropagated lychnis flos-cuculi and the biological activity of plant. Molecules 2021; 26(4): 904.
[http://dx.doi.org/10.3390/molecules26040904] [PMID: 33572129]

[268] Maliński MP, Kikowska MA, Soluch A, Kowalczyk M, Stochmal A, Thiem B. Phytochemical screening, phenolic compounds and antioxidant activity of biomass from *Llychnis flos-cuculi l. In vitro* cultures and intact plants. Plants 2021; 10(2): 206.
[http://dx.doi.org/10.3390/plants10020206] [PMID: 33499074]

[269] Wang MY, West BJ, Jensen CJ, *et al. Morinda citrifolia* (Noni): A literature review and recent advances in Noni research. Acta Pharmacol Sin 2002; 23(12): 1127-41.
[PMID: 12466051]

[270] Baque MA, Hahn EJ, Paek KY. Growth, secondary metabolite production and antioxidant enzyme response of *Morinda citrifolia* adventitious root as affected by auxin and cytokinin. Plant Biotechnol Rep 2010; 4(2): 109-16.
[http://dx.doi.org/10.1007/s11816-009-0121-8]

[271] Hagendoorn MJM, Van Der Plas LHW, Segers GJ. Accumulation of anthraquinones in *Morinda citrifolia* cell suspensions. Plant Cell Tissue Organ Cult 1994; 38(2-3): 227-34.
[http://dx.doi.org/10.1007/BF00033881]

[272] Hagendoorn L. Intergroup biases in multiple group systems: The perception of ethnic hierarchies. Eur Rev Soc Psychol 1995; 6(1): 199-228.
[http://dx.doi.org/10.1080/14792779443000058]

[273] Quevedo CV, Perassolo M, Giulietti AM, Talou JR. Enhancement of anthraquinone production in *Morinda citrifolia* cell suspension cultures after stimulation of the proline cycle with two proline analogs. Biotechnol Lett 2012; 34(3): 571-5.
[http://dx.doi.org/10.1007/s10529-011-0806-2] [PMID: 22109937]

[274] Perassolo M, Smith ME, Giulietti AM, Rodríguez Talou J. Synergistic effect of methyl jasmonate and cyclodextrins on anthraquinone accumulation in cell suspension cultures of *Morinda citrifolia* and *Rubia tinctorum.* Plant Cell Tissue Organ Cult 2016; 124(2): 319-30.
[http://dx.doi.org/10.1007/s11240-015-0896-y]

[275] Abdullah MA, Ariff AB, Marziah M, Ali AM, Lajis NH. Strategies to overcome foaming and wall-growth during the cultivation of *Morinda elliptica* cell suspension culture in a stirred-tank bioreactor. Plant Cell Tissue Organ Cult 2000; 60(3): 205-12.
[http://dx.doi.org/10.1023/A:1006495107778]

[276] Ahmed S, Hahn EJ, Paek KY. Aeration volume and photosynthetic photon flux affect cell growth and secondary metabolite contents in bioreactor cultures of *Morinda citrifolia.* J Plant Biol 2008; 51(3): 209-12.
[http://dx.doi.org/10.1007/BF03030700]

[277] Wang MY, Su C. Cancer preventive effect of *Morinda citrifolia* (Noni). Ann N Y Acad Sci 2001;

952(1): 161-8.
[http://dx.doi.org/10.1111/j.1749-6632.2001.tb02737.x] [PMID: 11795436]

[278] Sharma SN, Jha Z, Sinha RK. Establishment of *in vitro* adventitious root cultures and analysis of andrographolide in *Andrographis paniculata.* Nat Prod Commun 2013; 8(8): 1934578X1300800.
[http://dx.doi.org/10.1177/1934578X1300800803] [PMID: 24079163]

[279] Komaraiah P, Kishor PBK, Carlsson M, Magnusson K-E, Mandenius C-F. Enhancement of anthraquinone accumulation in *Morinda citrifolia* suspension cultures. Plant Sci 2005; 168(5): 1337-44.
[http://dx.doi.org/10.1016/j.plantsci.2005.01.017]

[280] Baque MA, Shiragi MHK, Moh SH. Production of biomass and bioactive compounds by adventitious root suspension cultures of *Morinda citrifolia* (L.) in a liquid-phase airlift balloon-type bioreactor. Vitr Cell Dev Biol - Plant 2013; 49: 737-49.
[http://dx.doi.org/10.1007/s11627-013-9555-3]

[281] Purwianingsih W, Hidayat RY, Rahmat A. Increasing anthraquinone compounds on callus leaf *Morinda citrifolia* (L.) by elicitation method using chitosan shell of shrimps (*Penaeus monodon*). J Phys Conf Ser 2019; 1280: 022001.
[http://dx.doi.org/10.1088/1742-6596/1280/2/022001]

[282] Ohta S, Yatazawa M. Nicotiana tabacum L. (Tobacco): *In Vitro* production of nicotine. In: Bajaj YPS, Ed. Medicinal and Aromatic Plants II Biotechnology in Agriculture and Forestry. Springer 1989; 7.

[283] Dawson R. Biosynthesis of the nicotiana alkaloids. In: Brode WR, Ed. Science in Progress. CT: Yale Univ Press New Haven 1962; Vol. 12: pp. 117-43.

[284] Benveniste P, Hirth L, Ourisson G. La biosynthèse des stérols dans les tissus de tabac cultivés *in vitro*—II. Phytochemistry 1966; 5(1): 45-58.
[http://dx.doi.org/10.1016/S0031-9422(00)85080-3]

[285] Mizukasi S, Tanabe Y, Noguchi M, Tamaki E. p-coumaroylputrescine, caffeoylputrescine and feruloylputrescine from callus tissue culture of Nicotiana tabacum. Phytochemistry 1971; 10(6): 1347-50.
[http://dx.doi.org/10.1016/S0031-9422(00)84339-3]

[286] Mizusa S, Tanabe Y, Noguchi M. A new aromatic amide, caffeoyl-putrescine from callus tissue cultures of *Nicotiana tabacum.* Agric Biol Chem 1970; 34(6): 972-3.
[http://dx.doi.org/10.1080/00021369.1970.10859716]

[287] Bunsupa S, Katayama K, Ikeura E, *et al.* Lysine decarboxylase catalyzes the first step of quinolizidine alkaloid biosynthesis and coevolved with alkaloid production in leguminosae. Plant Cell 2012; 24(3): 1202-16.
[http://dx.doi.org/10.1105/tpc.112.095885] [PMID: 22415272]

[288] Häkkinen ST, Moyano E, Cusidó RM, Palazón J, Piñol MT, Oksman-Caldentey KM. Enhanced secretion of tropane alkaloids in *Nicotiana tabacum* hairy roots expressing heterologous hyoscyamine-6β-hydroxylase. J Exp Bot 2005; 56(420): 2611-8.
[http://dx.doi.org/10.1093/jxb/eri253] [PMID: 16105856]

[289] Zayed R, Wink M. Induction of pyridine alkaloid formation in transformed root cultures of *Nicotiana tabacum.* Z Naturforsch C J Biosci 2009; 64(11-12): 869-74.
[http://dx.doi.org/10.1515/znc-2009-11-1219] [PMID: 20158160]

[290] Hildreth SB, Gehman EA, Yang H, *et al.* Tobacco nicotine uptake permease (NUP1) affects alkaloid metabolism. Proc Natl Acad Sci 2011; 108(44): 18179-84.
[http://dx.doi.org/10.1073/pnas.1108620108] [PMID: 22006310]

[291] Zhao B. Alkaloid production by hairy root cultures. phd thesis. Utah: Utah state univeristy logan 2014.

[292] Ritala A, Dong L, Imseng N, *et al.* Evaluation of tobacco (*Nicotiana tabacum* L. cv. Petit Havana SR1) hairy roots for the production of geraniol, the first committed step in terpenoid indole alkaloid

pathway. J Biotechnol 2014; 176: 20-8.
[http://dx.doi.org/10.1016/j.jbiotec.2014.01.031] [PMID: 24530945]

[293] Kumar LMP, Indira M. Trends in Fertilizer Consumption and Foodgrain Production in India: A Co-integration Analysis. SDMIMD Journal of Management 2017; 8(2): 45-50.
[http://dx.doi.org/10.18311/sdmimd/2017/18025]

[294] Capdesuñer Y, García-Brizuela J, Mock HP, Hernández KV, de la Torre MH, Santiesteban-Toca CE. Accessing to the *Nicotiana tabacum* leaf antimicrobial activity: *In-silico and in-vitro* investigations. Plant Physiol Biochem 2019; 139: 591-9.
[http://dx.doi.org/10.1016/j.plaphy.2019.04.015] [PMID: 31030027]

[295] Kumar M, Jha S, Mitra A. Targeted profiling reveals metabolic perturbations in cryptogein-cotransformed hairy root cultures of *Nicotiana tabacum*. Acta Physiol Plant 2020; 42(11): 166.
[http://dx.doi.org/10.1007/s11738-020-03155-4]

[296] Isah T, Mujib A. Camptothecin from *Nothapodytes nimmoniana*: review on biotechnology applications. Acta Physiol Plant 2015; 37(6): 106.
[http://dx.doi.org/10.1007/s11738-015-1854-3]

[297] Khadke S, Kuvalekar A. Direct somatic embryogenesis and plant regeneration from leaf and stem explants of *Nothapodytes foetida*: A critically endangered plant species Nutrigenomics and Functional Foods Laboratory, Interactive Research School for Health Affairs (IRSHA), Sures. Int J Plant, AnimEnviron Sci 2013; 257-64.

[298] Govindachari TR, Viswanathan N. Alkaloids of *Mappia foetida*. Phytochemistry 1972; 11(12): 3529-31.
[http://dx.doi.org/10.1016/S0031-9422(00)89852-0]

[299] Namdeo AG, Sharma A. HPLC analysis of camptothecin content in various parts of *Nothapodytes foetida* collected on different periods. Asian Pac J Trop Biomed 2012; 2(5): 389-93.
[http://dx.doi.org/10.1016/S2221-1691(12)60062-8] [PMID: 23569936]

[300] Patwardhan A. Domestication of *Nothapodytes nimmoniana* (grah.). Mabb An endangered medicinal tree from Western Ghats of India. rufford small grants Found UK 2006; pp. 7-15.

[301] Saha S, Sengupta C. An efficient method for micropropagation of *Ocimum basilicum* L. Indian J Plant Physiol 2010.

[302] Imad HH, Lena FH, Sabreen AK. Analysis of bioactive chemical compounds of *Aspergillus niger* by using gas chromatography-mass spectrometry and fourier-transform infrared spectroscopy. J Pharmacogn Phytother 2015; 7(8): 132-63.
[http://dx.doi.org/10.5897/JPP2015.0354]

[303] Labra M, Miele M, Ledda B, Grassi F, Mazzei M, Sala F. Morphological characterization, essential oil composition and DNA genotyping of *Ocimum basilicum* L. cultivars. Plant Sci 2004; 167(4): 725-31.
[http://dx.doi.org/10.1016/j.plantsci.2004.04.026]

[304] Tada H, Murakami Y, Omoto T, Shimomura K, Ishimaru K. Rosmarinic acid and related phenolics in hairy root cultures of *Ocimum basilicum*. Phytochemistry 1996; 42(2): 431-4.
[http://dx.doi.org/10.1016/0031-9422(96)00005-2]

[305] Tchoumbougnang F, Zollo PHA, Avlessi F, *et al.* Variability in the chemical compositions of the essential oils of five *Ocimum* species from tropical african area. J Essent Oil Res 2006; 18(2): 194-9.
[http://dx.doi.org/10.1080/10412905.2006.9699064]

[306] Verma RS, Padalia RC, Chauhan A, Thul ST. Exploring compositional diversity in the essential oils of 34 Ocimum taxa from Indian flora. Ind Crops Prod 2013; 45: 7-19.
[http://dx.doi.org/10.1016/j.indcrop.2012.12.005]

[307] Zheljazkov VD, Cantrell CL, Evans WB, Ebelhar MW, Coker C. Yield and composition of *Ocimum basilicum* L. and *Ocimum sanctum* L. grown at four locations. HortScience 2008; 43(3): 737-41.
[http://dx.doi.org/10.21273/HORTSCI.43.3.737]

[308] Marzouk AM. Hepatoprotective triterpenes from hairy root cultures of Ocimum basilicum L. Z Naturforsch C J Biosci 2009; 64(3-4): 201-9.
[http://dx.doi.org/10.1515/znc-2009-3-409] [PMID: 19526713]

[309] Rady MR, Nazif NM. Rosmarinic acid content and RAPD analysis of *in vitro* regenerated basil (*Ocimum americanum*) plants. Fitoterapia 2005; 76(6): 525-33.
[http://dx.doi.org/10.1016/j.fitote.2005.04.001] [PMID: 16112496]

[310] Strazzer P, Guzzo F, Levi M. Correlated accumulation of anthocyanins and rosmarinic acid in mechanically stressed red cell suspensions of basil (*Ocimum basilicum*). J Plant Physiol 2011; 168(3): 288-93.
[http://dx.doi.org/10.1016/j.jplph.2010.07.020] [PMID: 20943285]

[311] Moschopoulou G, Kintzios S. Achievement of thousand-fold accumulation of rosmarinic acid in immobilized cells of sweet basil (*Ocimum basilicum* L.) by ten-fold increase of the volume of the immobilization matrix. J Biol Res 2011; 15: 59-65.

[312] Kintzios S, Kollias H, Straitouris E, Makri O. Scale-up micropropagation of sweet basil (*Ocimum basilicum* L.) in an airlift bioreactor and accumulation of rosmarinic acid. Biotechnol Lett 2004; 26(6): 521-3.
[http://dx.doi.org/10.1023/B:BILE.0000019561.89044.30] [PMID: 15127795]

[313] Mathew R, Sankar DP. Growth characteristics of cell suspension cultures for secondary metabolite production in *Ocimum basilicum* L *Ocimum sanctum* L and *Ocimum gratissimum* L. J Pharm Res 2011; 4: 3323-6.

[314] Osman A, El-Kadafy A, Sewedan E, Moubarak M, Abdel-Rahman M. The effect of polyethylene glycol (peg) on calluses of sweet basil (*Ocimum basilicum* L.). Scientific Journal of Flowers and Ornamental Plants 2020; 7(4): 447-59.
[http://dx.doi.org/10.21608/sjfop.2020.134610]

[315] Srivastava S, Cahill DM, Conlan XA, Adholeya A. A novel *in vitro* whole plant system for analysis of polyphenolics and their antioxidant potential in cultivars of *Ocimum basilicum*. J Agric Food Chem 2014; 62(41): 10064-75.
[http://dx.doi.org/10.1021/jf502709e] [PMID: 25275827]

[316] Srivastava S, Conlan XA, Cahill DM, Adholeya A. Rhizophagus irregularis as an elicitor of rosmarinic acid and antioxidant production by transformed roots of *Ocimum basilicum* in an *in vitro* co-culture system. Mycorrhiza 2016; 26(8): 919-30.
[http://dx.doi.org/10.1007/s00572-016-0721-4] [PMID: 27485855]

[317] Mathew R, Deepa Sankar P. Comparison of major secondary metabolites quantified in elicited cell cultures, non-elicited cell cultures, callus cultures and field grown plants of *Ocimum*. Int J Pharm Pharm Sci 2014; 6: 102-6.

[318] Nazir M, Tungmunnithum D, Bose S, *et al.* Differential Production of Phenylpropanoid Metabolites in Callus Cultures of *Ocimum basilicum* L. with Distinct *In Vitro* Antioxidant Activities and *In Vivo* Protective Effects against UV stress. J Agric Food Chem 2019; 67(7): 1847-59.
[http://dx.doi.org/10.1021/acs.jafc.8b05647] [PMID: 30681331]

[319] Bhuvaneshwari K, Gokulanathan A, Jayanthi M, *et al.* Can *Ocimum basilicum* L. and *Ocimum tenuiflorum* L. *in vitro* culture be a potential source of secondary metabolites? Food Chem 2016; 194: 55-60.
[http://dx.doi.org/10.1016/j.foodchem.2015.07.136] [PMID: 26471526]

[320] Pavingerová D, Gális I, Ondřej M. Tissue culture and transformation of*Oenothera biennis*. Biol Plant 1996; 38(1): 27-32.
[http://dx.doi.org/10.1007/BF02879628]

[321] Thiem B, Skrzypczak L, Lamer-Zarawska E. Micropropagation of selected *Oenothera* species and preliminary studies on their secondary metabolites. Acta Soc Bot Pol 2014; 68(1): 15-20.

[http://dx.doi.org/10.5586/asbp.1999.003]

[322] Huang Y, Huang C. Nutraceutical and specialty lipids and their co-products. Taylor and francis 2006.

[323] Martinez LD, de Halac IN. Organogenesis of anther-derived calluses in long-term cultures of *Oenothera hookeri* de Vries. Plant Cell Tissue Organ Cult 1995; 42(1): 91-6.
[http://dx.doi.org/10.1007/BF00037686]

[324] Ghasemnezhad A, Honermeier B. Seed yield, oil content and fatty acid composition of *Oenothera biennis* L. affected by harvest date and harvest method. Ind Crops Prod 2007; 25(3): 274-81.
[http://dx.doi.org/10.1016/j.indcrop.2006.12.005]

[325] Ghasemzadeh A. Global issues of food production. Agrotechnology 2012; 1(2): 1-2.
[http://dx.doi.org/10.4172/2168-9881.1000e102]

[326] Yongqing X, Fenglan L, Baozhong H. Megasporogenesis and female gamete development in Oenothera biennis L. J Anhui Agric Sci 2011.

[327] Hafez RF, Ghadimzadeh M, Moghaddam AF, Jafari M. Micropropagation and regeneration potentiality of evening primrose (*Oenothera biennis* L .). Indian Journal of Fundamental and Applied Life Sciences 2015; 5: 36-42.

[328] Choi SM, Son SH, Yun SR. Pilot-scale culture of adventitious roots of ginseng in a bioreactor system. Plant Cell Tissue Organ Cult 2000; 97: 131-41.
[http://dx.doi.org/10.1023/A]

[329] Palazón J, Mallol A, Eibl R, Lettenbauer C, Cusidó RM, Piñol MT. Growth and ginsenoside production in hairy root cultures of *Panax ginseng* using a novel bioreactor. Planta Med 2003; 69(4): 344-9.
[http://dx.doi.org/10.1055/s-2003-38873] [PMID: 12709902]

[330] Ali M, Hahn EJ, Paek KY. Methyl jasmonate and salicylic acid induced oxidative stress and accumulation of phenolics in *Panax ginseng* bioreactor root suspension cultures. Molecules 2007; 12(3): 607-21.
[http://dx.doi.org/10.3390/12030607] [PMID: 17851415]

[331] Jeong G-T, Park D-H, Ryu H-W. Production of antioxidant compounds by culture of *panax ginseng* c.a. meyer hairy roots. In: Davison BH, Evans BR, Finkelstein M, McMillan JD, Eds. Twenty-Sixth symposium on biotechnology for fuels and chemicals.
[http://dx.doi.org/10.1007/978-1-59259-991-2_96]

[332] Liu H, Lu X, Hu Y, Fan X. Chemical constituents of *Panax ginseng* and *Panax notoginseng* explain why they differ in therapeutic efficacy. Pharmacol Res 2020; 161: 105263.
[http://dx.doi.org/10.1016/j.phrs.2020.105263] [PMID: 33127555]

[333] Dewir YH, Chakrabarty D, Wu CH, Hahn EJ, Jeon WK, Paek KY. Influences of polyunsaturated fatty acids (PUFAs) on growth and secondary metabolite accumulation in *Panax ginseng* C.A. Meyer adventitious roots cultured in air-lift bioreactors. S Afr J Bot 2010; 76(2): 354-8.
[http://dx.doi.org/10.1016/j.sajb.2009.10.008]

[334] Sivakumar G, Yu KW, Lee JS, *et al.* Tissue cultured mountain ginseng adventitious roots ™: Safety and toxicity evaluation. Eng Life Sci 2006; 6(4): 372-83.
[http://dx.doi.org/10.1002/elsc.200520139]

[335] Baeg IH, So SH. The world ginseng market and the ginseng (Korea). J Ginseng Res 2013; 37(1): 1-7.
[http://dx.doi.org/10.5142/jgr.2013.37.1] [PMID: 23717152]

[336] Chen S, Wang Z, Huang Y, *et al.* Ginseng and anticancer drug combination to improve cancer chemotherapy: A critical review. Evid Based Complement Alternat Med 2014; 2014: 1-13.
[http://dx.doi.org/10.1155/2014/168940] [PMID: 24876866]

[337] Liu H, Lv C, Lu J. Panax ginseng C. A. Meyer as a potential therapeutic agent for organ fibrosis disease. Chin Med 2020; 15(1): 124.

[http://dx.doi.org/10.1186/s13020-020-00400-3] [PMID: 33292321]

[338] Langhansova L, Langhansova L, Dvorakova M. Increased ginsenosides production by elicitation of *in vitro* cultivated *Panax ginseng* adventitious roots. Med Aromat Plants 2014; 3(1): 1-5.
[http://dx.doi.org/10.4172/2167-0412.1000147]

[339] Kochan E, Szymczyk P, Kuźma Ł, Szymańska G. Nitrogen and phosphorus as the factors affecting ginsenoside production in hairy root cultures of *Panax quinquefolium* cultivated in shake flasks and nutrient sprinkle bioreactor. Acta Physiol Plant 2016; 38(6): 149.
[http://dx.doi.org/10.1007/s11738-016-2168-9]

[340] Chen K, Liu J, Ji R, *et al.* Biogenic synthesis and spatial distribution of endogenous phytohormones and ginsenosides provide insights on their intrinsic relevance in *Panax ginseng.* Front Plant Sci 2019; 9: 1951.
[http://dx.doi.org/10.3389/fpls.2018.01951] [PMID: 30687354]

[341] Dantas LA, Melo AM, Pereira PS, Souza LA, Vasconcelos Filho SC, Silva FG. Histochemical screening of leaves compared to *in situ* and *in vitro* calluses of *Solanum aculeatissimum* Jacq. J Agric Sci 2017; 9(7): 80.
[http://dx.doi.org/10.5539/jas.v9n7p80]

[342] Pinto JR, Marshall JD, Dumroese RK, Davis AS, Cobos DR. Establishment and growth of container seedlings for reforestation: A function of stocktype and edaphic conditions. For Ecol Manage 2011; 261(11): 1876-84.
[http://dx.doi.org/10.1016/j.foreco.2011.02.010]

[343] Kittipongpatana N, Hock RS, Porter JR. Production of solasodine by hairy root, callus, and cell suspension cultures of *Solanum aviculare* forst. Plant Cell Tissue Organ Cult 1998; 52(3): 133-43.
[http://dx.doi.org/10.1023/A:1005974611043]

[344] Weissenberg M. Isolation of solasodine and other steroidal alkaloids and sapogenins by direct hydrolysis-extraction of Solanum plants or glycosides therefrom. Phytochemistry 2001; 58(3): 501-8.
[http://dx.doi.org/10.1016/S0031-9422(01)00185-6] [PMID: 11557084]

[345] Bhatnagar P, Bhatnagar M, Nath AK, Sharma DR. Production of solasodine by *Solanum laciniatum* using plant tissue culture technique. Indian J Exp Biol 2004; 42(10): 1020-3.
[PMID: 15511009]

[346] Bhalsing SR, Maheshwari VL. *In vitro* culture and regeneration of *Solanum khasianum* and extraction of solasodine. J Plant Biochem Biotechnol 1997; 6(1): 39-40.
[http://dx.doi.org/10.1007/BF03263007]

[347] Šutković J, Ler D. *In vitro* production of solasodine alkaloid in *Solanum nigrum* under salinity stress. J Phytol Phytophysiol 2011; 3: 1-52.

[348] Jacob A, Malpathak N. Plantlet regeneration enhances solasodine productivity in hairy root cultures of *Solanum khasianum Clarke*. Vitr Cell Dev Biol - Plant 2005; 41: 291-5.
[http://dx.doi.org/10.1079/IVP2005637]

[349] Dantas LA, Rosa M, Resende EC, *et al.* Spectral quality as an elicitor of bioactive compound production in *Solanum aculeatissimum* JACQ cell suspension. J Photochem Photobiol B 2020; 204: 111819.
[http://dx.doi.org/10.1016/j.jphotobiol.2020.111819] [PMID: 32062388]

[350] Leonard E, Runguphan W, O'Connor S, Prather KJ. Opportunities in metabolic engineering to facilitate scalable alkaloid production. Nat Chem Biol 2009; 5(5): 292-300.
[http://dx.doi.org/10.1038/nchembio.160] [PMID: 19377455]

[351] Chinh VT, Quang BH, Choudhary RK, Xia NH, Lee J. Stephania subpeltata H. S. Lo (Menispermaceae): A new record for the flora of vietnam. Korean J Plant Taxon 2016; 46(3): 288-94.
[http://dx.doi.org/10.11110/kjpt.2016.46.3.288]

[352] Jiang Y, Liu M, Liu H, Liu S. A critical review: Traditional uses, phytochemistry, pharmacology and

toxicology of Stephania tetrandra S Moore (Fen Fang Ji). Springer Netherlands 2020.

[353] Stévigny C, Bailly C, Quetin-Leclercq J. Cytotoxic and antitumor potentialities of aporphinoid alkaloids. Curr Med Chem Anticancer Agents 2005; 5(2): 173-82.
[http://dx.doi.org/10.2174/1568011053174864] [PMID: 15777224]

[354] Chen KS, Ko FN, Teng CM, Wu YC. Antiplatelet of vasorelaxing actions of some benzylisoquinoline and phenanthrene alkaloids. J Nat Prod 1996; 59(5): 531-4.
[http://dx.doi.org/10.1021/np960354x] [PMID: 8778245]

[355] Kongkiatpaiboon S, Duangdee N, Prateeptongkum S, Chaijaroenkul W. Acetylcholinesterase inhibitory activity of alkaloids isolated from *Stephania venosa.* Nat Prod Commun 2016; 11(12): 1934578X1601101.
[http://dx.doi.org/10.1177/1934578X1601101208] [PMID: 30508338]

[356] Kitisripanya T, Komaikul J, Tawinkan N, Atsawinkowit C, Putalun W. Dicentrine production in callus and cell suspension cultures of *Stephania venosa.* Nat Prod Commun 2013; 8(4): 1934578X1300800.
[http://dx.doi.org/10.1177/1934578X1300800408] [PMID: 23738448]

[357] Kuo CL, Chang JY, Chang HC. *In vitro* production of benzylisoquinoline from *Stephania tetrandra* through callus culture under the influence of different additives. Bot Stud 2011; 52: 285-94.

[358] Gorpenchenko T, Grigorchuk V, Bulgakov D, Tchernoded G, Bulgakov V. Tempo-spatial pattern of stepharine accumulation in stephania glabra morphogenic tissues. Int J Mol Sci 2019; 20(4): 808.
[http://dx.doi.org/10.3390/ijms20040808] [PMID: 30781887]

[359] Gorpenchenko TY, Grigorchuk VP, Fedoreyev SA, Tarbeeva DV, Tchernoded GK, Bulgakov VP. Stepharine production in morphogenic cell cultures of *Stephania glabra* (ROXB.) Miers. Plant Cell Tissue Organ Cult 2017; 128(1): 67-76.
[http://dx.doi.org/10.1007/s11240-016-1083-5]

[360] Christen AA, Bland J, Gibson DM. Cell cultures as a means to produce taxol. Proc Am Assoc Cancer Res 1989; 30.

[361] Malik S, Cusidó RM, Mirjalili MH, Moyano E, Palazón J, Bonfill M. Production of the anticancer drug taxol in *Taxus baccata* suspension cultures: A review. Process Biochem 2011; 46(1): 23-34.
[http://dx.doi.org/10.1016/j.procbio.2010.09.004]

[362] Zhao C, Song G, Fu C, *et al.* A systematic approach to expound the variations in taxane production under different dissolved oxygen conditions in *Taxus chinensis* cells. Plant Cell Rep 2016; 35(3): 541-59.
[http://dx.doi.org/10.1007/s00299-015-1902-x] [PMID: 26620815]

[363] Tao X, Lipsky PE. The Chinese anti-inflammatory and immunosuppressive herbal remedy Tripterygium wilfordii Hook F. Rheum Dis Clin North Am 2000; 26(1): 29-50.

[364] Brinker AM, Ma J, Lipsky PE, Raskin I. Medicinal chemistry and pharmacology of genus Tripterygium (Celastraceae). Phytochemistry 2007; 68(6): 732-66.
[http://dx.doi.org/10.1016/j.phytochem.2006.11.029] [PMID: 17250858]

[365] Liu Z, Ma L, Zhou GB. The main anticancer bullets of the Chinese medicinal herb, thunder god vine. Molecules 2011; 16(6): 5283-97.
[http://dx.doi.org/10.3390/molecules16065283] [PMID: 21701438]

[366] Cascão R, Fonseca JE, Moita LF. Celastrol: A spectrum of treatment opportunities in chronic diseases. Front Med 2017; 4: 69.
[http://dx.doi.org/10.3389/fmed.2017.00069] [PMID: 28664158]

[367] Miao G peng, Zhu C shu, Feng J tao. Aggregate cell suspension cultures of *Tripterygium wilfordii* Hook. f. for triptolide, wilforgine, and wilforine production. Plant Cell Tissue Organ Cult 2013; 112: 109-16.
[http://dx.doi.org/10.1007/s11240-012-0211-0]

[368] Zhu C, Miao G, Guo J, *et al.* Establishment of *Tripterygium wilfordii* Hook. f. Hairy root culture and optimization of its culture conditions for the production of triptolide and wilforine. J Microbiol Biotechnol 2014; 24(6): 823-34.
[http://dx.doi.org/10.4014/jmb.1402.02045] [PMID: 24651642]

[369] Song Y, Chen S, Wang X, *et al.* A novel strategy to enhance terpenoids production using cambial meristematic cells of *Tripterygium wilfordii* Hook. f. Plant Methods 2019; 15(1): 129.
[http://dx.doi.org/10.1186/s13007-019-0513-x] [PMID: 31719835]

[370] Lange BM, Fischedick JT, Lange MF, Srividya N, Šamec D, Poirier BC. Integrative approaches for the identification and localization of specialized metabolites in Tripterygium roots. Plant Physiol 2017; 173(1): 456-69.
[http://dx.doi.org/10.1104/pp.15.01593] [PMID: 27864443]

[371] Zhang B, Chen M, Pu S, *et al.* Identification of secondary metabolites in *Tripterygium wilfordii* hairy roots and culture optimization for enhancing wilforgine and wilforine production. Ind Crops Prod 2020; 148: 112276.
[http://dx.doi.org/10.1016/j.indcrop.2020.112276]

[372] Debnath SC, Goyali JC. *In vitro* propagation and variation of antioxidant properties in micropropagated vaccinium berry plants—A review. Molecules 2020; 25(4): 788.
[http://dx.doi.org/10.3390/molecules25040788] [PMID: 32059466]

[373] Fang Y, Smith MAL, Pepin M. Producing Cell Cultures of Ohelo (*Vaccinium pahalae*). In Vitro 1999; 5476-6.

[374] Cüce M, Bekїrcan T, Sökmen A. Phenolic constituents of *vaccinium* species from both natural resources and micropropagated plantlets. International Journal of Secondary Metabolite 2018; 5(4): 304-11.
[http://dx.doi.org/10.21448/ijsm.445551]

[375] Goyali JC, Igamberdiev AU, Debnath SC. Propagation methods affect fruit morphology and antioxidant properties but maintain clonal fidelity in lowbush blueberry. HortScience 2015; 50(6): 888-96.
[http://dx.doi.org/10.21273/HORTSCI.50.6.888]

[376] Georgieva M, Badjakov I, Dincheva I. *In vitro* propagation of wild Bulgarian small berry fruits (Bilberry, lingonberry, raspberry and strawberry). Bulg J Agric Sci 2016; 22: 46-51.

[377] Ghosh A, Igamberdiev AU, Debnath SC. Thidiazuron-induced somatic embryogenesis and changes of antioxidant properties in tissue cultures of half-high blueberry plants. Sci Rep 2018; 8(1): 16978.
[http://dx.doi.org/10.1038/s41598-018-35233-6] [PMID: 30451961]

[378] Ali M, Abbasi BH, Ali GS. Elicitation of antioxidant secondary metabolites with jasmonates and gibberellic acid in cell suspension cultures of *Artemisia absinthium* L. Plant Cell Tissue Organ Cult 2015; 120(3): 1099-106.
[http://dx.doi.org/10.1007/s11240-014-0666-2]

[379] Hayat K, Ali S, Ullah S, Fu Y, Hussain M. Green synthesized silver and copper nanoparticles induced changes in biomass parameters, secondary metabolites production, and antioxidant activity in callus cultures of *Artemisia absinthium* L. Green Processing and Synthesis 2021; 10(1): 61-72.
[http://dx.doi.org/10.1515/gps-2021-0010]

[380] Balasubramani S, Ranjitha Kumari BD, Moola AK, *et al.* Enhanced Production of β-Caryophyllene by Farnesyl Diphosphate Precursor-Treated Callus and Hairy Root Cultures of *Artemisia vulgaris* L. Front Plant Sci 2021; 12: 634178.
[http://dx.doi.org/10.3389/fpls.2021.634178] [PMID: 33859659]

[381] Jiao jiao J, Feng Q, Sun H feng. Response of bioactive metabolite and biosynthesis related genes to methyl jasmonate elicitation in *Codonopsis pilosula*. Molecules 2019; 24(3): 533.
[http://dx.doi.org/10.3390/molecules24030533]

[382] Açikgöz MA, Kara ŞM, Aygün A, Özcan MM, Bati Ay E. Effects of methyl jasmonate and salicylic acid on the production of camphor and phenolic compounds in cell suspension culture of endemic Turkish yarrow(*Achilleagypsicola*) species. Turk J Agric For 2019; 43(3): 351-9.
[http://dx.doi.org/10.3906/tar-1809-54]

[383] Mendoza D, Cuaspud O, Arias JP, Ruiz O, Arias M. Effect of salicylic acid and methyl jasmonate in the production of phenolic compounds in plant cell suspension cultures of *Thevetia peruviana*. Biotechnol Rep 2018; 19: e00273.
[http://dx.doi.org/10.1016/j.btre.2018.e00273] [PMID: 29998072]

[384] Liu J, Gao F, Ren J, Lu X, Ren G, Wang R. A novel AP2/ERF transcription factor CR1 regulates the accumulation of vindoline and serpentine in *Catharanthus roseus*. Front Plant Sci 2017; 8: 2082.
[http://dx.doi.org/10.3389/fpls.2017.02082] [PMID: 29270185]

[385] Li M, Peebles CAM, Shanks JV, San KY. Effect of sodium nitroprusside on growth and terpenoid indole alkaloid production in *Catharanthus roseus* hairy root cultures. Biotechnol Prog 2011; 27(3): 625-30.
[http://dx.doi.org/10.1002/btpr.605] [PMID: 21567990]

[386] Sobhani Najafabadi A, Khanahmadi M, Ebrahimi M, Moradi K, Behroozi P, Noormohammadi N. Effect of different quality of light on growth and production of secondary metabolites in adventitious root cultivation of *Hypericum perforatum*. Plant Signal Behav 2019; 14(9): 1640561.
[http://dx.doi.org/10.1080/15592324.2019.1640561] [PMID: 31291819]

[387] Ebadollahi R, Jafarirad S, Kosari-Nasab M, Mahjouri S. Effect of explant source, perlite nanoparticles and TiO$_2$/perlite nanocomposites on phytochemical composition of metabolites in callus cultures of *Hypericum perforatum*. Sci Rep 2019; 9(1): 12998.
[http://dx.doi.org/10.1038/s41598-019-49504-3] [PMID: 31506546]

[388] Gadzovska-Simic S, Tusevski O, Antevski S, *et al.* Secondary metabolite production in Hypericum perforatum L. cell suspensions upon elicitation with fungal mycelia from *Aspergillus flavus*. Arch Biol Sci 2012; 64(1): 113-21.
[http://dx.doi.org/10.2298/ABS1201113G]

[389] Gadzovska Simic S, Tusevski O, Maury S, Delaunay A, Joseph C, Hagège D. Effects of polysaccharide elicitors on secondary metabolite production and antioxidant response in *Hypericum perforatum* L. shoot cultures. ScientificWorldJournal 2014; 2014: 1-10.
[http://dx.doi.org/10.1155/2014/609649] [PMID: 25574489]

[390] Ahmadi Moghadam Y, Piri K, Bahramnejad B, Ghiasvand T. Dopamine production in hairy root cultures of *Portulaca oleracea* (Purslane) using *Agrobacterium rhizogenes*. J Agric Sci Technol 2014; 16: 409-20.

[391] Amini SA, Shabani L, Afghani L, Jalalpour Z, Sharifi-Tehrani M. Squalestatin-induced production of taxol and baccatin in cell suspension culture of yew (*Taxus baccata* L.). Turk J Biol 2014; 38: 528-36.
[http://dx.doi.org/10.3906/biy-1401-47]

[392] Sabater-Jara AB, Onrubia M, Moyano E, *et al.* Synergistic effect of cyclodextrins and methyl jasmonate on taxane production in *Taxus x media* cell cultures. Plant Biotechnol J 2014; 12(8): 1075-84.
[http://dx.doi.org/10.1111/pbi.12214] [PMID: 24909837]

[393] Fulzele D, Satdive R, Kamble S. Improvement of anticancer drug camptothecin production by gamma irradiation on callus Cultures of *Nothapodytes foetida*. Intl J Pharma Res Allied 2015; 4: 19-27.

[394] Chauhan R, Keshavkant S, Quraishi A. Enhanced production of diosgenin through elicitation in micro-tubers of *Chlorophytum borivilianum* Sant et Fernand. Ind Crops Prod 2018; 113: 234-9.
[http://dx.doi.org/10.1016/j.indcrop.2018.01.029]

[395] Miclea I, Suhani A, Zahan M, Bunea A. Effect of jasmonic acid and salicylic acid on growth and biochemical composition of *in-vitro*-propagated *Lavandula angustifolia* mill. Agronomy (Basel) 2020;

10(11): 1722.
[http://dx.doi.org/10.3390/agronomy10111722]

[396]   Gupta K, Garg S, Singh J, Kumar M. Enhanced production of napthoquinone metabolite (shikonin) from cell suspension culture of *Arnebia* sp. and its up-scaling through bioreactor. 3 Biotech 2014; 4: 263-73.
[http://dx.doi.org/10.1007/s13205-013-0149-x]

[397]   Hazra S, Bhattacharyya D, Chattopadhyay S. Methyl jasmonate regulates podophyllotoxin accumulation in *Podophyllum hexandrum* by altering the ROS-responsive podophyllotoxin pathway gene expression additionally through the down regulation of few interfering miRNAs. Front Plant Sci 2017; 8: 164.
[http://dx.doi.org/10.3389/fpls.2017.00164] [PMID: 28261233]

[398]   Saeed S, Ali H, Khan T, Kayani W, Khan MA. Impacts of methyl jasmonate and phenyl acetic acid on biomass accumulation and antioxidant potential in adventitious roots of *Ajuga bracteosa* Wall ex Benth., a high valued endangered medicinal plant. Physiol Mol Biol Plants 2017; 23(1): 229-37.
[http://dx.doi.org/10.1007/s12298-016-0406-7] [PMID: 28250598]

[399]   Khojasteh A, Mirjalili MH, Palazon J, Eibl R, Cusido RM. Methyl jasmonate enhanced production of rosmarinic acid in cell cultures of *Satureja khuzistanica* in a bioreactor. Eng Life Sci 2016; 16(8): 740-9.
[http://dx.doi.org/10.1002/elsc.201600064]

[400]   Belchi-Navarro S, Pedreño MA, Corchete P. Methyl jasmonate increases silymarin production in *Silybum marianum* (L.) Gaernt cell cultures treated with β-cyclodextrins. Biotechnol Lett 2011; 33(1): 179-84.
[http://dx.doi.org/10.1007/s10529-010-0406-6] [PMID: 20872165]

[401]   Hao X, Shi M, Cui L, Xu C, Zhang Y, Kai G. Effects of methyl jasmonate and salicylic acid on tanshinone production and biosynthetic gene expression in transgenic *Salvia miltiorrhiza* hairy roots. Biotechnol Appl Biochem 2015; 62(1): 24-31.
[http://dx.doi.org/10.1002/bab.1236] [PMID: 24779358]

[402]   Bonfill M, Mangas S, Moyano E, Cusido RM, Palazón J. Production of centellosides and phytosterols in cell suspension cultures of *Centella asiatica.* Plant Cell Tissue Organ Cult 2011; 104(1): 61-7.
[http://dx.doi.org/10.1007/s11240-010-9804-7]

[403]   Chodisetti B, Rao K, Gandi S, Giri A. Improved gymnemic acid production in the suspension cultures of *Gymnema sylvestre* through biotic elicitation. Plant Biotechnol Rep 2013; 7(4): 519-25.
[http://dx.doi.org/10.1007/s11816-013-0290-3]

[404]   Hou M, Wang R, Zhao S, Wang Z. Ginsenosides in *Panax* genus and their biosynthesis. Acta Pharm Sin B 2021; 11(7): 1813-34.
[http://dx.doi.org/10.1016/j.apsb.2020.12.017] [PMID: 34386322]

[405]   Zhang R, Tan S, Zhang B, Hu P, Li L. Cerium-promoted ginsenosides accumulation by regulating endogenous methyl jasmonate biosynthesis in hairy roots of *Panax ginseng*. Molecules 2021; 26(18): 5623.
[http://dx.doi.org/10.3390/molecules26185623] [PMID: 34577094]

[406]   Kim YS, Han JY, Lim S. Overexpressing Arabidopsis jasmonic acid carboxyl methyltransferase (AtJMT) results in stimulation of root growth and ginsenoside heterogeneity in *Panax ginseng*. Plant Omics 2012; 5: 28-32.

[407]   Gadzovska S, Maury S, Delaunay A, Spasenoski M, Joseph C, Hagège D. Jasmonic acid elicitation of *Hypericum perforatum* L. cell suspensions and effects on the production of phenylpropanoids and naphtodianthrones. Plant Cell Tissue Organ Cult 2007; 89(1): 1-13.
[http://dx.doi.org/10.1007/s11240-007-9203-x]

[408]   Gangopadhyay M, Dewanjee S, Bhattacharya S. Enhanced plumbagin production in elicited *Plumbago indica* hairy root cultures. J Biosci Bioeng 2011; 111(6): 706-10.

[http://dx.doi.org/10.1016/j.jbiosc.2011.02.003] [PMID: 21382748]

[409] Sivanandhan G, Rajesh M, Arun M, *et al.* Effect of culture conditions, cytokinins, methyl jasmonate and salicylic acid on the biomass accumulation and production of withanolides in multiple shoot culture of *Withania somnifera* (L.) Dunal using liquid culture. Acta Physiol Plant 2013; 35(3): 715-28. [http://dx.doi.org/10.1007/s11738-012-1112-x]

CHAPTER 12

Harnessing the Potential of Plant Tissue Culture Techniques for the Herbal Industry

Dechen Dolker[1], Kuldeep Kaur[1], Shashikanta Behera[1], Panchsheela Nogia[1], Sakshi Rawat[1], Vaishali Kumari[1] and Pratap Kumar Pati[1,2,*]

[1] *Department of Biotechnology, Guru Nanak Dev University, Amritsar-143 005, Punjab, India*

[2] *Department of Agriculture, Guru Nanak Dev University, Amritsar, Punjab, India*

Abstract: Over the past few years, there has been a tremendous global shift of preference toward herbal medicine because of its affordability, accessibility, efficacy, and lesser side effects. The pharmacological and healing properties of the herbs are due to the presence of a wide array of secondary metabolites. These metabolites are biosynthesized through defined pathways and stored in various parts of the plant, like leaf, root, rhizome, bark, and floral parts. In recent years due to the growing realization of the pharmaceutical properties of medicinal plants, they have been subjected to indiscriminate exploitation. Further, the lack of agrotechnology in many cases and the nonavailability of broad genetic diversity provide impediments to their largescale cultivation and improvement. This situation has created a huge gap between the demand and supply of medicinal plants all over the world. Hence, rapidly propagating high valued medicinal plants through unconventional technologies is warranted and will provide high dividends to farmers and the herbal industry. Further, generating large-scale healthy, genetically uniform plants with defined chemical content will facilitate pre-clinical and translational studies. Therefore, efforts in the development of robust *in vitro* propagation systems for herbal plants can address the core concern of their conservation and large-scale utilization. Studies on cell suspension, hairy root culture, and genetic transformation have provided the desired impetus in metabolic engineering and enhanced their commercial value. The present article highlights some of these developments and provides a futuristic perspective on the subject.

Keywords: Cell suspension culture, Hairy root culture, Herbal medicine, Medicinal plants, Metabolic engineering, Micropropagation, Secondary metabolites.

* **Corresponding author Pratap Kumar Pati:** Department of Biotechnology, Guru Nanak Dev University, Amritsar-143 005, Punjab, India; & Department of Agriculture, Guru Nanak Dev University, Amritsar, Punjab, India; E-mail: pkpati@yahoo.com

Mohammad Anis & Mehrun Nisha Khanam (Eds.)

INTRODUCTION

The herbal industry greatly relies on herbs that contain active ingredients derived from plant parts such as leaves, roots, or flowers to treat diseases and enhance general wellbeing [1 - 3]. Since ancient times, herbs have been considered an important part of society, well-known for their culinary as well as medicinal uses. Traditional herbal medicines form a major part of the healthcare system all over the world and have become a rising global commercial enterprise [4 - 6]. At present, almost 80% population in developing countries rely largely on herbal medicines for their basic healthcare requirements [7 - 9]. The past decade has witnessed a tremendous surge in the acceptance and renewed interest in the use of herbal medicines, owing to their safety and health-promoting effects, which has led to the rapid growth of the herbal drug industry [10, 11]. Medicinal plants are also gaining greater attention from the scientific community for novel drug discovery and development. The extensive exploitation of herbs and other plant-based natural products has resulted in a huge gap between their demand and availability [12]. In addition to that, information regarding cultivation practice is only available for a few medicinal plants (less than 10%) and agro-technology is available for about 1% of the total plants known globally, which further limits their cultivation [13]. An emerging concern is the rapid extinction of plant species worldwide, with experts predicting that we are losing at least one potential major drug every two years. Out of an estimated 422,000 medicinal and aromatic plant (MAP) species identified worldwide, 12.5% (52000) of them are used medicinally, and 8% (4160) of them are considered threatened species [14, 15]. To meet the escalating demand for herbal medicines and products, biotechnological interventions through plant cell, tissue, and organ culture offer a sustainable method for addressing some of the challenges in the propagation of valuable medicinal plants. *In vitro* propagation is a promising alternative that will facilitate the efficient and rapid mass propagation of plants to obtain uniform plant materials throughout the year, independent of the environmental conditions [16, 17]. Further, the therapeutically important secondary metabolites, which are otherwise synthesized in low amounts in plants, can be engineered to increase yields as well as to synthesize target compounds using *in vitro* systems and lay the foundation for their large-scale production in bioreactors [18, 19].

THE ECONOMIC IMPORTANCE OF HERBAL MEDICINE

The global market for herbal medicine and herbal products is estimated to have an annual growth rate of up to 15%, representing a significant share of the total world pharmaceutical market [20]. The international herbal medicine market was estimated at US$ 60 billion in 2010 and is expected to flourish with good growth potential to reach US$ 5 trillion by 2050 [21]. The annual turnover of herbal medicines increased around 5-15% from the past decade in the year 2000 to an estimated US$ 30 billion in various developed countries, including the United States (USA), Australia, Canada, and parts of Europe. In Asia, with the increasing human population and commercial trade, the demand for herbal products almost doubled during the late 1990s [22]. In India, the export of herbal extracts and herbal products accounted for US$ 456.12 million during the year 2017-2018, with a growth rate of 12.23% over the previous year [23], while the annual herbal drug production in China is worth US$ 48 billion with the export of US$ 3.6 billion [24]. The demand for herbal products also increased as a result of the emergence of natural cosmetics, functional foods, herbal supplements, fragrances, and various other botanical products that represent multibillion-dollar industries. As per previous estimates, only 6% of existing plant species have been investigated for their potential medicinal properties [25 - 27]. However, with the advanced scientific developments, the percentage of characterized species is likely to be higher, but still, a large number of plants need to be studied for their potent bioactivities. Hence, there is a promising potential for future discoveries from plant-derived products for various industrial applications, including novel drug development.

The present article discusses the challenges of the herbal industry and possible technological interventions to address these pending issues. It is strongly realized that the large-scale production of medicinal plants and their bioactive compounds is essential to cater to the need of herbal industries. The use of *in vitro* propagation techniques, the establishment of cell suspension and hairy root culture system, and metabolic engineering are the key focus areas that hold promise in this direction.

LARGE SCALE PLANT PROPAGATION THROUGH PLANT TISSUE CULTURE TECHNIQUES

Plant tissue culture is considered a promising tool for the propagation of a large number of plants for commercial purposes [28]. It refers to the cultivation of plant cells, tissues, and organs on an artificial nutrient media under aseptic and optimum conditions [29]. Compared to conventional methods of propagation, it offers several unique advantages such as enormous multiplicative capacity, efficient ex-situ conservation of endangered plants, production of healthy and disease-free plants throughout the year, and use of cell, tissue and organ culture for the production of various bioactive compounds which is otherwise a difficult task. In the context of medicinal plants, the use of plant cell, tissue and organ culture techniques becomes more relevant due to the huge commercial angle attached to it. For a long time, many researchers have been working on the propagation of medicinal plants employing plant tissue culture protocols (Table **1**)

[30 - 61]. However, new challenges in optimizing microenvironment, nutrient requirements, and cost reduction have allowed the researchers to bring innovative practices into the propagation system. Regardless of the plant, an effective micropropagation protocol involves distinct and interrelated steps. These are (a) Establishment of aseptic cultures, (b) Shoot multiplication, (c) Rooting of *in vitro* grown microshoots, and (d) Acclimatization of *in vitro* regenerated plants.

Table 1. *In vitro* **propagation of important medicinal plants through meristem culture.**

Plant Species	Explant	Shooting Medium	Response	Shoots/Explant	Rooting Medium	References
Acacia catechu	Shoot apices	MS + BA (1.5 mg/l) + KN (1.5 mg/l)	Shoot bud induction	12	¼ MS + IAA (3.0 mg/l)	[30]
Citrus aurantifolia	Nodal explant	MS+ BA (1.0 mg/l) + KN (0.5 mg/l)	Shoot bud induction	8	MS + IAA (1.0 mg/l)	[31]
Atropa acuminafa	Shoot tip	RT + BA (1 mg/l) + IBA (1 mg/l)	Shoot proliferation	5.8	RT + IBA (1.0 mg/l)	[32]
Tylophora indica	Nodal explant	MS + BA (2.5 µM) + NAA (0.5 µM)	Shoot proliferation	8.6	½ MS + IBA (0.5 µM)	[33]
Asparagus racemosus	Nodal explant	MS + 2iP (3.69 µM)	Multiple shoot formation	3.5	½ MS + NAA (1.61 µM) + KIN (0.46 µM) + ADS (98.91 µM) + malt extract (500 mg/l) + PG (198.25 µM)	[34]
Salvia officinalis	Shoot tip	MS liquid + BA (0.45 mg/l) + IAA (0.1 mg/l)	Shoot bud induction	3	NI	[35]
Saraca asoca	Nodal explants	MS + BA (0.5 mg/l)	Multiple shoot formation	11.71	MS + IBA (4.0 mg/l)	[36]

Plant Species	Explant	Shooting Medium	Response	Shoots/Explant	Rooting Medium	References
Emblica officinalis	Nodal explant	MS + BA (4.0 mg/l) + NAA (0.5 mg/l)	Multiple shoot formation	3.20	MS + IBA (2.0 mg/l) + BA (0.5 mg/l)	[37]
Catharanthus roseus	Nodal explant	MS + BA (0.5 mg/l) + NAA (1.0 mg/l)	Multiple shoot formation	35.10	½ MS + IBA (0.1 mg/l)	[38]
Stemona tuberosa	Nodal explant	MS + BA (3.0 mg/l) + NAA (0.5 mg/l)	Multiple shoot formation	25.87	½ MS + NAA (1.0 mg/l)	[39]
Wattakaka volubilis	Nodal explant	MS + BA (0.6 mg/l) + NAA (0.2 mg/l)	Multiple shoot formation	23.4	½ MS + IBA (0.6 mg/l)	[40]
Uraria picta	Nodal explant	MS + BA (1.0 mg/l)	Shoot multiplication	20	½ MS + IBA (1.5 mg/l)	[41]
Berberis aristata	Nodal segment	WPM + BA (8.88 µM) + NAA (1.34 µM) + CH (500 mg/l) + GA$_3$ (1.44 µM)	Shoot multiplication	26.67	WPM + IBA (100 µM)	[42]
Hedychium coronarium	Rhizome	MS + BA (2.0 mg/l) + NAA (0.5 mg/l)	Simultaneous multiple shoot proliferation and rooting	3.6	*	[43]
Stevia rebaudiana	Nodal explant	MS + TDZ (0.2 mg/l)	Shoot multiplication	5.8	½ MS	[44]
Withania somnifera	Cotyledonary node	MS + BA (1.0 mg/l)	Shoot multiplication	25	½ MS + IBA (1.0 mg/l)	[45]
Aloe vera	Shoot tip	MS + BA (4.0 mg/l) + IAA (1.0 mg/l)	Shoot multiplication	58.88	MS + IAA (1.0 mg/l) + BA (4.0 mg/l)	[46]
Withania ashwagandha	Nodal explant	MS + BA (5.0 mg/l) + KN (1.0 mg/l)	Shoot multiplication	19	½ MS + IBA (2.0 mg/l)	[47]

(Table 1) cont.....

Plant Species	Explant	Shooting Medium	Response	Shoots/Explant	Rooting Medium	References
Bacopa monnieri	Nodal explant	MS + BA (3.0 mg/l) + GA$_3$ (1.0 mg/l)	Shoot multiplication	114.2	½ MS + IBA (0.2 mg/l)	[48]
Aconitum heterophyllum	Shoot tip	MS + KIN (0.25 mg/l) + IAA (0.25 mg/l)	Shoot multiplication	NI	MS + IAA (1.0 mg/l)	[49]
Withania somnifera	Nodal explant	MS + BA (0.5 mg/l) + NAA (1.5 mg/l)	Multiple shoot formation	5.3	MS + IBA (2.0 mg/l)	[50]
Cinchona officinalis	Nodal explant	B5 + BA (5.0 mg/l) + IBA (3.0 mg/l)	Multiple shoot formation	5.3	NI	[51]
Tinospora cordifolia	Nodal explant	MS + BA (4.44 µM) + 2iP (2.45µM)	Multiple shoot formation	7.9	½ MS + IBA (2.45 µM)	[52]
Symplocos racemosa	Nodal explant	MS + BA (3.0 mg/l) + 2,4-D (0.5 mg/l) + GA$_3$ (2.0 mg/l)	Multiple shoot formation	5.7	½ WPM + IBA (6.0 mg/l)	[53]
Rhodiola imbricata	*In vitro* seedlings	MS + TDZ (1.0 µM)	Multiple shoot formation	7.87	MS + NAA (0.5 µM)	[54]
Hedychium coronarium	Rhizomatic bud	MS + TDZ (0.8 mg/l) MS + GA$_3$ (1.0 mg/l)	Simultaneous multiple shoot proliferation and rooting	15.8	*	[55]
Hedychium coronarium	Axenic cotyledonary node	MS + mT (3.0 mg/l)	Simultaneous multiple shoot proliferation and rooting	48.5	*	[56]
Vitex agnus-castus	Nodal explant	MS + BA (2.0 mg/l) + KN (0.1 mg/l)	Shoot induction	5.7	½ MS + IBA (0.1 mg/l)	[57]

(Table 1) cont.....

Plant Species	Explant	Shooting Medium	Response	Shoots/Explant	Rooting Medium	References
Dioscorea deltoidea	Nodal explant	MS + BA (2.0 mg/l) + IBA (1.0 mg/l)	Shoot bud induction	3.86	MS + NAA (2.0 mg/l)	[58]
Withania somnifera	Nodal explant	MS + BA (5.0 μM) + NAA (0.5 μM) + KN (10.0 μM)	Multiple shoot formation	7.06	1/6 AN strength in MS	[59]
Ruta graveolens	*In vitro* seedling	MS + BA (1.5 mg/l)	Multiple shoot formation	4.2	MS + NAA (0.9 mg/l)	[60]
Curcuma amada	Rhizomatic bud	MS + mT (3.0 mg/l)	Simultaneous multiple shoot proliferation and rooting	19.8	*	[61]

Simultaneously, shooting and rooting occur on the same medium, 2iP- 2-Isopentenyl adenine, ½ MS - Half-strength Murashige and Skoog (1962) medium, ADS - Adenine sulfate, AN - Ammonium nitrate, BA - N^6-Benzyladenine, GA$_3$ - Gibberellic acid, IAA - Indole-3-acetic acid, IBA - Indole-3-butyric acid, KN - Kinetin, MS - Murashige and Skoog (1962) medium, mT - meta-Topolin, NAA - α-naphthalene acetic acid, NI - No information, PG - Phloroglucinol, RT - Revised tobacco medium, TDZ - Thidiazuron, WPM - Lloyd and McCown (1980) Woody Plant Medium.

Establishment of Aseptic Cultures

The establishment of aseptic culture is the first stage for a successful *in vitro* propagation protocol. Various factors such as explant, sterilization process, medium and culture conditions largely contribute to the establishment of aseptic cultures for any plant species. The type, size, and physiological stage of explants play a vital role in the initiation of successful *in vitro* propagation of medicinal plants. Different types of explants such as shoot tip, node, rhizome, rhizomatic bud, *in vitro* seedling, and the axenic cotyledonary node have been used for multiple shoot proliferation in various medicinal plants depending on the aim of the experiments. However, nodal explant has been frequently used for multiple shoot proliferation in several medicinal plants, including *Stevia rebaudiana*, *Bacopa monnieri*, *Withania somnifera*, *Tinospora cordifolia*, *Symplocos racemosa*, and *Dioscorea deltoidea* (Table **1**). Healthy and optimum-sized explants showed a better response for multiple shoot proliferation compared to diseased and larger-sized explants of medicinal plants. The chances of contamination are reported to be higher in large-sized explants of plants, including *Sapium sebiferum* [62] and *Cannabis sativa* [63]. Juvenile explants showed maximum shoot proliferation in comparison to older or matured explants.

The explants obtained from field-grown plants are infected with different disease-causing pathogens. Thus, it is required to sterilize the explants before inoculating on the culture medium for *in vitro* shoot proliferation. Different types of sterilizing agents, such as liquid detergent, fungicide, sodium hypochlorite, mercuric chloride, and ethyl alcohol, were used to remove bacterial and fungal contamination from the explants of medicinal plants to establish aseptic culture [64 - 66]. The types and concentrations of surface sterilizing agents used vary from one medicinal plant to the other. Different types and concentrations of liquid detergents were used for the pre-sterilization of different explants, for example, 5.0% of teepol was used for seed explants in *Withania somnifera* [67] and 2.5% of teepol was used for pre-sterilization of nodal explants in *Withania somnifera* [68, 69]. Different concentrations of tween-20 (1.0-10%) were also reported for pre-sterilization of explant in several medicinal plants. In the case of *Withania somnifera,* a higher concentration of tween-20 (10%) was used for pre-sterilization of its axillary bud [70]. For the removal of fungal contamination from explant, 2.0% of bavistin (fungicide) was also used in different medicinal plants, including *Symplocos racemosa*, *Hedychium coronarium*, and *Curcuma amada*. In general, 0.1% of mercuric chloride was used for surface sterilization of the explant of *Hedychium coronarium*, *Symplocos racemosa*, and *Paederia foetida* [71]. Whereas, 0.04%, 0.08%, and 0.2% of mercuric chloride were used for surface sterilization of explant in *Rhodiola imbricata* [72] and *Withania somnifera* [73, 74], respectively.

Shoot Multiplication

Through Meristem Culture

There are different types of culture media formulations such as Murashige and Skoog (MS) (1962) medium, Gamborg's B5 (1968) medium, Lloyd and McCown (1980) Woody Plant medium, and Nitsch and Nitsch (NN) (1969) medium, which have been used in tissue culture for *in vitro* shoot proliferation of medicinal plants. Among all these, the MS medium is one of the most frequently used media for *in vitro* shoot multiplication of medicinal plants (Tables **1** and **2**). [75 - 87]. MS medium contains all plant macronutrients, micronutrients, vitamins, and some organic compounds, which are essential for plant growth and development [88]. Carbon source has a key role in the morphogenesis of tissues by providing energy as well as maintaining the osmotic balance between plant cells and external conditions in the culture medium. Sucrose (3%) has been commonly used as a carbon source for *in vitro* shoot proliferation of several plants, including *Catharanthus roseus* [89]. Whereas the higher concentration of sucrose, *i.e.*, 4% and 6% have also been reported for shoot multiplication of *Withania somnifera* [90].

Table 2. *In vitro* **shoot organogenesis using different explants of important medicinal plants.**

Plant	Explant	Mode of Regeneration	Shooting Medium	Shooting (%)	Shoots/Explants	Rooting Medium	References
Asparagus racemosus	Shoot segment	Indirect	MS + IAA (0.5 mg/l) + BA (1.0 mg/l)	NI	NI	½ MS + IBA (0.5 mg/l)	[75]
Aloe vera	Stem	Indirect	MS + 2,4-D (1.0 mg/l) + KN (0.2 mg/l) MS + 2,4-D (0.02 mg/l) + KN (1.0 mg/l)	NI	15.5	NI	[76]
Aconitum heterophyllum	Leaf and Petiole	Indirect	MS + BA (1.0 mg/l) + NAA (0.1 mg/l) ¼ MS + (IBA (1.0 mg/l)	NI	NI	MS + IBA (1.0 mg/l)	[77]
Acacia catechu	Cultured cotyledons	Indirect	MS + BA (2.0 mg/l) + KN (2.0 mg/l)	NI	NI	Dipped in sterilized IAA solution (10 mg/l) for 24 h ½ MS + AC (0.02%)	[78]

(Table 2) cont.....

Plant	Explant	Mode of Regeneration	Shooting Medium	Shooting (%)	Shoots/Explants	Rooting Medium	References
Salvia officinalis	Shoot tip	Indirect	MS + TDZ (4.5 µM) + Ascorbic acid (0.45 mM) MS + BAP (4.4 µM) + Ascorbic acid (0.45 mM)	78.90	7.70	MS + IBA (4.9 µM)	[79]
Catharanthus roseus	Petiole	Direct	MS + BA (2.2 µM) + NAA (5.3 µM)	19.1	5.7	½ MS + IBA (2.2 µM)	[80]
Urginea maritima	Bulb scales	Direct	MS + TDZ (0.55 mg/l)	89.67	3.58	NI	[81]
Emblica officinalis	Root explant	Indirect	MS + BA (1.0 µM)	66.67	55	NI	[82]
Typhonium trilobatum	corm buds	Indirect	MS + BA (0.5 mg/l) + NAA (2.0 mg/l) MS + BA (5.0 mg/l) + NAA (1.0 mg/l)	85	11	MS + IAA (0.4 mg/l)	[83]
Sauropus androgynus	Leaf	Indirect	MS + BA (2.0 mg/l) + IAA (0.5 mg/l)	90	NI	MS + IAA (1.0 mg/l)	[84]
Berberis aristata	Leaf	Indirect	WPM + TDZ (0.5 µM)	NI	17.6	½ WPM + IBA (9.8 µM)	[85]

(Table 2) cont.....

Plant	Explant	Mode of Regeneration	Shooting Medium	Shooting (%)	Shoots/Explants	Rooting Medium	References
Aconitum balfourii	Leaf	Indirect	MS + TDZ (0.5 mg/l)	86.67	7.8	MS + IAA (0.25 mg/l) + NAA (0.25 mg/l)	[86]
Rauwolfia tetraphylla	Leaf	Indirect	MS + TDZ (0.25 mg/l) + BA (2.0 mg/l)	NI	25	MS + IAA (1.0 mg/l) + IBA (1.0 mg/l)	[87]

µM - Micro molar, 2,4-D - 2,4-dichlorophenoxyacetic acid, ½ MS - Half-strength Murashige and Skoog (1962) medium, AC - Activated charcoal, BA - N^6-Benzyladenine, GA_3 - Gibberellic acid, IAA - Indole--acetic acid, IBA - Indole-3-butyric acid, KN - Kinetin, MS - Murashige and Skoog (1962) medium, mg/l - milli gram per liter, NAA - α-naphthalene acetic acid, NI - No information, TDZ - Thidiazuron, WPM - Lloyd and McCown (1980) Woody Plant Medium.

The type and concentration of gelling agents and the status of culture media (semi-solid or solid) influence the shoot multiplication in plants. Agar has been frequently used for the solidification of culture medium. 0.7% of agar was used commonly for solidifying culture medium in plants like *Bacopa monnieri, Dioscorea deltoidea, Symplocos racemosa, Hedychium coronarium,* and *Withania somnifera* (Table **1**). The cost of gelling agents used in plant tissue culture is high and constitutes almost 70-80% of the total culture medium-cost. For commercial-scale production of *in vitro* plants, factors such as low-cost, high productivity, ease of use and maintenance, automation and optimization of the culture environment are critical. A liquid culture system can thus be optimized for large-scale cost-efficient *in vitro* plant propagation. Moreover, a liquid culture medium offers several advantages over a solid culture medium for commercial propagation of medicinal plants, including uniform culture conditions, faster growth, sterilization by microfiltration, ease of use, and renewal of media composition [91]. The micropropagation of medicinal plants, including *Arnebia euchroma* [92] and *Mentha × piperita* [93], has been successfully carried out using a liquid culture system. The basal medium without a plant growth regulator is usually not favourable for large-scale multiple shoot production of medicinal plants. Hence, different types of cytokinins such as N^6-benzyladenine (BA), kinetin (KN), meta-Topolin (mT), thidiazuron (TDZ), zeatin (Z), 2-isopentenyl adenine (2-ip), and auxins such as indole-3-acetic acid (IAA), indole-3-butyric acid (IBA), α-naphthalene acetic acid (NAA) have been supplied alone or in combination in the basal medium for multiple shoot proliferation of medicinal plants (Table **1**).

Among the different plant growth regulators, cytokinins like BA, KN, TDZ supplemented MS basal medium for multiple shoot proliferation have been reported in various medicinal plants, including *Curcuma amada, Rhodiola imbricata*, *Saraca asoca, Stevia rebaudiana*, and *Withania somnifera*. In the past few years, another cytokinin *m*T has attracted the attention of researchers due to improved shoot proliferation, *in vitro* rooting and survival rate after acclimatization in various micropropagated medicinal plants such as *Hedychium coronarium, Curcuma amada*, and *Withania somnifera* (Table **1**). The use of cytokinin along with auxins has been shown to provide a synergetic effect on multiple shoot proliferation in several medicinal plants. In the case of *Catharanthus roseus, Emblica officinalis, Hedychium coronarium, Stemona tuberosa*, and *Tylophora indica,* plant shoot multiplication has been reported on BA + NAA supplemented medium, while in the case of *Atropa acuminafa* and *Cinchona officinalis*, shoot multiplication was observed on BA + IBA supplemented medium. Similarly, BA + IAA supplemented medium has also been reported for shoot multiplication of *Acontium heterophyllum, Aloe vera*, and *Salvia officinalis* (Table **1**). Gibberellic acid (GA_3) has been used in multiplication medium or MS medium for shoot elongation of several medicinal plants *i.e.,* cassava (*Manihot esculenta* Crantz), castor (*Rinus communis* L.), *Cichorium intybus* L., *Ficus religiosa* L [94 - 97]. GA_3 increases the osmotic uptake of nutrients, causing cell multiplication as well as elongation of cambium tissue of the internodal region, increasing the length of shoots [98].

Apart from growth regulators, the addition of several growth additives such as silver nitrate ($AgNO_3$), adenine sulphate (ADS), activated charcoal (AC), and phloroglucinol (PG) in the culture medium showed a promising effect on shoot proliferation and elongation, reduction of hyperhydricity, and prevention of phenolic secretion in different medicinal plants like *Bacopa monnieri* [99], *Curcuma longa* [100], *Gloriosa superba* [101], *Gymnema sylvestre* [102], *Prosopis cineraria* [103], *Prunus cerasus* [104], *Vitex negundo* [105], and *Withania coagulans* [106]. $AgNO_3$ plays an important role in multiple shoot formation by inhibiting ethylene synthesis [107]. PG has been supplied in a culture medium to prevent hyperdicity of *in vitro* shoots of medicinal plants by acting as a precursor in the lignin biosynthesis pathway [108]. Whereas AC plays a critical role in the micropropagation of medicinal plants due to its irreversible adsorption of phenolic compounds, toxic metabolites, as well as brown exudate accumulation in the culture medium [109].

Adventitious Shoot Organogenesis

Adventitious shoot organogenesis in medicinal plants involves the formation of shoots either directly from leaf, petiole, root, and stem or indirectly from callus derived from these explants on MS medium fortified with different combinations of auxins and cytokinins under *in vitro* conditions (Table **2**). Cytokinins are mostly considered effective plant growth regulators for shoot regeneration in different medicinal plant species, including *Aloe arborescens* [110, 111]. Generally, cytokinins are of two types, *i.e.*, adenine-type (BA, KN, and Z) and phenylurea-type (diphenylurea and thidiazuron) [112, 113]. Adenine-type cytokinins (BA and KN) have been used extensively for adventitious shoot regeneration of several medicinal plants, such as *Acacia catechu*, *Eblica officinalis*, *Paederia foetida*, and *Withania somnifera*. While phenylurea-type (TDZ) has also been used in some medicinal plants including *Aconitum balfourii*, *Berberis aristata*, *Rauwolfia tetraphylla*, and *Urginea maritima*. Furthermore, the combination of cytokinin (BA) along with auxins (IAA, IBA, and NAA) has been documented in some medicinal plants for adventitious shoot regeneration (Table **2**).

Rooting of *in vitro* Regenerated Shoots

In micropropagation protocol, *in vitro* rooting is the most critical step for successful plant regeneration and establishment in the soil. The use of basal medium (½ MS or MS) has been reported for promoting the rooting of *in vitro* regenerated shoots of several medicinal plants including *Stevia rebaudiana* and *Accacia catechu*. However, the rooting response was found to be more efficient when the culture medium is supplemented with auxins. Auxin alone, particularly NAA, IBA or IAA supplemented ½ MS or MS medium has been used by several researchers for rooting of *in vitro* regenerated shoots of medicinal plants such as *Acacia catechu*, *Asparagus racemosa*, *Atropa acuminafa*, *Catharanthus roseus*, *Citrus aurantifolia*, *Tylophora indica*, *Typhonium trilobatum*, *Saraca asoca*, *Symplocos racemosa*, *Uraria picta*, *Withania somnifera* (Tables **1** and **2**). It has been observed that IBA is one of the most commonly used auxins, which has been successfully implemented for rooting of *in vitro* regenerated shoots in several medicinal plants (Tables **1** and **2**).

Somatic Embryogenesis

Somatic embryogenesis (SE) is a tissue-culture technique for the production of somatic embryos, which is further used in the propagation and genetic improvement of several plant species [114]. During SE, somatic cells are reprogrammed to undergo many cellular and metabolic changes to form embryogenic cells that develop into somatic embryos [115]. Somatic embryos can form a variety of differentiated cell types, including cotyledon segments, roots, leaves, petioles, corm slices, and bulb scales in various high-value medicinal plants (Table **3**) [116 - 128]. The endogenous levels of PGRs in tissues decide whether the induction of somatic embryos can happen spontaneously on a hormone-free medium or if it requires exogenous phytohormones in a culture medium. The process of SE can be either direct (no intermediate callusing phase) or indirect, which implies the formation of disorganized callus tissue [129]. In *Desmodium motorium,* cotyledon segments were used to induce embryogenic calli on MS medium augmented with IAA (2.9 µM) and BA (4.44 and 8.88 µM), and somatic embryos were induced on hormone-free MS medium. In majority of the medicinal plants, MS medium supplemented with different PGRs mainly auxins (2,4-D, NAA, and picloram) alone or in combination with different cytokinins (BAP, KN, and TDZ) induces the formation of somatic embryos in *Silybum marianum, Ledebouria revolute, Merwilla plumbea, Ajuga bracteosa, Bacopa monnieri* and *Hypoxis hemerocallidea.* Apart from PGRs, various growth additives like spermidine, coconut water, and haemoglobin were also tried for somatic embryogenesis. The influence of different concentrations (2.5, 5, 7.5, 10, 12.5, and 15 µM) of copper nanoparticles (Cu-NPs) on somatic embryogenesis was investigated in *Ocimum basilicum* and the highest induction rate of somatic embryos was achieved at 5.0 µM of Cu-NPs (Table **3**). Apart from primary somatic embryogenesis, where somatic embryos are induced from explant cells, the new somatic embryos could also be formed from the existing somatic embryos during secondary somatic embryogenesis [130].

Table 3. Somatic embryogenesis in important medicinal plants.

Plant Species	Explant	Medium	Response	Somatic Embryos Induction (%)	References
Desmodium motorium	Embryogenic calli from cotyledon segments	MS	Somatic embryogenesis	-	[116]
Withania somnifera	Calli from cotyledonary leaf	MS + KN (3.0 mg/l)	Somatic embryogenesis	97.33	[117]
Merwilla plumbea	Calli from leaf	MS (liquid) + Picloram (0.4 µM) + TDZ (0.9 µM) + Haemoglobin (150 mg/l)	Somatic embryogenesis	-	[118]
Wedelia calendulacea	Calli from leaf	MS + 2,4-D (0.5 mg/l)	Somatic embryogenesis	76	[119]
Curcuma longa	Leaf	MS + 2,4-D (4.49 µM) MS + BA (1.32 µM)	Somatic embryogenesis	91.1	[120]

Plant Species	Explant	Medium	Response	Somatic Embryos Induction (%)	References
Ledebouria revoluta	Calli from bulb scale	MS + TDZ (3.0 mg/l) + NAA (0.75 mg/l) + Spermidine (1.75 mM)	Somatic embryogenesis	46.70/500 mg callus	[121]
Bacopa monnieri	Leaf explants	MS + BA (12.5 µM) + 2, 4-D (1.0 µM) + Sucrose (250 mM)	Somatic embryogenesis	77.77	[122]
Silybum marianum	Embryonic calli from petiole	B5 + 2,4-D (0.5 mg/l) + TDZ (1.5 mg/l)	Somatic embryogenesis	77	[123]
Hypoxis hemerocallidea	Corm slices	MS + 2,4-D (15.0 µM) + BA (2.5 µM)	Somatic embryogenesis	30.56	[124]
Peucedanum japonicum	Calli from root	MS + ABA (4.0 mg/l)	Somatic embryogenesis	30	[125]
Ajuga bracteosa	Non-embryonic calli from leaf	MS + BA (2.0 mg/l) + 2, 4-D (1.0 mg/l)	Somatic embryogenesis	92.75	[126]
Ocimum basilicum	Calli from leaf	Modified culture medium + Copper nanoparticles (5.0 µM)	Somatic embryogenesis	84	[127]
Minthostachys verticillata	Calli from leaf	MS + Coconut water (2.5%)	Somatic embryogenesis	100	[128]

µM - Micro molar, 2,4-D - 2,4-dichlorophenoxyacetic acid, ABA - Abscisic acid, B5 - Gamborg's B5 (1968) medium, BA - N[6]-Benzyladenine, KN - Kinetin, MS - Murashige and Skoog (1962) medium, mg/l - milli gram per liter, NAA - α-naphthalene acetic acid, NI - No information, TDZ - Thidiazuron.

Acclimatization

Acclimatization is the last and very important step in plant tissue culture for the successful field establishment of *in vitro* regenerated plants. Normally, a large number of *in vitro* grown plants are unable to survive outside the *in vitro* conditions when they are transferred in field environments [131]. The environment outside the greenhouse has considerably high light intensity, lower relative humidity, and variations in temperature that are stressful to *in vitro* regenerated plants compared to culture room conditions [132]. Thus, *in vitro* regenerated plants are successfully established in the soil by following different steps like transferring to a small pot containing potting substrates and covering with a polyethylene bag to maintain humidity. Later small holes are punched in the polyethylene bag to gradually reduce the humidity. Subsequently, these plants are transferred to shade condition followed by transfer to field establishment. Different types of potting substrates have been used for the successful acclimatization of *in vitro* regenerated medicinal plants. A mixture of garden soil and sand (1:1) has been preferred for the successful acclimatization of *Hedychium coronarium, Symplocos racemosa, Curcuma amada, Paederia foetida* (Table **1**).

BIOTECHNOLOGICAL   APPROACHES   FOR   SECONDARY METABOLITE PRODUCTION

Cell Suspension Culture and Its Potential in the Herbal Industry

Plants produce a large number of secondary metabolites (Table **4**) [133 - 193] and (Table **5**) [194 - 243] which are used as raw materials for pharmaceuticals, insecticides, cosmetics, flavorings, fragrances, and food industries [244]. These secondary metabolites are traditionally collected from plants grown in their natural habitats [245]. Unregulated harvesting of such important medicinal plants from their natural habitat may ultimately lead to their extinction [246]. Thus, for commercial utilization of secondary metabolites in the herbal industry, large-scale cultivation of these medicinal plants is required, which is often time-consuming and needs proper cultivation practices. There are several limitations, including regional, seasonal and environmental restrictions for the production of commercially important secondary metabolites in uniform quality and quantity around the year [247]. Moreover, the chemical synthesis of secondary metabolites is also difficult due to their complex structure and thus increases the cost of production [248]. Therefore, it is challenging to fulfill the commercial demand for secondary metabolites through chemical synthesis or metabolite extraction from natural habitat-grown plants. In this context, biotechnological intervention through cell suspension culture can provide an alternative method for the production of pharmaceutically and industrially important secondary metabolites around the year.

Table 4. Cell suspension culture system of medicinal plants for secondary metabolite production.

| Plant Species | Secondary Metabolite | Culture Medium | Culture Conditions | | References |
			Photo Period	Type of Culture	
Papaver somniferum	Codeine	LS	Continuous light	Shake flask	[133]
Salvia miltiorrhiza	Cryptotanshinon	MS + Sucrose (30 g/l)	Dark	Shake flask	[134]

(Table 4) cont.....

Plant Species	Secondary Metabolite	Culture Medium	Culture Conditions		References
			Photo Period	**Type of Culture**	
Dioscorea deltoidea	Diosgenin	MS + 2,4-D (0.1 mg/l)	Dark	Shake flask	[135]
Fumaria capreolata	Isoquinoline alkaloids	LS	NI	NI	[136]
Ailanthus altissima	Alkaloids	MS + Sucrose (50 g/l) + KN (0.1 mg/l) + 2,4-D (1.0 mg/l)	Continuous light	Shake flask	[137]
Picrasma quassioides	Quassin	B5 + Glucose (20 g/l) + KN (0.5 mg/l) + 2,4-D (1.0 mg/l)	Continuous light	Shake flask	[138]
Rauwolfia serpentina	Reserpine	LS + KN (1.0 μM) + 2,4-D (1.0 μM)	Dark	Shake flask	[139]
Catharanthus roseus	Vinblastine	MS + Sucrose (30 g/l) + BA (0.5 mg/l) + NAA (0.5 mg/l)	Dark	Shake flask	[140]
Coptis japonica	Berberine	LS + BA (0.1 μM) + NAA (10 μM)	Dark	Shake flask	[141]
Camellia sinensis	Theamine	MS + Sucrose (30 g/l) + KN (0.1 mg/l) + IBA (2.0 mg/l)	Dark	Shake flask	[142]
Cephaelis ipecacuanha	Emetine	MS + Sucrose (60 g/l) + IBA (1.0 mgl) + IAA (0.5 mg/l)	NI	NI	[143]
Digitalis lanata	Digoxin	MS + Glucose (33 g/l) + KH_2PO_4 (340 mg/l) + Glycine (4.0 mg/l)	Continuous light	Shake flask	[144]
Cornus kousa	Polyphenols	MS + BA (1.0 mg/l) + 2,4-D (2.0 mg/l)	NI	NI	[145]
Mucuna pruriens	L-dihydroxyphenylalanine	MS + BA (1.0 mg/l) + IAA (1.0 mg/l) + Saccharose (40 g/l)	Continuous light	Shake flask	[146]

(Table 4) cont.....

Plant Species	Secondary Metabolite	Culture Medium	Culture Conditions		References
			Photo Period	Type of Culture	
Panax ginseng	Ginsenosides	MS + Sucrose (30 g/l) + KN (0.1 mg/l) + 2,4-D (1.0 mg/l)	Dark	Shake flask	[147]
Sanguinaria canadensis	Sanguinarine	MS + Sucrose (30 g/l) + BA (0.5 mg/l) + 2,4-D (0.1 mg/l)	Continuous light	Shake flask	[148]
Salvia miltiorrhiza	Tanshinone	B5 + Sucrose (30 g /l)	Dark	Shake flask	[149]
Solanum malacoxylon	Cholecalciferol	B5	16h light	Shake flask	[150]
Glehnia littoralis	Furanocoumarin	LS + KN (1.0 mg/l) + 2,4-D (1.0 mg/l)	Dark	Shake flask	[151]
Lycium chinense	Cerebroside	MS + KN (0.1 ppm) + 2,4-D (1.0 ppm)	Dark	Shake flask	[152]
Cinchona robusta	Robustaquinones	B5 + Sucrose (20 g/l) + KN (0.2 mg/l) + 2,4-D (1.0 mg/l) + Cysteine (50 mg/l)	Continuous light	Shake flask	[153]
Coleus forskolii	Forskolin	B5 + Sucrose (30 g/l)	Dark	Shake flask	[154]
Lithospermum erythrorhizon	Shikonin	LS + KN (10 µM) + IAA (10 µM)	Dark	Shake flask	[155]
Papaver somniferum	Morphine	LS	Continuous light	Shake flask	[156]
Piqueria trinervia	Antifungal monoterpene	MS + NAA (1.0 mg/l) + BA (1.0 mg/l)	NI	Shake flask	[157]
Taxus brevifolia	Taxol	B5 + Sucrose (30 g/l) + 2,4-D (10 µM) + KN (4.0 µM) + GA$_3$ (1.0 µM)	Dark	Shake flask	[158]

(Table 4) cont.....

Plant Species	Secondary Metabolite	Culture Medium	Culture Conditions		References
			Photo Period	Type of Culture	
Bacopa monnieri	Bacoside	MS + Sucrose (30 g/l) + KN (0.5 mg/l) + NAA (1.0 mg/l) + CH (1.0 g/l)	Dark	Shake flask	[159]
Catharanthus roseus	Ajmalicine	MS + Sucrose (40 g/l) + KN (0.1 mg/l) + IAA (1.0 mg/l) + NAA (1.0 mg/l)	Darkness	Shake flask	[160]
Hypericum perforatum	Hypericin	MS + Sucrose (30 g/l) + KN (0.11 µM) + 2,4-D (0.9 µM)	Dark and light	Shake flask	[161]
Podophyllum hexandrum	Podophyllotoxin	MS + Glucose (30 g/l) + Sucrose (30 g/l) + IAA (1.4 mg/l) + Pectinase (1.5 mg/l) + PVP (10 g/l)	16 h light	Bioreactor	[162]
Ammi majus	Coumarins	B5 + Sucrose (30 g/l)	16h light	Shake flask	[163]
Capsicum frutescens	Capsaicin	MS + KN (2.3 µM) + 2,4-D (7.6 µM)	Continuous light	Shake flask	[164]
Crocus sativus	Crocin	B5 + CH (300 mg/l) + BA (0.5 mg/l) + NAA (2.0 mg/l) + IAA (2.0 mg/l)	Darkness	Shake flask	[165]
Plumbago rosea	Plumbagin	Heller + NAA (0.25 mg/l) + IBA (5.0 mg/l) + BA (0.05 mg/l)	16 h light	Shake flask	[166]
Eucommia ulmoides	Chlorogenic acid	MS + Sucrose (30 g/l) + LH (300 mg/l) + 2,4-D (2.0 mg/l)	NI	Shake flask	[167]
Caesalpinia pulcherrima	Homoisoflavonoids	MS + BA (1.0 µM) + 2,4-D (10 µM)	Dark	Shake flask	[168]

(Table 4) cont.....

Plant Species	Secondary Metabolite	Culture Medium	Culture Conditions		References
			Photo Period	**Type of Culture**	
Perilla frutescens	Anthocyanin	MS + Sucrose (30 g/l) + BA (0.5 mg/l) + 2,4-D (0.2 mg/l)	16h light	Shake flask	[169]
Saussurea medusa	Jaceosidin	MS + Sucrose (30 g/l) + Glucose (10 g/l) + myo-inositol (100 mg/l) + BA (0.5 mg /l) + NAA (2.0 mg/l)	Continuous light	Shake flask	[170]
	Hispidulin				
Silybum marianum	Silymarin	MS + Sucrose (30 g/l) + 2,4-D (1.0 mg/l) + BA (0.5 mg/l)	Dark	Shake flask	[171]
Camptotheca acuminata	Camptothecin	B5 + Sucrose (40 g/l) + KN (0.5 mg/l)+ 2,4-D (1.0 mg/l)	16h light	Shake flask	[172]
Anchusa officinalis	Rosmarinic acid	B5 + Sucrose (30 g/l) + 2,4-D (1.0 mg/l) + KIN (0.1 mg/l)	Continuous light	Shake flask	[173]
Cistanche salsa	Phenylethanoid Glycosides	MS + Glucose (40 g/l) + IAA (3.0 mg/l)	Dark	Shake flask	[174]
Morinda elliptica	Anthraquinones	B5 + Sucrose (20 g/l) + KN (0.2 mg/l) + 2,4-D (2.0 mg/l) + NAA (0.5 mg/l) + IAA (0.5 mg/l)	16h light	Shae flask	[175]
Artemisia annua	Artemisinin	MS + Sucrose (30 g/l) + KN (0.1 mg/l) + NAA (0.1 mg/l)	16h light	Shake flask	[176]
Calophyllum inophyllum	Dipyranocoumarins	WPM + Sucrose (20 g/l)	Continuous light	Shake flask	[177]
Ginkgo biloba	Ginkgolides	MS + Sucrose (30 g/l) + NAA (3.5 mg/l)	Dark	Shake flask	[178]

(Table 4) cont.....

Plant Species	Secondary Metabolite	Culture Medium	Culture Conditions		References
			Photo Period	**Type of Culture**	
Psoralea corylifolia	Phytoestrogens	MS + BA (4.40 μM) + IAA (5.7 μM)	16 h light	Shake flask	[179]
Eriobotrya japonica	Triterpene	MS + Sucrose (30 g/l) + BA (2.5 mg/l) + NAA (1.0 mg/l)	Dark	Shake flask	[180]
Withania somnifera	Withanolide A	MS + Sucrose (30 g/l)	16 h light	Shake flask	[181]
Cephalotaxus fortune	Abietane diterpenoids ·	MS + Sucrose (30 g/l) + KN (0.1 mg/l) + 2,4-D (2.0 mg/l)	Darkness	Shake flask	[182]
Gymnema sylvestre	Gymnemic acid	MS + BA (0.5 mg/l) + IAA (1.5 mg/l)	16h light	Shake flask	[183]
Vitis vinifera	Resveratrol	B5 + Sucrose (30 g/l) + CH (250 mg/l) + KN (0.2 mg/l)+ NAA (0.1 mg/l)	Dark	Shake flask	[184]
Withania somnifera	Withanolide A	MMS + 2,4-D (2.0 mg/l) + KN (0.5 mg/l)	16h light	Shake flask	[185]
Helianthus tuberosus	Inulin	MS + NAA (1.0 mg/l) + BA (1.0 mg/l)	NI	NI	[186]
Larrea divaricata	Phenolic compound	MS + BA (5.0 μM) + 2,4-D (9.0 μM)	16 h light	Shake flask	[187]
Panax ginseng	Ginsenoside	MS + Sucrose (30 g/l) + KN (0.25 mg/l)	Dark	Shake flask	[188]
Eurycoma longifolia	Eurycomanone	MS + Sucrose (30 g/l) + KN (1.0 mg/l) + NAA (1.25 mg/l)	8 h light	Shake flask	[189]

(Table 4) cont.....

Plant Species	Secondary Metabolite	Culture Medium	Culture Conditions		References
			Photo Period	Type of Culture	
Salvia leriifolia	Caffeic acid and Salvianolic acid B	MS + Sucrose (40 g/l) + BA (5.0 mg/l) + NAA (5.0 mg/l)	16 h light	Shake flask	[190]
	Rosmarinic acid	MS + Sucrose (50 g/l) + BA (5.0 mg/l) + NAA (5.0 mg/l)			
Lonicera japonica	Chlorogenic acid	MS + Sucrose (30 g/l) + BA (1.5 mg/l) + NAA (0.2 mg/l) + 2,4-D (0.1 mg/l)	Dark	Shake flask	[191]
Panax ginseng	Ginsenoside	MS + Sucrose (40 g/l) + 2,4-D (1.0 mg/l)	Dark	Shake flask	[192]
Clinacanthus nutans	Phenolics	MS + 2,4-D (0.25 mg/l) + BA (0.25 mg/l)	16 h light	Shake flask	[193]

µM - Micro molar, 2,4-D - 2,4-dichlorophenoxyacetic acid, B5 - Gamborg's B5 (1968) medium, BA - N⁶-Benzyladenine, CH- Casein hydrolysate, g/l - gram per liter, GA_3 - Gibberellic acid, h - Hour(s), IAA - Indole-3-acetic acid, IBA - Indole-3-butyric acid, KH_2PO_4 - Potassium dihydrogen phosphate, KN - Kinetin, LS - Linsmaier and Skoog (1965) medium, LH - Lactalbumin hydrolysate, mg/l - milligram per liter, MMS - Modified Murashige and Skoog's (1962) medium, MS - Murashige and Skoog's (1962) medium, NAA - α-Napthaleneacetic acid, NI - No information, ppm - parts per million, PVP - Polyvinylpyrrolidone, WPM - Lloyd and McCown (1980) Woody Plant Medium.

Table 5. Secondary metabolite production through cell suspension culture using elicitors of medicinal plants.

Plant Species	Secondary Metabolites Enhanced	Culture Medium	Elicitors	Elicitation Duration	Fold or % of SMs Enhanced	References
Thalictrum rugosum	Berberine	B5 + 2,4-D (4.5 µM)	Carbohydrate fraction of yeast extract	NI	4	[194]
Eschscholtzia californica	Benzophenanthridine alkaloids	B5 + Sucrose (20 g/l) + KN (0.5 µM) + 2,4-D (5.0 µM)	Yeast extract	NI	3.5	[195]
Salvia miltiorrhiza	Cryptotanshinone	B5 + Sucrose (20 g/l)	Carbohydrate fraction of yeast extract	5 d	*	[196]

(Table 5) cont.....

Plant Species	Secondary Metabolites Enhanced	Culture Medium	Elicitors	Elicitation Duration	Fold or % of SMs Enhanced	References
Taxus chinensis	Taxol	B5 + Sucrose (30 g/l) + NAA (10 μM)	Mycelia extract of fungus isolated from the inner bark of *Taxus chinensis* + Salicylic acid	50 h	7.5	[197]
Cupressus lusitanica	β- Thujaplicin	MB5 + Sucrose (30 g/l) + BA (0.01 μM) + NAA (10 μM)	Yeast extract + Ferrous ion	7d	3-4	[198]
Catharanthus roseus	Ajmalicine	MS + Sucrose (30 g/l) + KN (0.1 mg/l) + NAA (2.0 mg/l) + IAA (2.0 mg/l)	Mycelia homogenate of *Aspergillum niger* + Tetramethyl ammonium bromide	NI	4	[199]
Catharanthus roseus	Ajmalicine	MS + Sucrose (30 g/l) + KN (4.60 μM) + 2,4-D (9.05 μM)	Cell free of filtrate *Trichoderma viride*	48 h	3	[200]
Taxus chinensis	Paclitaxel	MMS + LH (200 mg/l) + BA (1.0 mg/l) + NAA (5.0 mg/l)	Hydrolysate filtrate of an endophytic fungus of *Taxus*	22 d	>70	[201]
Taxus chinensis var *mairei*	Taxol	MB5 + Sucrose (25 g/l) + BA (0.15 mg/l) + NAA (2.0 mg/l)	Mycelia extract of *Fusarium oxysporum*	96 h	3	[202]
Taxus media	Taxane	B5 + Sucrose (30 g/l) + Picloram (2.0 mg/l) + KN (0.1 mg/l)	Methyl jasmonate	28 d	2.82	[203]
			Arachidonic acid		3.73	
Catharanthus roseus	Ajmalicine	MS + Sucrose (30 g/l) + KN (0.1 mg/l) + IAA (2.0 mg/l)	Nitric oxide	4 d	1.6	[204]
	Catharanthine			4 d	2.9	

(Table 5) cont.....

Plant Species	Secondary Metabolites Enhanced	Culture Medium	Elicitors	Elicitation Duration	Fold or % of SMs Enhanced	References
Morinda citrifolia	Anthraquinone	B5 + Sucrose (20 g/l) + CH (2.0 g/l) + NAA (1.86 mg/l) + NaH$_2$PO$_4$ (0.17 g/l)	Salicylic acid	14 d	3.06	[205]
Morinda elliptica	Anthraquinone	B5 + Sucrose (20 g/l) + NAA (1.86 mg/l)	Jasmonic acid	5 d	2.9	[206]
Eleutherococcus sessiliflorus	Eleutheroside B	MS	Methyl jasmonate	6 w	3.5	[207]
	Eleutheroside E			6 w	2.6	
	Chlorogenic acids			6 w	3.2	
Linum album	Podophyllotoxins	MS + NAA (0.4 mg/l)	Co-culture with *Sebacina vermifera*	24 h	3.9	[208]
	6-Methoxy podophyllotoxin				7.6	
Rubia tinctorum	Anthraquinone	MS + Sucrose (30 g/l) + IAA (1.0 mg/l) + KIN (0.2 mg/l) + NAA (0.2 mg/l)	Salicylic acid	7 d	1.11	[209]
Withania somnifera	Withaferin A	MS + Sucrose (50 g/l)	Cell extract of *Verticilium dahaliae* + Copper sulfate	4 d	13.8	[210]
Linum album	Podophyllotoxins	MS + NAA (0.4 mg/l)	Co-culture with *Sebacina vermifera*	24 h	3.76	[211]
	6-Methoxy podophyllotoxin				8.74	
Calendula officinalis	Oleanolic acid	MS + BA (0.2 mg/l) + 2,4-D (0.4 mg/l)	Jasmonic acid	72 h	9.4	[212]
Papaver somniferum	Sanguinarine	MS + Glycine (3.0 mg/l) + CH (1.0 g/l)	Methyl jasmonate	48 h	10.8	[213]
Euphorbia pekinensis	Isoeuphpekinensin	MS + Sucrose (30 g/l) + BA (2.0 mg/l) + NAA (0.4 mg/l)	Mycelia extract of *Fusarium* sp.	6d	5.81	[214]
	Euphol				3.56	

(Table 5) cont.....

Plant Species	Secondary Metabolites Enhanced	Culture Medium	Elicitors	Elicitation Duration	Fold or % of SMs Enhanced	References
Gymnema sylvestre	Gymnemic acid	MS + BA (0.5 mg/l) + IAA (1.5 mg/l)	Cell extract of *Aspergillus niger*	-	9	[215]
Calophyllum inophyllum	Inophyllum A	WPM	Dried cell powder of *Phoma* sp.	45-50 d	751	[216]
	Inophyllum B		Dried cell powder of *Nigrospora sphaerica*		414	
	Inophyllum C		Culture filtrate of *Nigrospora sphaerica*		928	
	Inophyllum P				750	
Catharanthus roseus	Alkaloid	MS + BA (0.1 mg/l) + 2,4-D (0.5 mg/l)	Co-culture with *Fusarium oxysporum*	36 h	48%	[217]
Taxus media	Taxane	B5 + Sucrose (30 g/l) + myo-Inositol (0.01%) + KN (1.0 mg/l) + 2,4-D (4.0 mg/l) + GA$_3$ (0.1 mg/l)	Methyl jasmonate	12 d	2.6	[218]
Hypericum perforatum	Anthocyanins	B5 + BA (0.5 mg/l) + 2,4-D (1.0 mg/l) + NAA (0.1 mg/l) + Sucrose (30 g/l)	Mycelia extract of *Aspergillus flavus*	14 d	4	[219]
Teucrium chamaedrys	Teucriosides	MS + Sucrose (30 g/l) + KN (0.2 mg/l) + 2,4-D (0.5 mg/l) + Phytagel (3 g/l)	Methyl jasmonate	14 d	5	[220]
Andrographis Paniculata	Andrographolides	MS + BA (0.5 mg/l) + 2,4-D (1.0 mg/l)	Mycelia powder of *Aspergillus niger*	10 d	6.94	[221]

(Table 5) cont.....

Plant Species	Secondary Metabolites Enhanced	Culture Medium	Elicitors	Elicitation Duration	Fold or % of SMs Enhanced	References
Panax ginseng	Ginsenoside	67-V + KN (0.25 mg/l) + 2,4-D (1.5 mg/l) + IAA (1.0 mg/l) + NAA (0.1 mg/l)	N-dicyclohexylcarbodiimide	11 d	3.0	[222]
Withania somnifera	Withanolide A	MS + Sucrose (50 g/l)	*Gracilaria edulis* (sea weed) extract	6 w	0.69	[223]
	Withanone			6 w	0.64	
	Withanolide B			6 w	0.64	
	Withanoferin A			6 w	0.6	
Papaver somnifera	Sanguinarine	MS + 2,4-D (1.0 mg/l)	Culture filtrate of *Trichoderma harzianum* + shikimate	5d	4	[224]
Psoralea corylifolia	Psoralen	MMS	Mycelia with spores extract of *Aspergillus niger*	72 h	9	[225]
Linum album	Podophyllotoxin	MS + KN (0.5 mg/l) + NAA (1.0 mg/l)	Culture filtrate of *Fusarium graminearum*	5 d	3	[226]
	Lariciresinol				2	
	Total phenolics			3 d	2	
Hypericum perforatum	Hypericin	MS	Mycelia extract of *Fusarium oxysporum* f. sp. *Lini*	1-21 d	3-4	[227]
	Pseudohypericin			1-21 d	3-4	
	Total flavonols			21 d	8	
	Total anthocyanins			7 d	5	
	Total phenolics			4 d	3.5	
	Total flavonoids			7 d	9	
Peganum harmala	Harmaline	MS + BA (1.0 mg/l) + NAA (0.5 mg/l)	Mycelium homogenate of *Aspergillus flavus*	15 d	1.69	[228]
	Harmine		*Saccharomyces cerevisiae*		1.68	
Melissa officinalis	Hydroxycinnamic acid derivatives	MS + Sucrose (30 g/l) + KN (1.5 mg/l) + 2,4-D (0.5 mg/l)	Hydrolyzate of *Botrytis cinerea*	72 h	3	[229]
Agastache rugosa	Rosmarinic acid	½ MS + Sucrose (30 g/l)	Yeast extract	-	18.5	[230]
Panax quinquefolius	Total Ginsenosides	MMS + NAA (5.4 µM) + KN (1.2 µM)	Culture filtrate of *Trichoderma atroviridae*	5 d	3.2	[231]

(Table 5) cont.....

Plant Species	Secondary Metabolites Enhanced	Culture Medium	Elicitors	Elicitation Duration	Fold or % of SMs Enhanced	References
Lantana camara	Ursolic acid	MS + BA (5.0 µM) + 2,4-D (1.0 µM) + NAA (1.0 µM)	Filter sterilized culture filtrate of *Piriformospora indica*	2 d	3.5	[232]
	Oleanolic acid				5.6	
	Betulinic acid				7.8	
Argemone Mexicana	Sanguinarine	MS + Sucrose (20 g/l) + BA (0.5 mg/l) + NAA (1.5 mg/l)	Yeast extract	48 h	> 8	[233]
Gymnema sylvestre	Gymnemic acid	MS + KN (1.0 mg/l) + 2,4-D (2.0 mg/l)	Consortium of dried mycelia powder of *Xylaria* sp. and *Polyancora globosa*	72 h	10.45	[234]
Ophiorrhiza mungos	Camptothecin	MS + Sucrose (30 g/l) + KN (0.5 mg/l) + NAA (3.0 mg/l) + 2,4-D (1.0 mg/l)	Carbohydrate fraction of yeast extract	10 d	13.3	[235]
Calligonum polygonoides	Catechin	MS	Crude yeast extract	48 h	4	[236]
	Isoquercitrin				2.4	
	Astragalin				1.7	
Epicoccum nigrum	Paclitaxel	MS + BA (0.2 mg/l) + GA₃ (2.0 mg/l) + 2,4-D (2.0 mg/l)	Filter sterilized cell extract of *Corylus avellanahs*	12 d	11.5	[237]
Artemisia annua	Artemisinin	MS + Sucrose (30 g/l) + KN (0.1 mg/l) + NAA (0.1 mg/l)	Sorbitol	19 d	8.67	[238]
Ocimum bacilicum	Chicoric acid	MS + Sucrose (30 g/l) + KN (0.5 mg/l) + NAA (2.5 mg/l)	Yeast extract	10 d	0.92	[239]
	Rosmarinic acid			10 d	1.25	
Leucas aspera	Triperpenoid saponin	MS + 2,4-D (2.0 mg/ L) + Picloram (0.2 mg/l)	Methyl jasmonate	24 d	1.68	[240]

Plant Species	Secondary Metabolites Enhanced	Culture Medium	Elicitors	Elicitation Duration	Fold or % of SMs Enhanced	References
Gymnema sylvestre	Deacylgymnemic acid	MS + KN (1.0 mg/l) + 2,4-D (3.0 mg/l)	Sodium nitroprusside	96 h	6.1	[241]
	Gymnemic acid XVII		Sodium nitroprusside	48 h	5.2	
	Gymnemagenin		Salicylic acid	48 h	4.12	
	Gymnemic acid IV		Salicylic acid	96 h	5.11	
Gymnema sylvestre	Gymnemic acid	MS + BA (2.0 mg/l) + NAA (2.0 mg/l) + Picloram (0.5 mg/l) + CH (100 mg/l)	Silver nitrate	12 d	3.8	[242]
Ruta graveolens	Rutin	MS + Sucrose (30 g/l) + IAA (1.5 mg/l) + BA (0.3 mg/l)	Mannitol	16 d	3	[243]

% - Percent, *- increased, ½ MS - Half strength Murashige and Skoog's (1962) medium, 2,4-D - 2,4-dichlorophenoxyacetic acid, 67-V - Veliky and Martin (1970) medium, μM - Micro molar, B5 - Gamborg's B5 (1968) medium, BA - N^6-Benzyladenine, CH- Casein hydrolysate, d - day(s), GA_3 - Gibberellic acid, g/l-gram per liter, h - hours, IAA - Indole-3-acetic acid, KN- Kinetin, LH - Lactoabumin hydrolysate, MB5 - Modified Gamborg's B5 (1968) medium, mg/l- milligram per liter, MMS - Modified Murashige and Skoog's (1962) medium, MS- Murashige and Skoog's (1962) medium, NAA- α-Napthaleneacetic acid, NaH_2PO_4 - Sodium dihydrogen phosphate, NI - No information, sp. - species, SMs - Secondary metabolites, w - week (s), WPM - Lloyd and McCown (1980) Woody Plant Medium.

Cell suspension culture is established by transferring an inoculum of friable callus in a liquid medium to obtain single cells. These cells divide rapidly and can produce a large quantity of valuable secondary metabolites [249]. Cell suspension culture is a simple and cost-effective method which has been extensively used to overcome the problems of large-scale production of secondary metabolites. The secondary metabolites produced *via* suspension culture are identical to those present in the mother or donor plant. This technology has shown a new avenue for the production of high-value natural products like diosgenin, reserpine, vinblastine, berberine, ginsenoside, rosamarinic acid, paclitaxel, and artemisinin instead of propagating the whole plant (Tables **4** and **5**). The cell suspension culture is considered to have more potential for commercial application in comparison to plant tissue or organ cultures. The advantages of cell suspension culture include (a) It is independent of seasonal and environmental changes as well as geographical restrictions, (b) It provides uniform quality and quantity of natural products in a short period, (c) It is possible to synthesize novel compounds in cultured cells, that usually do not occur in the native plant (d) Ease of handling and scaling up, and (e) Enhanced uptake of nutrients and higher yield of bioactive compounds [250, 251].

There are different factors associated with cell suspension culture for the production of important secondary metabolites, such as the selection of cell line, culture conditions (photoperiod), culture medium, types and concentrations of carbon source and growth regulators, and aeration of cultures (Tables **4** and **5**). For the initiation of cell suspension culture, a callus culture needs to be established first, which must be repeatedly subcultured more than four times for callus proliferation. The proliferated callus has been used for initiating cell suspension culture. However, repeated subculturing of the cell line might also lead to variations due to genetic changes in the culture or physiological conditions. The duration of the photoperiod (*i.e.*, continuous dark, continuous light, 16 h light, 8 h light) is varied according to the cell line as well as the production of desirable secondary metabolites in the cell suspension culture. It has been commonly observed that the cell suspension cultures of several medicinal plants were incubated in dark conditions for the production of secondary metabolites (Table **4**).

Different types of medium such as MS liquid medium, modified MS liquid medium, B5 liquid medium, modified B5 liquid medium, Linsmair and Skoog (LS) (1965) liquid medium, Heller medium, and WPM liquid medium have been used for cell suspension culture of several medicinal plants (Tables **4** and **5**). However, MS medium was found to be a more preferable medium for cell suspension culture and secondary metabolite production, followed by B5 medium (Tables **4** and **5**). The use of LS medium has also been reported in cell suspension culture of some medicinal plants, including *Papaver somniferum*, *Rauwolfia serpentine* and *Coptis japonica* (Table **4**). Sucrose has been reported as a suitable carbon source in a varied concentration from 20 g/l to 60 g/l for secondary metabolite production of medicinal plants through cell suspension culture. However, the use of sucrose at a concentration of 30 g/l has been frequently reported by many workers in cell suspension cultures of different medicinal plants. Besides sucrose, glucose has also been used as a carbon source in the cell suspension culture of medicinal plants, including *Cistanche salsa*. Saccharose (40 g/l) has been used as a carbon source in the cell suspension culture of *Mucuna pruriens* for the production of L-dihydroxyphenylalanine. Moreover, the combination of sucrose and glucose has also been used as a carbon source in the cell suspension culture of *Podophyllum hexandrum* and *Saussurea medusa* to produce podophyllotoxin and hispidulin, respectively (Table **4**).

It has been observed that plant growth regulator-free basal medium is not sufficient for the establishment of cell suspension culture and secondary metabolite production of all medicinal plant species. Hence, the addition of plant growth regulators in the basal culture medium is essential to promote cell division and differentiation in cell suspension culture. Different types, concentrations as well as combinations of cytokinins (BA, KN, Z), auxins (IBA, IAA, NAA, 2, 4-D), and GA$_3$ have been tested in cell suspension culture for the production of secondary metabolites (Tables **4** and **5**). Basal culture medium containing KN alone has been used in *Panax ginseng* for the production of ginsenoside. The combination of BA along with NAA in culture medium has been frequently used for cell suspension culture in *Eriobotrya japonica*, *Ginkgo biloba*, *Helianthus tuberosus*, and *Salvia leriifolia* (Table **4**).

Besides all the aforementioned factors, elicitation is also considered to be an important factor for enhancing secondary metabolite accumulation in the cell suspension culture of medicinal plants [252]. The phenomenon of inducing enhanced biosynthesis of secondary metabolites by using various elicitors is called elicitation. Elicitors are defined as 'a biotic or abiotic substance which, when applied in small concentrations to a living system or supplied on optimum culture medium, enhances the biosynthesis of secondary metabolites [253]. There are two categories of elicitors; (i) biotic elicitors (*i.e.*, yeast extract, fungal spores, seaweeds, endophytes, mannan, cellulose, chitosan, alginate, and pectin, *etc.*) and (ii) abiotic elicitors (*i.e.*, thermal stress, light, UV irradiation, heavy metal salts, inorganic salts, osmotic stress, sorbitol, methyl jasmonate, salicylic acid, silver nitrate, and sodium nitroprusside, *etc.*) based on their nature of origin. To increase the production of secondary metabolites in cells, various types of elicitors, including yeast extract, mycelia homogenate, chitosan, silver nitrate, jasmonic acid, methyl jasmonate, salicylic acid, *etc.*, have been used by several researchers in cell suspension culture of medicinal plants (Table **4**). Some workers have reported the enhancement of secondary metabolites through cell suspension culture by adding a single elicitor on optimum culture medium, while others have reported the use of multiple elicitors (Table **5**). Moreover, the age or growth stage of cell culture and duration of elicitation also plays an important role in secondary metabolite enhancement [253]. The content of ajmalicine was increased almost 3 fold in *Catharanthus roseus* cells treated with *Trichoderma viride* cell filtrate for 48 hours. The use of methyl jasmonate as an elicitor in the culture medium of *Papaver somniferum* resulted in 10.8 fold enhanced production of sanguinarine in comparison to control. Likewise, in *Taxus media,* almost 2.6 fold increased production of taxane was reported after 12 days of culture on methyl jasmonate supplied medium compared to control (Table **5**).

Production of Bioactive Compounds of Medicinal Plants Using Hairy Root Culture System

Hairy root technology has been exploited for the production of various pharmaceutically important secondary metabolites in several medicinal plants, including *Atropa belladonna, Datura stramonium, Catharanthus roseus, and Withania somnifera* (Table **6**) [254 - 272]. Hairy root culture, also called transformed root culture, is induced by infecting the wounded plant tissues with pathogenic gram-negative soil bacterium *Agrobacterium rhizogenes,* causing the growth of very fine adventitious roots [273]. Hairy roots are capable of producing equal or even higher amounts of bioactive compounds compared to normal roots [274]. There are several distinctive features exhibited by hairy roots, such as faster growth, autotrophy in plant hormones, production of high levels of secondary metabolites, and genetic and biochemical stability, which impart significant advantages compared to the intact plant and undifferentiated cell culture [275, 276]. Moreover, the hairy roots resemble normal roots in terms of their anatomy and metabolic activity, producing similar types of secondary metabolites [277]. For induction of hairy roots, various explants such as stem, leaf, cotyledon, and petiole have been used in different medicinal plants such as *Artemisia vulgaris, Salvia miltiorrhiza, Panax ginseng, Hyoscyamus reticulates* (Table **6**). Various factors such as culture medium and its composition (*i.e.,* types and concentrations of nitrogen and carbon sources), plant growth regulators, culture conditions (*i.e.,* temperature, light, and relative humidity) [278], infection time, plant species, type of explant, *Agrobacterium* strain [279], incubation time, inoculum of bacterial cell density [280], elicitors, and precursors [281] have largely contributed to the efficient transformation. The age, hormonal balance, and wound response of the host tissue were also found to be important factors responsible for the specificity of *Agrobacterium* transformation [282]. The optimum time required for the induction of hairy roots varies from two weeks to three weeks depending on the plant species [283].

Table 6. Secondary metabolites production through hairy root culture of medicinal plants.

Plant	Agrobacterium Strain	Secondary Product	Explant	Culture Medium	Elicitor	Content of Secondary Metabolites	References
Atropa belladona	*A. rhizogenes* 15834	Atropine	Stems	MS	-	0.37% DW	[254]
		Scopolamine				0.024% DW	
Panax ginseng	*A. rhizogenes* A4	Ginsenoside	Callus	MS	-	0.95% per DW	[255]
Catharanthus roseus	*A. rhizogenes* 15834	Vinblastine	Seedlings	½ B5 + Sucrose (30 g/l)	-	0.05μg/g	[256]

(Table 6) cont.....

Plant	Agrobacterium Strain	Secondary Product	Explant	Culture Medium	Elicitor	Content of Secondary Metabolites	References
Catharanthus roseus	*A. rhizogenes* 15834	Catharanthine	Seedlings	½ B5 + Sucrose (30 g/l)	-	2 mg/ g DW	[257]
		Ajmalicine				4 mg/g	
		Serpentine				2 mg/g	
		Vindoline				0.4 mg/g	
Panax ginseng	*A. rhizogenes* A4	Ginsenoside	Rhizomes	SH	Methyl jasmonate	124.18 mg/ l	[258]
Solanum tuberosum	*A. rhizogenes*	Rishitin	Potato tuber discs	MS + Sucrose (30 g/l)	*Rhizoctonia bataticola* extract + β-cyclodextrin	213 µg/ g DW	[259]
		Lubimin				171 µg/ g DW	
Salvia miltiorrhiza	*A. rhizogenes* 15834	Tanshinones	Plantlets	MS + Sucrose (30 g/l)	Yeast elicitor	87.5 mg/l	[260]
Linum album	*A. rhizogenes* LBA 9402	Podophyllotoxin	Leaf	MS	Fungal extract *Fusarium graminearum*	190 µg/ g DW	[261]
		Lariciresinol				260 µg/ g DW	
		6-methoxy podophyllotoxin			*Trichoderma viride*	160 µg/ g DW	
Tribulus terrestris	*A. rhizogenes* 15834	Harmine	Leaf	MS	-	1.7 µg/g DW	[262]
Isatis tinctoria	*A. rhizogenes* LBA9402	Flavonoids	Petioles	½ MS	-	438.10 µg/g DW	[263]
Silybum marianum	*A. rhizogenes* AR15834	Silymarin	Cotyledon, leaf	MS + sucrose (30 g/l)	*Trichoderma harzanium* strain KHB	0.45 mg/g DW	[264]
					Trichoderma harzanium strain G46-7	0.33 mg/g DW	
Withania somnifera	*A. rhizogenes* R1000	Withanolide A	Leaf	MS	*Gracilaria edulis*	5.23 mg/g DW	[265]
		Withaferin A				2.24 mg/g DW	
		Withanone				4.83 mg/g DW	
Datura stramonium	*A. rhizogenes* A4	Hyoscyamine	Hypocotyl	½ B5 + Sucrose (30 g/l)	Salicylic acid and acetylsalicylic acid	12.31mg/g DW	[266]
Hyoscyamus reticulatus	*A. rhizogenes* A7	Hyoscyamine	Cotyledon	MS + sucrose (30 g/l)	Iron oxide nanoparticles	43.82%	[267]
		Scopolamine				20.3%	

Plant	Agrobacterium Strain	Secondary Product	Explant	Culture Medium	Elicitor	Content of Secondary Metabolites	References
Ocimum tenuiflorum	*A. rhizogenes* LBA 9402	Ursolic acid	Leaf	MS	Yeast extract (50 mg/l)	1.56 mg/g DW	[268]
		Eugenol				0.41 mg/g DW	
Daucus carota	*Rhizobium rhizogenes* A4	Anthocyanin	Tap root discs and hypocotyl segments	½ MS	Ethephon	82%	[269]
		Hydroxycinnamic acid				>20%	
Salvia przewalskii	*A. rhizogenes* ATCC 15834	Rosmarinic acid	leaf	MS	Methyl jasmonate	67.1273 mg/g DW	[270]
		Salvianolic acid B				21.4448 mg/g DW	
		Cryptotanshione				0.0674 mg/g DW	
		Tanshinone IIA				0.3791mg/g DW	
Artemisia vulgaris	*A. rhizogenes* A4	β-caryophyllene	Leaf	MS	Farnesyl diphosphate	2.92 mg/ml	[271]
	A. rhizogenes R1000					2.80 mg/ml	
Salvia virgata	*A. rhizogenes* ATCC15834	Rosmarinic acid	Leaf	MS + Sucrose (30 g/l)	Methyl jasmonate	18.45 mg/g DW	[272]
		Salvianolic acid A				2.11 mg/g DW	
		Total flavonoid				5.09 mg QUE/g DW	
		Total phenol				123.6 mg GAE/g DW	

% - Percentage, ½ MS - Half strength Murashige and Skoog (1962) medium, ½ B5 - Half strength Gamborg's B5 (1968) medium, ATCC - American Type Culture Collection, g/l - gram per liter, MS - Murashige and Skoog (1962) medium, SH - Schenk and Hildebrandt (1972) Medium, mg/g DW - milligram per gram of dry weight, mg QUE/g DW - milligram Quercetin equivalent per gram of dry weight, mg GAE/g DW - milligram Galic acid equivalent per gram of dry weight, mg/ml - milli gram per milli liter, μg/g DW – microgram per gram of dry weight.

Culture medium has been shown to significantly affect the growth as well as biomass of hairy roots, which eventually affects secondary metabolite production [284, 285]. Different types of media were tested for the hairy root cultures of *Artemisia annua* for artemisinin production. B5 medium supplemented with 3% sucrose has been frequently used for the highest metabolite yield; however, some studies have also reported the use of MS medium [286 - 289]. Enhanced production of kutkoside and picroside I (1.1 and 1.3 times, respectively) have been reported on ½ B5 medium compared to B5 medium in hairy root culture of

Picrorhiza kurroa [290]. Among different culture media tested (*i.e.*, ½ MS, MS, ½ B5, and B5), ½ MS medium supplemented with 3.5% sucrose was found to be the best for the growth of hairy root with enhanced ajmalicine content in *Rauwolfia serpentine* [291]. The positive effects of MS medium have been reported in hairy root cultures of several medicinal plants such as *Anethum graveolens* [292], and *Plumbago zeylanica* [293]. Whereas only a few reports are available for successful hairy root culture establishment using NN medium, including *Swertia chirata* [294]. Hairy roots can be cultured without the exogenous addition of plant growth regulators, as the bacterial t-DNA carries genes encoding for the plant growth hormones [295]. However, the presence of a growth regulator is shown to affect the organogenesis, root growth as well as production of secondary metabolites. The accumulation of loganic acid and gentiopicroside enhanced 6.6 fold and 1.8 fold, respectively, in the presence of Z (1 mg/l) and NAA (1 mg/l) compared to the roots of greenhouse-grown plants [296]. Stem segments with leaves were more suitable for hairy root formation than stem segments without leaves due to the presence of several meristematic cells in young leaves [297]. Different *Agrobacterium* strains, such as *A. rhizogenes* 15834, *A. rhizogenes* A4, *A. rhizogenes* 15834, *A. rhizogenes* R1000, have been used for hairy root induction in several medicinal plants (Table **6**). *A. rhizogenes* strains including A4GUS, LBA9402, R1000, and ATCC11325 were used for the establishment of hairy root culture in *Gentiana macrophylla*. The secondary metabolite production (secoiridoid glucoside gentiopicroside) was found to vary in these four different strains and the highest transformation rate was observed with strain R1000 [298]. The transformation efficiency and production of artemisinin were shown to differ in hairy roots induced by different *Agrobacterium* strains in *Artemisia annua* [299]. Hence, it is imperative to say that the *Agrobacterium* transformation efficiency is plant species-dependent and must be determined experimentally. Acetosyringone is a phenolic compound, which serves as a nutrient source for the *Agrobacterium* and is known to enhance transformation efficiency. The transformation rate was enhanced by adding acetosyringone into the nutrient medium during co-cultivation in *Momordica charantia* [300], *Cucumis sativus* [301], *Arabidopsis thaliana* [302], and Citrus cultivars [303]. Various researchers working on hairy root culture of medicinal plants have used different types of elicitors, such as yeast extract, fungal extract, methyl jasmonate, salicylic acid, iron oxide nanoparticles, *etc.*, to enhance the production of specific secondary metabolites (Table **6**). Elicitation-based hairy root culture is an efficient strategy to overcome various challenges associated with the large-scale production of commercially important bioactive compounds. Hairy root cultures are mostly preferred for elicitation because of their genetic stability, high growth rate, and uniform production of secondary metabolites after elicitation. However, different parameters such as types and concentrations of elicitor and treatment duration need to be optimized for a better response of elicitation. The elicitation of a culture medium with 0.1 mM methyl jasmonate resulted in the accumulation of a large quantity of asiaticoside (7.12 mg/g DW) from hairy root cultures of *Centella asiatica* [304]. Similarly, the elicitation of a culture medium with jasmonic acid and AlCl$_3$ was found to be beneficial for the improved production of hyoscyamine and scopolamine, which increased up to 83% and 43%, respectively [305].

In another study, tanshinone production was enhanced 10 fold after adding 50 g/l sorbitol and 100 mg/l polysaccharide fraction of yeast extract in the hairy root culture of *Salvia miltiorrhiza* [306]. Elicitation of *Orthosiphon aristatus* culture with yeast extract resulted in a more than a 4 fold increase with 17.99 mg/g DW phenolic acids compared to 4.03 mg/g DW in the control culture [307]. Scale-up of hairy root production using different types of bioreactors such as basket bubble, airlift, and liquid-dispersed bioreactors have been exploited for commercial production of secondary metabolites because of their low shear stress and better aeration [308].

Metabolic Engineering for Enhanced Production of Pharmaceutically Important Compounds

Plant metabolic engineering has gained importance in recent years for the enhanced production of specific secondary metabolites. The key aspect of metabolic engineering in plants involves the identification of the rate-limiting enzymes of the biosynthetic pathway and their modulation. Various strategies, such as the overexpression of key genes and transcription factors, have been used by several researchers to overproduce pharmaceutically important metabolites [309, 310]. Identification of specific promoters and their regulation is also attempted by many researchers [311, 312]. While studying the effect of overexpression of the *Arabidopsis thaliana* gene (*AtCPK1*), encoding for a calcium-dependent protein kinase, a substantial increase in the anthraquinone content was reported in *Rubia cordifolia* [313]. Similarly, overexpression of the tobacco *pmt* gene in *Datura metel* and *Hyoscyamus muticus* resulted in a higher accumulation of tropane alkaloids as compared to control [314]. Further, it was also observed that overexpressing the bacterial isochorismate synthase gene in *Rubia peregrine* led to an increase in the production of anthraquinone and total alizarin by 20% and 30%, respectively [315]. In addition to key pathway genes, several transcription factors have also been studied for their regulatory role in secondary metabolite production. For example, overexpressing the CrMYC1 transcription factor, which regulates the biosynthesis of terpenoid indole alkaloid in *Catharanthus roseus,* led to a 2.5 and 3 fold enhanced production of vinblastine and catharanthine, respectively, compared with control plants [316]. Apart from overexpression studies, the gene silencing approach and redirection of pathways have also been successfully explored for targeted metabolic engineering. For instance, RNAi mediated silencing of *quinolinate phosphoribosyl transferase (QTP)* gene in *Duboisia leichhardtii* was reported for attaining the enhanced biosynthesis of pharmaceutically valued tropane alkaloid scopolamine with the additional advantage of reduced nicotine content. Their common intermediate precursor methylpyrollinium cation was diverted towards the production of scopolamine by silencing the *QTP* gene, which in general, is responsible for the biosynthesis of nicotine [317]. Further, in-silico approaches, synthetic biology and integrated omics technology have been explored for their potential benefit to engineer plants for higher production of specific metabolites [318, 319]. The utilization of computational tools has helped in promoter prediction and analysis, investigation of the biosynthetic pathway, and reconstruction of metabolic pathways, unraveling the mechanisms of plant secondary metabolite synthesis and their regulation [320]. One such example is the improved production of a streptogramin antibiotic pristinamycin II (PII) using a combinatorial approach which includes the duplication of PII biosynthetic gene cluster and systemic manipulation of the regulatory genes in *Streptomyces pristinaespiralis* [321].

In recent years, there has been an expansion of interest in metabolic engineering through the emerging approach of engineering secondary metabolite transporters. In medicinal plants, various secondary metabolite transporters such as ATP Binding Cassette (ABC), multidrug and toxic compound extrusion (MATE), purine uptake permease (PUP), and nitrate and peptide transporter family (NPF) have been identified. The modulation of expression of these transporters could play a very important role in systemic metabolic engineering in medicinal plants. Plant secondary metabolites are synthesized only in specific plant parts and then either transported to the storage locations or the site of their functional activation. This type of source to sink tissue mobilization of secondary metabolites is majorly driven by various transporters belonging to the ABC, MATE, PUP, and NPF families [322]. The engineering of transporters is one of the emerging areas for enhancing the secondary metabolite content in medicinally important plants [323, 324], which will accelerate the availability and supply of bioactive compounds for herbal industries. It is also the most viable option to control the metabolite production in a tissue-specific manner that would certainly help reduce the overall cost of metabolite extraction. Recently a large number of secondary metabolite transporters have been identified due to the combinatorial usage of various bioinformatics and experimental approaches [325, 326]. However, their functional characterization and substrate specificity analysis remain immensely challenging. Being an evolving area, only limited reports are available for the successful implementation of transporter engineering to enhance secondary metabolites in the plants, but this certainly provides insights for potential future opportunities

[327]. The manipulation of transport pathways can be attained either in the native plant systems or in heterologous host organisms to achieve the long-term goal of secondary metabolite engineering. The classical example of transporter engineering in a native plant system includes a high valued medicinal plant *Catharanthus roseus,* which is known to possess anti-carcinogenic properties due to the presence of various monoterpene indole alkaloids such as vinblastine, vincristine, and their monomeric precursors namely catharanthine and vindoline. The overexpression of a transporter named CrTPT2 in the hairy roots of *C. roseus* has shown five-fold higher accumulation of catharanthine [328]. The compound catharanthine is biosynthesized in the leaf epidermis and then gets mobilized onto the leaf outer surface with the help of a transporter named CrTPT2. Virus-induced gene silencing (VIGS) based downregulation of CrTPT2 has led to tissue-specific enhanced accumulation of catharanthine in the leaf epidermis [329]. In addition to the traditional plant-based hosts, metabolic engineering is also considered to be achievable using heterologous microbial organisms with great benefits. To elucidate the missing links of complex biosynthetic pathways of plant secondary metabolites and for the large-scale production of pharmaceutically valued bioactive compounds, yeast and bacterial host systems have been successfully employed [330]. In a recent study, yeast engineering has been carried out for improving the *de novo* production of therapeutic tropane alkaloids, namely hyoscyamine and scopolamine, by incorporating the required transporters AbPUP1 and AbLP1 from *Atropa belladonna* and co-factor regeneration machinery to regulate the multi-step biosynthesis and transport pathways [331]. Similarly, *E. coli* has also been engineered with *Arabidopsis* AtDTX1 transporter for enhancing the production of reticuline which is an important metabolite intermediate from the alkaloid biosynthetic pathway [332].

CONCLUSION AND FUTURE PROSPECTS

The use of herbal medicines continues to expand rapidly throughout the world with a significant share of the population now resorting to herbal products for their healthcare. Indiscriminate collection and export of medicinal plants for industrial uses have placed many of these medicinal plants at risk of extinction. In this context, plant tissue culture offers a possible solution for the large-scale propagation of medicinal plants and the production of commercially important secondary metabolites. The exploitation of plant tissue and cell cultures for the production of valuable pharmaceuticals and natural products has developed into a huge market with considerable potential for the future. However, the challenge exists in the development of cost-efficient protocols and fine-tuning the prerequisites for the scale-up of production at the cellular or plant level. In recent years, there has been an addition of knowledge on various dimensions in culturing of plant cells, tissue, and organs under *in vitro* conditions. However, future research needs to be focused on the cost of production of tissue culture plants, optimization of the microenvironment, and their scale-up. Similarly, more and more studies are required for the identification of the precise biosynthetic routes and characterization of key genes and regulators of important secondary metabolites of medicinal plants to accomplish systemic metabolic engineering. Further, the exploration of small molecules which could effectively regulate the biosynthetic pathway could be critical in the future.

REFERENCES

[1]   Bent S. Herbal medicine in the United States: review of efficacy, safety, and regulation: grand rounds at University of California, San Francisco Medical Center. J Gen Intern Med 2008; 23(6): 854-9.
[http://dx.doi.org/10.1007/s11606-008-0632-y] [PMID: 18415652]

[2]   Pan SY, Litscher G, Gao SH, *et al.* Historical perspective of traditional indigenous medical practices: the current renaissance and conservation of herbal resources. Evid Based Complement Alternat Med 2014; 2014: 1-20.
[http://dx.doi.org/10.1155/2014/525340] [PMID: 24872833]

[3]   Available at: https://apps.who.int/iris/handle/10665/312342(2019).

[4]   Engebretson J. Culture and complementary therapies. Complement Ther Nurs Midwifery 2002; 8(4): 177-84.
[http://dx.doi.org/10.1054/ctnm.2002.0638] [PMID: 12463606]

[5]   Conboy L, Kaptchuk TJ, Eisenberg DM, Gottlieb B, Acevedo-Garcia D. The relationship between social factors and attitudes toward conventional and CAM practitioners. Complement Ther Clin Pract 2007; 13(3): 146-57.
[http://dx.doi.org/10.1016/j.ctcp.2006.12.003] [PMID: 17631257]

[6]   Evans M, Shaw A, Thompson EA, *et al.* Decisions to use complementary and alternative medicine (CAM) by male cancer patients: information-seeking roles and types of evidence used. BMC Complement Altern Med 2007; 7(1): 25.
[http://dx.doi.org/10.1186/1472-6882-7-25] [PMID: 17683580]

[7]   Bodeker C, Bodeker G, Ong CK, Grundy CK, Burford G, Shein K. WHO global atlas of traditional, complementary and alternative medicine. Geneva, Switzerland: World Health Organization 2005.

[8]   Tugume P, Nyakoojo C. Ethno-pharmacological survey of herbal remedies used in the treatment of paediatric diseases in Buhunga parish, Rukungiri District, Uganda. BMC Complement Altern Med 2019; 19(1): 353-61.
[http://dx.doi.org/10.1186/s12906-019-2763-6] [PMID: 31806007]

[9]   Gupta V, Guleri R, Gupta M, *et al.* Anti-neuroinflammatory potential of *Tylophora indica* (Burm. f) Merrill and development of an efficient *in vitro* propagation system for its clinical use. PLoS One 2020; 15(3): e0230142.
[http://dx.doi.org/10.1371/journal.pone.0230142] [PMID: 32210464]

[10]   Calixto JB. Efficacy, safety, quality control, marketing and regulatory guidelines for herbal medicines (phytotherapeutic agents). Braz J Med Biol Res 2000; 33(2): 179-89.
[http://dx.doi.org/10.1590/S0100-879X2000000200004] [PMID: 10657057]

[11]   Sen S, Chakraborty R. Revival, modernization and integration of Indian traditional herbal medicine in clinical practice: Importance, challenges and future. J Tradit Complement Med 2017; 7(2): 234-44.
[http://dx.doi.org/10.1016/j.jtcme.2016.05.006] [PMID: 28417092]

[12]   Subrat N, Iyer M, Prasad R. The ayurvedic medicine industry: Current status and 574 sustainability. Ecotech Services. New Delhi: International Institute for Environment and 575 Development 2002.

[13]   Kala CP, Dhyani PP, Sajwan BS. Developing the medicinal plants sector in northern India: challenges and opportunities. J Ethnobiol Ethnomed 2006; 2(1): 32.
[http://dx.doi.org/10.1186/1746-4269-2-32]

[14]   Walter KS, Gillett HJ. 1997 IUCN Red List of threatened plants - Gland. Switzerland: IUCN 1998.

[15]   Schippmann U, Leaman DJ, Cunningham AB. Impact of cultivation and gathering of 581 medicinal plants on biodiversity: global trends and issues. Biodiversity and the ecosystem 582 approach in agriculture, forestry and fisheries. Springer 2002.

[16]   Ramachandra Rao S, Ravishankar GA. Plant cell cultures: Chemical factories of secondary metabolites. Biotechnol Adv 2002; 20(2): 101-53.
[http://dx.doi.org/10.1016/S0734-9750(02)00007-1] [PMID: 14538059]

[17]   Debnath M, Malik C, Bisen P. Micropropagation: a tool for the production of high quality plant-based medicines. Curr Pharm Biotechnol 2006; 7(1): 33-49.
[http://dx.doi.org/10.2174/138920106775789638] [PMID: 16472132]

[18]   Hussain MS, Fareed S, Ansari S, Rahman MA, Ahmad IZ, Saeed M. Current approaches toward production of secondary plant metabolites. J Pharm Bioallied Sci 2012; 4(1): 10-20.
[http://dx.doi.org/10.4103/0975-7406.92725] [PMID: 22368394]

[19]   Marchev AS, Yordanova ZP, Georgiev MI. Green (cell) factories for advanced production of plant secondary metabolites. Crit Rev Biotechnol 2020; 40(4): 443-58.
[http://dx.doi.org/10.1080/07388551.2020.1731414] [PMID: 32178548]

[20]   Naoghare PK, Song JM. Chip-based high-throughput screening of herbal medicines. Comb Chem High Throughput Screen 2010; 13(10): 923-31.
[http://dx.doi.org/10.2174/138620710793360338] [PMID: 20883193]

[21]   Jadhav CA, Vikhe DN, Jadhav RS. Global and domestic market of herbal medicines: A review. Research Journal of Science and Technology 2020; 12(4): 327-30.
[http://dx.doi.org/10.5958/2349-2988.2020.00049.2]

[22]   Nirmal SA, Pal SC, Otimenyin SO, *et al.* Contribution of herbal products in global market. Pharm Rev 2013; 3: 95-104.

[23]   Export of Herbs and Herbal Products. Ministry of Commerce and Industry 2019.

[24]   Xu J, Xia Z. Traditional Chinese Medicine (TCM) – Does its contemporary business booming and globalization really reconfirm its medical efficacy & safety? Medicine in Drug Discovery 2019; 1: 100003.
[http://dx.doi.org/10.1016/j.medidd.2019.100003]

[25]   Verpoorte R. Pharmacognosy in the new millennium: leadfinding and biotechnology. J Pharm Pharmacol 2010; 52(3): 253-62.
[http://dx.doi.org/10.1211/0022357001773931] [PMID: 10757412]

[26]   Fabricant DS, Farnsworth NR. The value of plants used in traditional medicine for drug discovery. Environ Health Perspect 2001; 109(Suppl 1) (Suppl. 1): 69-75.
[http://dx.doi.org/10.1289/ehp.01109s169] [PMID: 11250806]

[27]   Cragg GM, Newman DJ. Natural products: A continuing source of novel drug leads. Biochim Biophys Acta, Gen Subj 2013; 1830(6): 3670-95.
[http://dx.doi.org/10.1016/j.bbagen.2013.02.008] [PMID: 23428572]

[28]   Shahzad A, Sharma S, Parveen S, *et al.* Historical perspective and basic principles of plant tissue culture. Plant biotechnology: principles and applications. Springer 2017; pp. 1-36.
[http://dx.doi.org/10.1007/978-981-10-2961-5_1]

[29]   Espinosa-Leal CA, Puente-Garza CA, García-Lara S. *In vitro* plant tissue culture: means for production of biological active compounds. Planta 2018; 248(1): 1-18.
[http://dx.doi.org/10.1007/s00425-018-2910-1] [PMID: 29736623]

[30] Kaur K, Kant U. Clonal propagation of *Acacia catechu* Willd. by shoot tip culture. Plant Growth Regul 2000; 31(3): 143-5.
[http://dx.doi.org/10.1023/A:1006362318265]

[31] Al-Khayri JM, Al-Bahrany AM. *In vitro* micropropagation of *Citrus aurantifolia* (lime). Curr Sci 2001; 81(9): 1242-6.

[32] Ahuja A, Sambyal M, Koul S. *In vitro* propagation and conservation of *Atropa acuminata* Royle ex Lindl - an indigenous threatened medicinal plant. J Plant Biochem Biotechnol 2002; 11(2): 121-4.
[http://dx.doi.org/10.1007/BF03263148]

[33] Faisal M, Ahmad N, Anis M. An efficient micropropagation system for *Tylophora indica*: an endangered, medicinally important plant. Plant Biotechnol Rep 2007; 1(3): 155-61.
[http://dx.doi.org/10.1007/s11816-007-0025-4]

[34] Bopana N, Saxena S. *In vitro* propagation of a high value medicinal plant: *Asparagus racemosus* Willd. *In Vitro* Cell Dev Biol Plant 2008; 44(6): 525-32.
[http://dx.doi.org/10.1007/s11627-008-9137-y]

[35] Grzegorczyk I, Wysokińska H. Liquid shoot culture of *Salvia officinalis* L. for micropropagation and production of antioxidant compounds; effect of triacontanol. Acta Soc Bot Pol 2011; 77(2): 99-104.
[http://dx.doi.org/10.5586/asbp.2008.013]

[36] Subbu RR, Chandraprabha A, Sevugaperumal R. *In vitro* clonal propagation of vulnerable medicinal plant, *Saraca asoca* (Roxb.) De Wilde. Indian J Nat Prod Resour 2008; 7(4): 338-41.

[37] Patidar DK, Tripathi MK, Tiwari R, Baghel BS, Tiwari S. *In vitro* propagation of *Emblica officinalis* from nodal segment culture. Agric Technol Thail 2010; 6(2): 245-56.

[38] Faheem M, Singh S, Tanwer BS, Khan M, Shahzad A. *In vitro* regeneration of multiplication shoots in *Catharanthus roseus* - an important medicinal plant. Adv Appl Sci Res 2011; 2(1): 208-313.

[39] Biswas A, Bari MA, Roy M, Bhadra SK. *In vitro* propagation of *Stemona tuberosa* Lour. -A rare medicinal plant through high frequency shoot multiplication using nodal explants. Plant Tissue Cult Biotechnol 2011; 21(2): 151-9.
[http://dx.doi.org/10.3329/ptcb.v21i2.10238]

[40] Vinothkumar D, Murugavelh S, Senthikumar M. Clonal propagation of *Wattakaka volubilis* through nodal explant culture. Ceylon J Sci Biol Sci 2011; 40(1): 53-8.
[http://dx.doi.org/10.4038/cjsbs.v40i1.3406]

[41] Parmar VR, Jasrai YT. Effect of thidiazuron (TDZ) on *in vitro* propagation of valuable medicinal plant: *Uraria picta* (Jacq.) Desv.ex DC. J Agric Res (Lahore) 2012; 53(4): 513-21.

[42] Pandey A, Brijwal L, Tamta S. *In vitro* propagation and phytochemical assessment of *Berberis chitria*: an important medicinal shrub of Kumaun Himalaya, India. J Med Plants Res 2013; 7(15): 930-7.

[43] Mohanty P, Behera S, Swain SS, Barik DP, Naik SK. Micropropagation of *Hedychium coronarium* J. Koenig through rhizome bud. Physiol Mol Biol Plants 2013; 19(4): 605-10.
[http://dx.doi.org/10.1007/s12298-013-0199-x] [PMID: 24431530]

[44] Lata H, Chandra S, Techen N, Wang YH, Khan IA. Molecular analysis of genetic fidelity in micropropagated plants of *Stevia rebaudiana* Bert. using ISSR marker. Am J Plant Sci 2013; 4(5): 964-71.
[http://dx.doi.org/10.4236/ajps.2013.45119]

[45] Nayak SA, Kumar S, Satapathy K, *et al. In vitro* plant regeneration from cotyledonary nodes of *Withania somnifera* (L.) Dunal and assessment of clonal fidelity using RAPD and ISSR markers. Acta Physiol Plant 2013; 35(1): 195-203.
[http://dx.doi.org/10.1007/s11738-012-1063-2]

[46] Molsaghi M, Moieni A, Kahrizi D. Efficient protocol for rapid *Aloe vera* micropropagation. Pharm Biol 2014; 52(6): 735-9.

[http://dx.doi.org/10.3109/13880209.2013.868494] [PMID: 24405115]

[47]   Mir BA, Mir SA, Koul S. *In vitro* propagation and withaferin A production in *Withania ashwagandha*, a rare medicinal plant of India. Physiol Mol Biol Plants 2014; 20(3): 357-64.
[http://dx.doi.org/10.1007/s12298-014-0243-5] [PMID: 25049463]

[48]   Behera S, Nayak N. An efficient micropropagation protocol of *Bacopa monnieri* (L.) Pennell through two-stage culture of nodal segments and *ex vitro* acclimatization. J Appl Biol Biotechnol 2015; 3(3): 16-21.

[49]   Belwal NS, Kamal B, Sharma V, Gupta S, Kumar Dobriyal A, Jadon VS. Production of genetically uniform plants from shoot tips of *Aconitum heterophyllum* Wall. – a critically endangered medicinal herb. J Hortic Sci Biotechnol 2016; 91(5): 529-35.
[http://dx.doi.org/10.1080/14620316.2016.1184434]

[50]   Autade RH, Fargade SA, Savant AR, Gangurde SS, Choudhary RS, Dighe SS. Micropropagation of Ashwagandha (*Withania somnifera*). Biosci Biotechnol Res Commun 2016; 9(1): 88-93.
[http://dx.doi.org/10.21786/bbrc/19.1/13]

[51]   Armijos-González R, Pérez-Ruiz C. *In vitro* germination and shoot proliferation of the threatened species *Cinchona officinalis* L (Rubiaceae). J For Res 2016; 27(6): 1229-36.
[http://dx.doi.org/10.1007/s11676-016-0272-8]

[52]   Mittal J, Mishra Y, Singh A, Batra A, Sharma MM. An efficient micropropagation of *Tinospora cordifolia* (Willd.) Miers ex Hook F & Thoms: A NMPB prioritized medicinal plant. Int J Biotechnol 2017; 16: 133-7.

[53]   Behera S, Barik DP, Naik SK. Micropropagation of *Symplocos racemosa* Roxb., a threatened medicinal tree of India. Curr Sci 2017; 113(4): 555-8.

[54]   Bhardwaj AK, Singh B, Kaur K, *et al.* In vitro propagation, clonal fidelity and phytochemical analysis of *Rhodiola imbricata* Edgew: a rare trans-Himalayan medicinal plant. Plant Cell Tissue Organ Cult 2018; 135(3): 499-513.
[http://dx.doi.org/10.1007/s11240-018-1482-x]

[55]   Behera S, Kamila PK, Rout KK, Barik DP, Panda PC, Naik SK. An efficient plant regeneration protocol of an industrially important plant, *Hedychium coronarium* J. Koenig and establishment of genetic & biochemical fidelity of the regenerants. Ind Crops Prod 2018; 126: 58-68.
[http://dx.doi.org/10.1016/j.indcrop.2018.09.058]

[56]   Behera S, Kar SK, Rout KK, Barik DP, Panda PC, Naik SK. Assessment of genetic and biochemical fidelity of field-established *Hedychium coronarium* J. Koenig regenerated from axenic cotyledonary node on meta-topolin supplemented medium. Ind Crops Prod 2019; 134: 206-15.
[http://dx.doi.org/10.1016/j.indcrop.2019.03.051]

[57]   Singh M, Chettri A, Pandey A, Sinha S, Singh KK, Badola HK. *In vitro* propagation and phytochemical assessment of *Aconitum ferox* wall: a threatened medicinal plant of Sikkim Himalaya. Proc Natl Acad Sci, India, Sect B Biol Sci 2020; 90(2): 313-21.
[http://dx.doi.org/10.1007/s40011-019-01104-x]

[58]   Nazir R, Gupta S, Dey A, *et al.* In vitro propagation and assessment of genetic fidelity in *Dioscorea deltoidea*, a potent diosgenin yielding endangered plant. S Afr J Bot 2021; 140: 349-55.
[http://dx.doi.org/10.1016/j.sajb.2020.07.018]

[59]   Kaur K, Singh P, Kaur K, Bhandawat A, Nogia P, Pati PK. Development of robust *in vitro* culture protocol for the propagation of genetically and phytochemically stable plants of *Withania somnifera* (L.) Dunal (Ashwagandha). Ind Crops Prod 2021; 166: 113428.
[http://dx.doi.org/10.1016/j.indcrop.2021.113428]

[60]   Al Shhab M, Shatnawi M, Abu-Romman S, Almajdalawi M, Odat N. Micropropagation and *in vitro* conservation of *Ruta graveolens* plants. Res Crops 2021; 22(2): 18-23.

[61]   Behera S, Monalisa K, Meher RK, *et al.* Phytochemical fidelity and therapeutic activity of

micropropagated *Curcuma amada* Roxb.: A valuable medicinal herb. Ind Crops Prod 2022; 176: 114401.
[http://dx.doi.org/10.1016/j.indcrop.2021.114401]

[62]   Hou J, Su P, Wang D, Chen X, Zhao W, Wu L. Efficient plant regeneration from *in vitro* leaves and petioles *via* shoot organogenesis in *Sapium sebiferum* Roxb. Plant Cell Tissue Organ Cult 2020; 142(1): 143-56.
[http://dx.doi.org/10.1007/s11240-020-01848-9]

[63]   Monthony AS, Page SR, Hesami M, Jones AMP. The past, present and future of *Cannabis sativa* tissue culture. Plants 2021; 10(1): 185-92.
[http://dx.doi.org/10.3390/plants10010185] [PMID: 33478171]

[64]   Acheampong S, Galyuon IK, Asare AT. Effects of sterilization protocols, benzylaminopurine and type of explants on growth initiation of pineapple [*Ananas comosus* (L.) Merr.] cultures. J Basic Appl Sci 2015; 1(3): 50-65.

[65]   Abbasi Z. A novel aseptic technique for micropropagation of *Aloe vera* mill. Adv Herb Med 2017; 3(3): 47-60.

[66]   Kaur K, Dolker D, Behera S, Pati PK. Critical factors influencing *in vitro* propagation and modulation of important secondary metabolites in *Withania somnifera* (L.) dunal. Plant Cell Tissue Organ Cult 2022; 149(1-2): 41-60.
[http://dx.doi.org/10.1007/s11240-021-02225-w] [PMID: 35039702]

[67]   Ray S, Jha S. Production of withaferin A in shoot cultures of *Withania somnifera*. Planta Med 2001; 67(5): 432-6.
[http://dx.doi.org/10.1055/s-2001-15811] [PMID: 11488457]

[68]   Sivanandhan G, Mariashibu TS, Arun M, *et al.* The effect of polyamines on the efficiency of multiplication and rooting of *Withania somnifera* (L.) Dunal and content of some withanolides in obtained plants. Acta Physiol Plant 2011; 33(6): 2279-88.
[http://dx.doi.org/10.1007/s11738-011-0768-y]

[69]   Sivanandhan G, Selvaraj N, Ganapathi A, Manickavasagam M. Enhanced biosynthesis of withanolides by elicitation and precursor feeding in cell suspension culture of *Withania somnifera* (L.) Dunal in shake-flask culture and bioreactor. PLoS One 2014; 9(8): e104005.
[http://dx.doi.org/10.1371/journal.pone.0104005] [PMID: 25089711]

[70]   Saritha KV, Naidu CV. *In vitro* flowering of *Withania somnifera* Dunal. An important antitumor medicinal plant. Plant Sci 2007; 172(4): 847-51.
[http://dx.doi.org/10.1016/j.plantsci.2006.12.016]

[71]   Behera B, Behera S, Jena PK, Barik DP, Naik SK. Adventitious shoot organogenesis and plant regeneration from internode explants of *Paederia foetida* L.: a valuable medicinal plant. Biosci Biotechnol Res Asia 2017; 14(3): 893-900.
[http://dx.doi.org/10.13005/bbra/2523]

[72]   Kumar Bhardwaj A, Naryal A, Bhardwaj P, *et al.* High efficiency *in vitro* plant regeneration and secondary metabolite quantification from leaf explants of *Rhodiola imbricata*. Pharmacogn J 2018; 10(3): 470-5.
[http://dx.doi.org/10.5530/pj.2018.3.77]

[73]   Kaur K, Kaur K, Bhandawat A, Pati PK. *In vitro* shoot multiplication using *meta*-Topolin and leaf-based regeneration of a withaferin A rich accession of *Withania somnifera* (L.) Dunal. Ind Crops Prod 2021; 171: 113872.
[http://dx.doi.org/10.1016/j.indcrop.2021.113872]

[74]   Sivanesan I, Murugesan K. An efficient regeneration from nodal explants of *Withania somnifera* Dunal. Asian J Plant Sci 2008; 7(6): 551-6.
[http://dx.doi.org/10.3923/ajps.2008.551.556]

[75]   Kumar Kar D, Sen S. Propagation of *Asparagus racemosus* through tissue culture. Plant Cell Tissue Organ Cult 1985; 5(1): 89-95.
[http://dx.doi.org/10.1007/BF00033574]

[76]   Roy SC, Sarkar A. *In vitro* regeneration and micropropagation of *Aloe vera* L. Sci Hortic (Amsterdam) 1991; 47(1-2): 107-13.
[http://dx.doi.org/10.1016/0304-4238(91)90032-T]

[77]   Giri A, Ahuja PS, Ajay Kumar PV. Somatic embryogenesis and plant regeneration from callus cultures of *Aconitum heterophyllum* Wall. Plant Cell Tissue Organ Cult 1993; 32(2): 213-8.
[http://dx.doi.org/10.1007/BF00029845]

[78]   Thakur M, Sharma DR, Kanwar K, Kant A. *In vitro* regeneration of *Acacia catechu* Willd. from callus and mature nodal explants--an improved method. Indian J Exp Biol 2002; 40(7): 850-3.
[PMID: 12597559]

[79]   Tawfik AA, Mohamed MF. Regeneration of salvia (*Salvia officinalis* L.) *via* induction of meristematic callus. *In Vitro* Cell Deve. Biol Plant 2007; 43(1): 21-7.

[80]   Dhandapani M, Kim DH, Hong SB. Efficient plant regeneration *via* somatic embryogenesis and organogenesis from the explants of *Catharanthus roseus*. *In Vitro* Cell Dev Biol Plant 2008; 44(1): 18-25.
[http://dx.doi.org/10.1007/s11627-007-9094-x]

[81]   Aasim M, Khawar KM, Özcan S. *In vitro* regeneration of red squill *Urginea maritima* (L.) Baker. using thidiazuron. Biotechnol Biotechnol Equip 2008; 22(4): 925-8.
[http://dx.doi.org/10.1080/13102818.2008.10817580]

[82]   Gour VS, Kant T. *In vitro* regeneration in *Emblica officinalis* from juvenile root-derived callus. J Indian Bot Soc 2010; 89: 34-6.

[83]   Paul KK, Bari MA. *In vitro* multiple shoot regeneration from corm bud explant in ghet kachu, *Typhonium trilobatum* schott - a medicinal aroid. Bangladesh J Sci Ind Res 2012; 47(2): 211-6.
[http://dx.doi.org/10.3329/bjsir.v47i2.11454]

[84]   Wee SL, Alderson PG, Yap WSP. Establishment of plantlet regeneration system from nodal, internodal and leaf explants of *Sauropus androgynus* (Sweet Shoot). Asian Journal of Biotechnology 2015; 7(2): 46-59.
[http://dx.doi.org/10.3923/ajbkr.2015.46.59]

[85]   Brijwal L, Pandey A, Tamta S. *In vitro* propagation of the endangered species *Berberis aristata* DC. *via* leaf-derived callus. *In Vitro* Cell Dev Biol Plant 2015; 51(6): 637-47.
[http://dx.doi.org/10.1007/s11627-015-9716-7]

[86]   Gondvai M, Chaturvedi P, Gaur AK. Thidiazuron induced high frequency establishment of callus cultures and plantlet regeneration in *Acontium balfourii* Stapf.: an endangered medicinal herb of North-West Himalayas. Indian J Biotechnol 2016; 15: 251-5.

[87]   Rohela GK, Jogam P, Bylla P, Reuben C. Indirect regeneration and assessment of genetic fidelity of acclimated plantlets by SCoT, ISSR, and RAPD markers in *Rauwolfia tetraphylla* L.: an endangered medicinal plant. BioMed Res Int 2019; 2019: 1-14.
[http://dx.doi.org/10.1155/2019/3698742] [PMID: 31111050]

[88]   Hussain A, Qarshi IA, Nazir H, Ullah I. Plant tissue culture: current status and 763 opportunities. Recent Adv Plant *In Vitro* Cult 2012; 1-28.
[http://dx.doi.org/10.5772/50568]

[89]   Pati PK, Kaur J, Singh P. A liquid culture system for shoot proliferation and analysis of pharmaceutically active constituents of *Catharanthus roseus* (L.) G. Don. Plant Cell Tissue Organ Cult 2011; 105(3): 299-307.
[http://dx.doi.org/10.1007/s11240-010-9868-4]

[90] Sivanesan I, Park SW. Optimizing factors affecting adventitious shoot regeneration, *in vitro* flowering and fruiting of *Withania somnifera* (L.) Dunal. Ind Crops Prod 2015; 76: 323-8.
[http://dx.doi.org/10.1016/j.indcrop.2015.05.014]

[91] Berthouly M, Etienne H. Temporary immersion system: a new concept for use liquid medium in mass propagation. Liquid culture systems for in vitro plant propagation. Springer 2005; pp. 165-95.
[http://dx.doi.org/10.1007/1-4020-3200-5_11]

[92] Malik S, Bhushan S, Sharma M, Ahuja PS. Biotechnological approaches to the production of shikonins: a critical review with recent updates. Crit Rev Biotechnol 2016; 36(2): 327-40.
[http://dx.doi.org/10.3109/07388551.2014.961003] [PMID: 25319455]

[93] Vaidya BN, Asanakunov B, Shahin L, Jernigan HL, Joshee N, Dhekney SA. Improving micropropagation of Mentha × piperita L. using a liquid culture system. *In Vitro* Cell Dev Biol Plant 2019; 55(1): 71-80.
[http://dx.doi.org/10.1007/s11627-018-09952-4]

[94] Bhagwat B, Vieiral LGF, Erickson LR. Stimulation of *in vitro* shoot proliferation from nodal explants of Cassava by thidiazuron, benzyladenine and gibberellic acid. Plant Cell Tissue Organ Cult 1996; 46(1): 1-7.
[http://dx.doi.org/10.1007/BF00039690]

[95] Sujatha M, Reddy TP. Differential cytokinin effects on the stimulation of *in vitro* shoot proliferation from meristematic explants of castor (*Ricinus communis* L.). Plant Cell Rep 1998; 17(6-7): 561-6.
[http://dx.doi.org/10.1007/s002990050442] [PMID: 30736636]

[96] Nandagopal S, Ranjitha Kumari BD. Adenine sulphate induced high frequency shoot organogenesis in callus and *in vitro* flowering of *Cichorium intybus* L. cv. Focus-a potent medicinal plant. Acta Agric Slov 2006; 87(2): 415-25.

[97] Siwach P, Gill AR. Enhanced shoot multiplication in *Ficus religiosa* L. in the presence of adenine sulphate, glutamine and phloroglucinol. Physiol Mol Biol Plants 2011; 17(3): 271-80.
[http://dx.doi.org/10.1007/s12298-011-0074-6] [PMID: 23573019]

[98] Barathkumar TR. Studies on influence of different seed treatments on dormancy 790 breaking in aonla (*Phyllanthus emblica* L.). J Pharm Phytochem SP2 131-3.2019;

[99] Antony Ceasar S, Lenin Maxwell S, Bhargav Prasad K, Karthigan M, Ignacimuthu S. Highly efficient shoot regeneration of *Bacopa monnieri* (L.) using a two-stage culture procedure and assessment of genetic integrity of micropropagated plants by RAPD. Acta Physiol Plant 2010; 32(3): 443-52.
[http://dx.doi.org/10.1007/s11738-009-0419-8]

[100] Ferrari MP, Antoniazzi D, Nascimento AB, Franz LF, Bezerra CS, Magalhaes HM. Evaluation of new protocol for *Curcuma longa* micropropagation: a medicinal and ornamental specie. J Med Plants Res 2016; 10(25): 67-376.

[101] Hassan AKMS, Roy SK. Micropropagation of *Gloriosa superba* L. through high frequency shoot proliferation. Plant Tissue Cult 2005; 15(1): 67-74.

[102] Komalavalli N, Rao MV. *In vitro* micropropagation of *Gymnema sylvestre* - a multipurpose medicinal plant. Plant Cell Tissue Organ Cult 2000; 61(2): 97-105.
[http://dx.doi.org/10.1023/A:1006421228598]

[103] Venkatachalam P, Jinu U, Gomathi M, *et al.* Role of silver nitrate in plant regeneration from cotyledonary nodal segment explants of *Prosopis cineraria* (L.) Druce.: A recalcitrant medicinal leguminous tree. Biocatal Agric Biotechnol 2017; 12: 286-91.
[http://dx.doi.org/10.1016/j.bcab.2017.10.017]

[104] Sarropoulou V, Dimassi-Theriou K, Therios I. Effect of the ethylene inhibitors silver nitrate, silver sulfate, and cobaltchloride on micropropagation and biochemical parameters in the cherryrootstocks CAB-6P and Gisela 6. Turk J Biol 2016; 40: 670-83.
[http://dx.doi.org/10.3906/biy-1505-92]

[105] Steephen M, Nagarajan S, Ganesh D. Phloroglucinol and silver nitrate enhances axillary shoot proliferation in nodal explants of *Vitex negundo* L. - an aromatic medicinal plant. Iran J Biotechnol 2010; 8(2): 82-9.

[106] Jain R, Sinha A, Kachhwaha S, Kothari SL. Micropropagation of *Withania coagulans* (Stocks) Dunal: a critically endangered medicinal herb. J Plant Biochem Biotechnol 2009; 18(2): 249-52.
[http://dx.doi.org/10.1007/BF03263330]

[107] Kumar V, Parvatam G, Ravishankar GA. AgNO₃ - a potential regulator of ethylene activity and plant growth modulator. Electron J Biotechnol 2009; 12(2): 0.
[http://dx.doi.org/10.2225/vol12-issue2-fulltext-1]

[108] Teixeira da Silva JA, Dobránszki J, Ross S. Phloroglucinol in plant tissue culture. *In Vitro* Cell Dev Biol Plant 2013; 49(1): 1-16.
[http://dx.doi.org/10.1007/s11627-013-9491-2]

[109] Thomas TD. The role of activated charcoal in plant tissue culture. Biotechnol Adv 2008; 26(6): 618-31.
[http://dx.doi.org/10.1016/j.biotechadv.2008.08.003] [PMID: 18786626]

[110] Velcheva M, Faltin Z, Vardi A, Eshdat Y, Perl A. Regeneration of *Aloe arborescensvia* somatic organogenesis from young inflorescences. Plant Cell Tissue Organ Cult 2005; 83(3): 293-301.
[http://dx.doi.org/10.1007/s11240-005-7192-1]

[111] Debiasi C, Silva CG, Pescador R. Micropropagação de babosa (*Aloe vera* L.). Rev Bras Plantas Med 2007; 9(1): 36-43.

[112] Aina O, Quesenberry K, Gallo M. Thidiazuron-induced tissue culture regeneration from quartered-seed explants of *Arachis paraguariensis*. Crop Sci 2012; 52(3): 1076-83.
[http://dx.doi.org/10.2135/cropsci2011.07.0367]

[113] Rana KL, Kour D, Kaur T, *et al.* Endophytic microbes: biodiversity, plant growth-promoting mechanisms and potential applications for agricultural sustainability. Antonie van Leeuwenhoek 2020; 113(8): 1075-107.
[http://dx.doi.org/10.1007/s10482-020-01429-y] [PMID: 32488494]

[114] Simonović ADM, M Trifunović-Momčilov M, Filipović BK, Marković MP, Bogdanović MD, Subotić AR. Somatic Embryogenesis in *Centaurium erythraea* Rafn- current status and perspectives: a review. Plants 2020; 10(1): 70-8.
[http://dx.doi.org/10.3390/plants10010070] [PMID: 33396285]

[115] Isah T. Induction of somatic embryogenesis in woody plants. Acta Physiol Plant 2016; 38(5): 118.
[http://dx.doi.org/10.1007/s11738-016-2134-6]

[116] Chitra Devi B, Narmathabai V. Somatic embryogenesis in the medicinal legume *Desmodium motorium* (Houtt.) Merr. Plant Cell Tissue Organ Cult 2011; 106(3): 409-18.
[http://dx.doi.org/10.1007/s11240-011-9937-3]

[117] Rani G, Virk GS, Nagpal A. Somatic embryogenesis in *Withania somnifera* (L.) Dunal. J Plant Biotechnol 2012; 6(2): 113-8.

[118] Baskaran P, Van Staden J. Somatic embryogenesis of *Merwilla plumbea* (Lindl.) Speta. Plant Cell Tissue Organ Cult 2012; 109(3): 517-24.
[http://dx.doi.org/10.1007/s11240-012-0118-9]

[119] Sharmin SA, Alam MJ, Sheikh MMI, *et al.* Somatic embryogenesis and plant regeneration in *Wedelia calendulacea* Less. an endangered medicinal plant. Braz Arch Biol Technol 2014; 57(3): 394-401.
[http://dx.doi.org/10.1590/S1516-8913201401840]

[120] Soundar Raju C, Aslam A, Shajahan A. High-efficiency direct somatic embryogenesis and plant regeneration from leaf base explants of turmeric (*Curcuma longa* L.). Plant Cell Tissue Organ Cult 2015; 122(1): 79-87.

[http://dx.doi.org/10.1007/s11240-015-0751-1]

[121] Haque SM, Ghosh B. High-frequency somatic embryogenesis and artificial seeds for mass production of true-to-type plants in *Ledebouria revoluta*: an important cardioprotective plant. Plant Cell Tissue Organ Cult 2016; 127(1): 71-83.
[http://dx.doi.org/10.1007/s11240-016-1030-5]

[122] Khilwani B, Kaur A, Ranjan R, Kumar A. Direct somatic embryogenesis and encapsulation of somatic embryos for *in vitro* conservation of *Bacopa monnieri* (L.) Wettst. Plant Cell Tissue Organ Cult 2016; 127(2): 433-42.
[http://dx.doi.org/10.1007/s11240-016-1067-5]

[123] Abbasi BH, Ali H, Yücesan B, Saeed S, Rehman K, Khan MA. Evaluation of biochemical markers during somatic embryogenesis in *Silybum marianum* L. 3 Biotech 2016; 6(1): 71.
[http://dx.doi.org/10.1007/s13205-016-0366-1]

[124] Kumar V, Moyo M, Van Staden J. Somatic embryogenesis in *Hypoxis hemerocallidea*: An important African medicinal plant. S Afr J Bot 2017; 108: 331-6.
[http://dx.doi.org/10.1016/j.sajb.2016.08.012]

[125] Chen CC, Agrawal DC, Lee MR, *et al.* Influence of LED light spectra on *in vitro* somatic embryogenesis and LC–MS analysis of chlorogenic acid and rutin in *Peucedanum japonicum* Thunb.: a medicinal herb. Bot Stud (Taipei, Taiwan) 2016; 57(1): 9.
[http://dx.doi.org/10.1186/s40529-016-0124-z] [PMID: 28597418]

[126] Rukh G, Ahmad N, Rab A, *et al.* Photo-dependent somatic embryogenesis from non-embryogenic calli and its polyphenolics content in high-valued medicinal plant of *Ajuga bracteosa*. J Photochem Photobiol B 2019; 190: 59-65.
[http://dx.doi.org/10.1016/j.jphotobiol.2018.11.012] [PMID: 30500677]

[127] Ibrahim AS, Fahmy AH, Ahmed SS. Copper nanoparticles elevate regeneration capacity of (*Ocimum basilicum* L.) plant *via* somatic embryogenesis. Plant Cell Tissue Organ Cult 2019; 136(1): 41-50.
[http://dx.doi.org/10.1007/s11240-018-1489-3]

[128] Bertero VG, Beznec A, Faccio P, *et al.* High-efficiency direct somatic embryogenesis and plant regeneration from leaf base explants of "peperina" (*Minthostachys verticillata*). In Vitro Cell Dev Biol Plant 2020; 56(6): 915-9.
[http://dx.doi.org/10.1007/s11627-020-10098-5]

[129] Phillips GC. *In vitro* morphogenesis in plants-recent advances. In Vitro Cell Dev Biol Plant 2004; 40(4): 342-5.
[http://dx.doi.org/10.1079/IVP2004555]

[130] Guan Y, Li SG, Fan XF, Su ZH. Application of somatic embryogenesis in woody plants. Front Plant Sci 2016; 7: 938.
[http://dx.doi.org/10.3389/fpls.2016.00938] [PMID: 27446166]

[131] asayesh ZM, Vahdati K, Aliniaeifard S. Investigation of physiological components involved in low water conservation capacity of *in vitro* walnut plants. Sci Hortic (Amsterdam) 2017; 224: 1-7.
[http://dx.doi.org/10.1016/j.scienta.2017.04.023]

[132] Kumar K, Rao IU. Morphophysiologicals problems in acclimatization of micropropagated plants in *ex vitro* conditions- a review. J Ornam Hortic Plant 2012; 2(4): 271-83.

[133] John Tam WH, Constabel F, Kurz WGW. Codeine from cell suspension cultures of *Papaver somniferum*. Phytochemistry 1980; 19(3): 486-7.
[http://dx.doi.org/10.1016/0031-9422(80)83215-8]

[134] Tsutomu N, Hitoshi M, Masao N, Hideko H, Kaisuke Y. Production of cryptotanshinone and ferruginol in cultured cells of *Salvia miltiorrhiza*. Phytochemistry 1983; 22(3): 721-2.
[http://dx.doi.org/10.1016/S0031-9422(00)86969-1]

[135] Tal B, Rokem JS, Gressel J, Goldberg I. The effect of chlorophyll-bleaching herbicides on growth,

carotenoid and diosgenin levels in cell suspension cultures of *Dioscorea deltoidea*. Phytochemistry 1984; 23(6): 1333-5.
[http://dx.doi.org/10.1016/S0031-9422(00)80456-2]

[136]   Rueffer M. The production of isoquinoline alkaloids by plant cell cultures. In: Phillipson JD, Roberts MF, Zenk LH, Eds. The chemistry and biology of isoquinoline alkaloids. Berlin: Springer 1985; pp. 265-80.
[http://dx.doi.org/10.1007/978-3-642-70128-3_18]

[137]   Crespi-Perellino N, Guicciardi A, Malyszko G, Arlandini E, Ballabio M, Minghetti A. Occurrence of indole alkaloids in *Ailanthus altissima* cell cultures. J Nat Prod 1986; 49(6): 1010-4.
[http://dx.doi.org/10.1021/np50048a007]

[138]   Scragg AH, Allan EJ. Production of the triterpenoid quassin in callus and cell suspension cultures of *Picrasma quassioides* Bennett. Plant Cell Rep 1986; 5(5): 356-9.
[http://dx.doi.org/10.1007/BF00268601] [PMID: 24248298]

[139]   Yamamoto O, Yamada Y. Production of reserpine and its optimization in cultured *Rauwolfia serpentina* Benth. cells. Plant Cell Rep 1986; 5(1): 50-3.
[http://dx.doi.org/10.1007/BF00269717] [PMID: 24247966]

[140]   Endo T, Goodbody A, Vukovic J, Misawa M. Biotransformation of anhydrovinblastine to vinblastine by a cell-free extract of *Catharanthus roseus* cell suspension cultures. Phytochemistry 1987; 26(12): 3233-4.
[http://dx.doi.org/10.1016/S0031-9422(00)82476-0]

[141]   Hara Y, Yoshioka T, Morimoto T, Fujita Y, Yamada Y. Enhancement of berberine production in suspension cultures of *Coptis japonica* by gibberellic acid treatment. J Plant Physiol 1988; 133(1): 12-5.
[http://dx.doi.org/10.1016/S0176-1617(88)80077-4]

[142]   Orihara Y, Furuya T. Production of theanine and other? -glutamyl derivatives by *Camellia sinensis* cultured cells. Plant Cell Rep 1990; 9(2): 65-8.
[http://dx.doi.org/10.1007/BF00231550] [PMID: 24226431]

[143]   Jha S, Sahu NP, Sen J, Jha TB, Mahato SB. Production of emetine and cephaeline from cell suspension and excised root cultures of *Cephaelis ipecacuanha*. Phytochemistry 1991; 30(12): 3999-4003.
[http://dx.doi.org/10.1016/0031-9422(91)83452-Q]

[144]   Kreis W, Reinhard E. 12β-Hydroxylation of digitoxin by suspension-cultured *Digitalis lanata* cells: Production of digoxin in 20-litre and 300-litre air-lift bioreactors. J Biotechnol 1992; 26(2-3): 257-73.
[http://dx.doi.org/10.1016/0168-1656(92)90011-W] [PMID: 1369154]

[145]   Ishimaru K, Arakawa H, Neera S. Polyphenol production in cell cultures of *Cornus kousa*. Phytochemistry 1993; 32(5): 1193-7.
[http://dx.doi.org/10.1016/S0031-9422(00)95090-8]

[146]   Pras N, Woerdenbag HJ, Batterman S, Visser JF, Uden W. *Mucuna pruriens*: Improvement of the biotechnological production of the anti-Parkinson drug L-dopa by plant cell selection. Pharm World Sci 1993; 15(6): 263-8.
[http://dx.doi.org/10.1007/BF01871128] [PMID: 8298586]

[147]   Zhong JJ, Bai Y, Wang SJ. Effects of plant growth regulators on cell growth and ginsenoside saponin production by suspension cultures of *Panax quinquefolium*. J Biotechnol 1996; 45(3): 227-34.
[http://dx.doi.org/10.1016/0168-1656(95)00170-0]

[148]   Archambault J, Williams RD, Bédard C, Chavarie C. Production of sanguinarine by elicited plant cell culture I. Shake flask suspension cultures. J Biotechnol 1996; 46(2): 95-105.
[http://dx.doi.org/10.1016/0168-1656(95)00184-0]

[149]   Chen H, Yuan JP, Chen F, Zhang YL, Jing-Yuan Song . Tanshinone production in Ti-transformed

Salvia miltiorrhiza cell suspension cultures. J Biotechnol 1997; 58(3): 147-56.
[http://dx.doi.org/10.1016/S0168-1656(97)00144-2] [PMID: 9470220]

[150]　Aburjai T, Bernasconi S, Manzocchi LA, Pelizzoni F. Effect of calcium and cell immobilization on the production of choleocalciferol and its derivatives by *Solanum malacoxylon* cell cultures. Phytochemistry 1997; 46(6): 1015-8.
[http://dx.doi.org/10.1016/S0031-9422(97)00408-1]

[151]　Kitamura Y, Ikenaga T, Ooe Y, Hiraoka N, Mizukami H. Induction of furanocoumarin biosynthesis in *Glehnia littoralis* cell suspension cultures by elicitor treatment. Phytochemistry 1998; 48(1): 113-7.
[http://dx.doi.org/10.1016/S0031-9422(97)00849-2] [PMID: 9621456]

[152]　Jang YP, Lee YJ, Kim YC, Huh H. Production of a hepatoprotective cerebroside from suspension cultures of *Lycium chinense.* Plant Cell Rep 1998; 18(3-4): 252-4.
[http://dx.doi.org/10.1007/s002990050566] [PMID: 30744230]

[153]　Schripsema J, Ramos-Valdivia A, Verpoorte R. Robustaquinones, novel anthraquinones from an elicited *Cinchona robusta* suspension culture. Phytochemistry 1999; 51(1): 55-60.
[http://dx.doi.org/10.1016/S0031-9422(98)00470-1]

[154]　Mukherjee S, Ghosh B, Jha S. Establishment of forskolin yielding transformed cell suspension cultures of *Coleus forskohlii* as controlled by different factors. J Biotechnol 2000; 76(1): 73-81.
[http://dx.doi.org/10.1016/S0168-1656(99)00181-9] [PMID: 10784298]

[155]　Yamamoto H, Yazaki K, Inoue K. Simultaneous analysis of shikimate-derived secondary metabolites in *Lithospermum erythrorhizon* cell suspension cultures by high-performance liquid chromatography. J Chromatogr, Biomed Appl 2000; 738(1): 3-15.
[http://dx.doi.org/10.1016/S0378-4347(99)00473-9] [PMID: 10778921]

[156]　Huang FC, Kutchan TM. Distribution of morphinan and benzo[c]phenanthridine alkaloid gene transcript accumulation in *Papaver somniferum.* Phytochemistry 2000; 53(5): 555-64.
[http://dx.doi.org/10.1016/S0031-9422(99)00600-7] [PMID: 10724180]

[157]　Saad I, Díaz E, Chávez I, Reyes-Chilpa R, Rubluo A, Jiménez-Estrada M. Antifungal monoterpene production in elicited cell suspension cultures of *Piqueria trinervia.* Phytochemistry 2000; 55(1): 51-7.
[http://dx.doi.org/10.1016/S0031-9422(00)00211-9] [PMID: 11021644]

[158]　Pan ZW, Wang HQ, Zhong JJ. Scale-up study on suspension cultures of *Taxus chinensis* cells for production of taxane diterpene. Enzyme Microb Technol 2000; 27(9): 714-23.
[http://dx.doi.org/10.1016/S0141-0229(00)00276-3] [PMID: 11064055]

[159]　Rahman LU, Verma PC, Singh D, Gupta MM, Banerjee S. Bacoside production by suspension cultures of *Bacopa monnieri* (L.) Pennell. Biotechnol Lett 2002; 24(17): 1427-9.
[http://dx.doi.org/10.1023/A:1019815018436]

[160]　ten Hoopen HJG, Vinke JL, Moreno PRH, Verpoorte R, Heijnen JJ. Influence of temperature on growth and ajmalicine production by *Catharantus roseus* suspension cultures. Enzyme Microb Technol 2002; 30(1): 56-65.
[http://dx.doi.org/10.1016/S0141-0229(01)00456-2]

[161]　Walker T, Pal Bais H, Vivanco JM. Jasmonic acid-induced hypericin production in cell suspension cultures of *Hypericum perforatum* L. (St. John's wort). Phytochemistry 2002; 60(3): 289-93.
[http://dx.doi.org/10.1016/S0031-9422(02)00074-2] [PMID: 12031448]

[162]　Chattopadhyay S, Srivastava AK, Bhojwani SS, Bisaria VS. Production of podophyllotoxin by plant cell cultures of *Podophyllum hexandrum* in bioreactor. J Biosci Bioeng 2002; 93(2): 215-20.
[http://dx.doi.org/10.1016/S1389-1723(02)80017-2] [PMID: 16233190]

[163]　Staniszewska I, Królicka A, Maliński E, Łojkowska E, Szafranek J. Elicitation of secondary metabolites in *in vitro* cultures of *Ammi majus* L. Enzyme Microb Technol 2003; 33(5): 565-8.
[http://dx.doi.org/10.1016/S0141-0229(03)00180-7]

[164]　Sudha G, Ravishankar GA. Putrescine facilitated enhancement of capsaicin production in cell

suspension cultures of *Capsicum frutescens*. J Plant Physiol 2003; 160(4): 339-46.
[http://dx.doi.org/10.1078/0176-1617-00928] [PMID: 12756913]

[165] Chen S, Wang X, Zhao B, Yuan X, Wang Y. Production of crocin using *Crocus sativus* callus by two-stage culture system. Biotechnol Lett 2003; 25(15): 1235-8.
[http://dx.doi.org/10.1023/A:1025036729160] [PMID: 14514073]

[166] Komaraiah P, Ramakrishna SV, Reddanna P, Kavi Kishor PB. Enhanced production of plumbagin in immobilized cells of *Plumbago rosea* by elicitation and *in situ* adsorption. J Biotechnol 2003; 101(2): 181-7.
[http://dx.doi.org/10.1016/S0168-1656(02)00338-3] [PMID: 12568747]

[167] Wang J, Liao X, Zhang H, Du J, Chen P. Accumulation of chlorogenic acid in cell suspension cultures of *Eucommia ulmoides*. Plant Cell Tissue Organ Cult 2003; 74(2): 193-5.
[http://dx.doi.org/10.1023/A:1023957129569]

[168] Zhao P, Iwamoto Y, Kouno I, Egami Y, Yamamoto H. Stimulating the production of homoisoflavonoids in cell suspension cultures of *Caesalpinia pulcherrima* using cork tissue. Phytochemistry 2004; 65(17): 2455-61.
[http://dx.doi.org/10.1016/j.phytochem.2004.08.004] [PMID: 15381409]

[169] Wang JW, Xia ZH, Chu JH, Tan RX. Simultaneous production of anthocyanin and triterpenoids in suspension cultures of *Perilla frutescens*. Enzyme Microb Technol 2004; 34(7): 651-6.
[http://dx.doi.org/10.1016/j.enzmictec.2004.02.004]

[170] Zhao DX, Fu CX, Han YS, Lu DP. Effects of elicitation on jaceosidin and hispidulin production in cell suspension cultures of *Saussurea medusa*. Process Biochem 2005; 40(2): 739-45.
[http://dx.doi.org/10.1016/j.procbio.2004.01.040]

[171] Sánchez-Sampedro MA, Fernández-Tárrago J, Corchete P. Yeast extract and methyl jasmonate-induced silymarin production in cell cultures of *Silybum marianum* (L.) Gaertn. J Biotechnol 2005; 119(1): 60-9.
[http://dx.doi.org/10.1016/j.jbiotec.2005.06.012] [PMID: 16054261]

[172] Pasqua G, Silvestrini A, Monacelli B, Mulinacci N, Menendez P, Botta B. Triterpenoids and ellagic acid derivatives from *in vitro* cultures of *Camptotheca acuminata* Decaisne. Plant Physiol Biochem 2006; 44(4): 220-5.
[http://dx.doi.org/10.1016/j.plaphy.2006.04.001] [PMID: 16762560]

[173] De-Eknamkul W, Ellis B. Rosmarinic acid production and growth characteristics of *Anchusa officinalis* cell suspension cultures. Planta Med 1984; 50(4): 346-50.
[http://dx.doi.org/10.1055/s-2007-969728] [PMID: 6505088]

[174] Liu JY, Guo ZG, Zeng ZL. Improved accumulation of phenylethanoid glycosides by precursor feeding to suspension culture of *Cistanche salsa*. Biochem Eng J 2007; 33(1): 88-93.
[http://dx.doi.org/10.1016/j.bej.2006.09.002]

[175] Chiang L, Abdullah MA. Enhanced anthraquinones production from adsorbent-treated *Morinda elliptica* cell suspension cultures in production medium strategy. Process Biochem 2007; 42(5): 757-63.
[http://dx.doi.org/10.1016/j.procbio.2007.01.005]

[176] Baldi A, Dixit VK. Yield enhancement strategies for artemisinin production by suspension cultures of *Artemisia annua*. Bioresour Technol 2008; 99(11): 4609-14.
[http://dx.doi.org/10.1016/j.biortech.2007.06.061] [PMID: 17804216]

[177] Pawar KD, Thengane SR. Influence of hormones and medium components on expression of dipyranocoumarins in cell suspension cultures of *Calophyllum inophyllum* L. Process Biochem 2009; 44(8): 916-22.
[http://dx.doi.org/10.1016/j.procbio.2009.03.005]

[178] Kang SM, Min JY, Kim YD, *et al.* Effect of biotic elicitors on the accumulation of bilobalide and

ginkgolides in *Ginkgo biloba* cell cultures. J Biotechnol 2009; 139(1): 84-8.
[http://dx.doi.org/10.1016/j.jbiotec.2008.09.007] [PMID: 18983879]

[179] Shinde AN, Malpathak N, Fulzele DP. Studied enhancement strategies for phytoestrogens production in shake flasks by suspension culture of *Psoralea corylifolia.* Bioresour Technol 2009; 100(5): 1833-9.
[http://dx.doi.org/10.1016/j.biortech.2008.09.028] [PMID: 19013062]

[180] Ho H, Liang K, Lin W, Kitanaka S, Wu J. Regulation and improvement of triterpene formation in plant cultured cells of *Eriobotrya japonica* Lindl. J Biosci Bioeng 2010; 110(5): 588-92.
[http://dx.doi.org/10.1016/j.jbiosc.2010.06.009] [PMID: 20656553]

[181] Nagella P, Murthy HN. Establishment of cell suspension cultures of *Withania somnifera* for the production of withanolide A. Bioresour Technol 2010; 101(17): 6735-9.
[http://dx.doi.org/10.1016/j.biortech.2010.03.078] [PMID: 20371175]

[182] Xu XH, Zhang W, Cao XP, Xue S. Abietane diterpenoids synthesized by suspension-cultured cells of *Cephalotaxus fortunei.* Phytochem Lett 2011; 4(1): 52-5.
[http://dx.doi.org/10.1016/j.phytol.2010.12.003]

[183] Praveen N, Murthy HN, Chung IM. Improvement of growth and gymnemic acid production by altering the macro elements concentration and nitrogen source supply in cell suspension cultures of *Gymnema sylvestre* R. Br. Ind Crops Prod 2011; 33(2): 282-6.
[http://dx.doi.org/10.1016/j.indcrop.2010.12.015]

[184] Yue X, Zhang W, Deng M. Hyper-production of 13C-labeled trans-resveratrol in *Vitis vinifera* suspension cell culture by elicitation and *in situ* adsorption. Biochem Eng J 2011; 53(3): 292-6.
[http://dx.doi.org/10.1016/j.bej.2010.12.002]

[185] Nagella P, Murthy HN. Effects of macroelements and nitrogen source on biomass accumulation and withanolide-A production from cell suspension cultures of *Withania somnifera* (L.) Dunal. Plant Cell Tissue Organ Cult 2011; 104(1): 119-24.
[http://dx.doi.org/10.1007/s11240-010-9799-0]

[186] Taha HS, Abd El-Kawy AM, Fathalla MAEK. A new approach for achievement of inulin accumulation in suspension cultures of Jerusalem artichoke (*Helianthus tuberosus*) using biotic elicitors. J Genet Eng Biotechnol 2012; 10(1): 33-8.
[http://dx.doi.org/10.1016/j.jgeb.2012.02.002]

[187] Palacio L, Cantero JJ, Cusidó RM, Goleniowski ME. Phenolic compound production in relation to differentiation in cell and tissue cultures of *Larrea divaricata* (Cav.). Plant Sci 2012; 193-194(19): 1-7.
[http://dx.doi.org/10.1016/j.plantsci.2012.05.007] [PMID: 22794913]

[188] Yu T, Rhee MH, Lee J, *et al.* Ginsenoside Rc from Korean red ginseng (*Panax ginseng* C.A. Meyer) attenuates inflammatory sysmpots of gastritis, hepatitis, and arthritis. Am J Chin Med 2016; 44(3): 595-615.
[http://dx.doi.org/10.1142/S0192415X16500336] [PMID: 27109153]

[189] Nhan NH, Loc NH. Production of eurycomanone from cell suspension culture of *Eurycoma longifolia.* Pharm Biol 2017; 55(1): 2234-9.
[http://dx.doi.org/10.1080/13880209.2017.1400077] [PMID: 29130786]

[190] Modarres M, Esmaeilzadeh Bahabadi S, Taghavizadeh Yazdi ME. Enhanced production of phenolic acids in cell suspension culture of *Salvia leriifolia* Benth. using growth regulators and sucrose. Cytotechnology 2018; 70(2): 741-50.
[http://dx.doi.org/10.1007/s10616-017-0178-0] [PMID: 29349583]

[191] Hu M, Hu Z, Du L, Du J, Luo Q, Xiong J. Establishment of cell suspension culture of *Lonicera japonica* Thunb and analysis its major secondary metabolites. Ind Crops Prod 2019; 137: 98-104.
[http://dx.doi.org/10.1016/j.indcrop.2019.05.024]

[192] Lee JW, Jo IH, Kim JU, Hong CE, Bang KH, Park YD. Determination of mutagenic sensitivity to

gamma rays in ginseng (*Panax ginseng*) dehiscent seeds, roots, and somatic embryos. Hortic Environ Biotechnol 2019; 60(5): 721-31.
[http://dx.doi.org/10.1007/s13580-019-00164-2]

[193]   Bong FJ, Yeou Chear NJ, Ramanathan S, Mohana-Kumaran N, Subramaniam S, Chew BL. The development of callus and cell suspension cultures of Sabah Snake Grass *(Clinacanthus nutans)* for the production of flavonoids and phenolics. Biocatal Agric Biotechnol 2021; 33: 101977.
[http://dx.doi.org/10.1016/j.bcab.2021.101977]

[194]   Funk C, Gügler K, Brodelius P. Increased secondary product formation in plant cell suspension cultures after treatment with a yeast carbohydrate preparation (elicitor). Phytochemistry 1987; 26(2): 401-5.
[http://dx.doi.org/10.1016/S0031-9422(00)81421-1]

[195]   Byun SK, Pedersen H. Two-phase air-lift production of benzophenanthridine alkaloids in cell suspensions of *Escherichia californica.* Biotechnol Bioeng 1994; 44: 14-20.
[http://dx.doi.org/10.1002/bit.260440104] [PMID: 18618441]

[196]   Chen H, Chen F. Effect of yeast elicitor on the secondary metabolism of Ti-transformed *Salvia miltiorrhiza* cell suspension cultures. Plant Cell Rep 2000; 19(7): 710-7.
[http://dx.doi.org/10.1007/s002999900166] [PMID: 30754810]

[197]   Yu LJ, Lan WZ, Qin WM, Xu HB. Effects of salicylic acid on fungal elicitor-induced membrane-lipid peroxidation and taxol production in cell suspension cultures of *Taxus chinensis.* Process Biochem 2001; 37(5): 477-82.
[http://dx.doi.org/10.1016/S0032-9592(01)00243-6]

[198]   Zhao J, Fujita K, Yamada J, Sakai K. Improved β-thujaplicin production in *Cupressus lusitanica* suspension cultures by fungal elicitor and methyl jasmonate. Appl Microbiol Biotechnol 2001; 55(3): 301-5.
[http://dx.doi.org/10.1007/s002530000555] [PMID: 11341310]

[199]   Zhao J, Zhu WH, Hu Q. Enhanced catharanthine production in *Catharanthus roseus* cell cultures by combined elicitor treatment in shake flasks and bioreactors. Enzyme Microb Technol 2001; 28(7-8): 673-81.
[http://dx.doi.org/10.1016/S0141-0229(01)00306-4] [PMID: 11339952]

[200]   Namdeo A, Patil S, Fulzele DP. Influence of fungal elicitors on production of ajmalicine by cell cultures of *Catharanthus roseus.* Biotechnol Prog 2002; 18(1): 159-62.
[http://dx.doi.org/10.1021/bp0101280] [PMID: 11822914]

[201]   Su X, Mei X, Gong W. Study of paclitaxel production from an antifungal variant of *Taxus* callus. Plant Cell Tissue Organ Cult 2002; 68(3): 215-23.
[http://dx.doi.org/10.1023/A:1013942719483]

[202]   Yuan YJ, Li C, Hu Z-D, Wu J-C, Zeng AP. Fungal elicitor-induced cell apoptosis in suspension cultures of *Taxus chinensis* var. *Mairei* for taxol production. Process Biochem 2002; 38(2): 193-8.
[http://dx.doi.org/10.1016/S0032-9592(02)00071-7]

[203]   Bonfill M, Palazón J, Cusidó RM, Joly S, Morales C, Teresa Piñol M. Influence of elicitors on taxane production and 3-hydroxy-3-methylglutaryl coenzyme A reductase activity in *Taxus media* cells. Plant Physiol Biochem 2003; 41(1): 91-6.
[http://dx.doi.org/10.1016/S0981-9428(02)00013-X]

[204]   Xu M, Dong J. Elicitor-induced nitric oxide burst is essential for triggering catharanthine synthesis in *Catharanthus roseus* suspension cells. Appl Microbiol Biotechnol 2005; 67(1): 40-4.
[http://dx.doi.org/10.1007/s00253-004-1737-9] [PMID: 15480633]

[205]   Komaraiah P, Kishor PBK, Carlsson M, Magnusson KE, Mandenius CF. Enhancement of anthraquinone accumulation in *Morinda citrifolia* suspension cultures. Plant Sci 2005; 168(5): 1337-44.
[http://dx.doi.org/10.1016/j.plantsci.2005.01.017]

[206] Chong TM, Abdullah MA, Lai OM, Nor'Aini FM, Lajis NH. Effective elicitation factors in *Morinda elliptica* cell suspension culture. Process Biochem 2005; 40(11): 3397-405.
[http://dx.doi.org/10.1016/j.procbio.2004.12.028]

[207] Shohael AM, Murthy HN, Hahn EJ, Lee HL, Paek KY. Increased eleutheroside production in *Eleutherococcus sessiliflorus* embryogenic suspension cultures with methyl jasmonate treatment. Biochem Eng J 2008; 38(2): 270-3.
[http://dx.doi.org/10.1016/j.bej.2007.07.010]

[208] Baldi A, Jain A, Gupta N, Srivastava AK, Bisaria VS. Co-culture of arbuscular mycorrhiza-like fungi (*Piriformospora indica* and *Sebacina vermifera*) with plant cells of *Linum album* for enhanced production of podophyllotoxins: a first report. Biotechnol Lett 2008; 30(9): 1671-7.
[http://dx.doi.org/10.1007/s10529-008-9736-z] [PMID: 18427926]

[209] Orban N, Boldizsar I, Szucs Z, Danos B. Influence of different elicitors on the synthesis of anthraquinone derivatives in *Rubia tinctorum* L. cell suspension cultures. Dyes Pigments 2008; 77(1): 249-57.
[http://dx.doi.org/10.1016/j.dyepig.2007.03.015]

[210] Baldi A, Singh D, Dixit VK. Dual elicitation for improved production of withaferin A by cell suspension cultures of *Withania somnifera*. Appl Biochem Biotechnol 2008; 151(2-3): 556-64.
[http://dx.doi.org/10.1007/s12010-008-8231-2] [PMID: 18449479]

[211] Baldi A, Farkya S, Jain A, *et al.* Enhanced production of podophyllotoxins by co-culture of transformed *Linum album* cells with plant growth-promoting fungi. Pure Appl Chem 2010; 82(1): 227-41.
[http://dx.doi.org/10.1351/PAC-CON-09-02-09]

[212] Wiktorowska E, Długosz M, Janiszowska W. Significant enhancement of oleanolic acid accumulation by biotic elicitors in cell suspension cultures of *Calendula officinalis* L. Enzyme Microb Technol 2010; 46(1): 14-20.
[http://dx.doi.org/10.1016/j.enzmictec.2009.09.002]

[213] Holková I, Bezáková L, Bilka F, Balažová A, Vanko M, Blanáriková V. Involvement of lipoxygenase in elicitor-stimulated sanguinarine accumulation in *Papaver somniferum* suspension cultures. Plant Physiol Biochem 2010; 48(10-11): 887-92.
[http://dx.doi.org/10.1016/j.plaphy.2010.08.004] [PMID: 20829053]

[214] Gao F, Yong Y, Dai C. Effects of endophytic fungal elicitor on two kinds of terpenoids production and physiological indexes in *Euphorbia pekinensis* suspension cells. J Med Plants Res 2011; 5(18): 4418-25.

[215] Devi CS, Srinivasan VM. *In vitro* studies on stimulation of gymnemic acid production using fungal elicitor in suspension and bioreactor based cell cultures of *Gymnema sylvestre* R. Br. Recent Res Sci Technol 2011; 3(4): 101-4.

[216] Pawar KD, Yadav AV, Shouche YS, Thengane SR. Influence of endophytic fungal elicitation on production of inophyllum in suspension cultures of *Calophyllum inophyllum* L. Plant Cell Tissue Organ Cult 2011; 106(2): 345-52.
[http://dx.doi.org/10.1007/s11240-011-9928-4]

[217] Tang Z, Rao L, Peng G, Zhou M, Shi G, Liang Y. Effects of endophytic fungus and its elicitors on cell status and alkaloid synthesis in cell suspension cultures of *Catharanthus roseus*. J Med Plants Res 2011; 5(11): 2192-200.

[218] Onrubia M, Moyano E, Bonfill M, Cusidó RM, Goossens A, Palazón J. Coronatine, a more powerful elicitor for inducing taxane biosynthesis in *Taxus media* cell cultures than methyl jasmonate. J Plant Physiol 2013; 170(2): 211-9.
[http://dx.doi.org/10.1016/j.jplph.2012.09.004] [PMID: 23102875]

[219] Gadzovska-Simic S, Tusevski O, Antevski S, *et al.* Secondary metabolite production in *Hypericum*

perforatum L. cell suspensions upon elicitation with fungal mycelia from *Aspergillus flavus*. Arch Biol Sci 2012; 64(1): 113-21.
[http://dx.doi.org/10.2298/ABS1201113G]

[220] Antognoni F, Iannello C, Mandrone M, *et al*. Elicited *Teucrium chamaedrys* cell cultures produce high amounts of teucrioside, but not the hepatotoxic neo-clerodane diterpenoids. Phytochemistry 2012; 81: 50-9.
[http://dx.doi.org/10.1016/j.phytochem.2012.05.027] [PMID: 22769437]

[221] Vakil MMA, Mendhulkar VD. Enhanced synthesis of andrographolide by *Aspergillus niger* and *Penicillium expansum* elicitors in cell suspension culture of *Andrographis paniculata* (Burm. f.) Nees. Bot Stud (Taipei, Taiwan) 2013; 54(1): 49-58.
[http://dx.doi.org/10.1186/1999-3110-54-49] [PMID: 28510886]

[222] Huang C, Qian ZG, Zhong JJ. Enhancement of ginsenoside biosynthesis in cell cultures of Panax ginseng by N,N'-dicyclohexylcarbodiimide elicitation. J Biotechnol 2013; 165(1): 30-6.
[http://dx.doi.org/10.1016/j.jbiotec.2013.02.012] [PMID: 23467002]

[223] Sivanandhan G, Kapil Dev G, Jeyaraj M, *et al*. A promising approach on biomass accumulation and withanolides production in cell suspension culture of *Withania somnifera* (L.) Dunal. Protoplasma 2013; 250(4): 885-98.
[http://dx.doi.org/10.1007/s00709-012-0471-x] [PMID: 23247920]

[224] Verma P, Khan SA, Mathur AK, Ghosh S, Shanker K, Kalra A. Improved sanguinarine production *via* biotic and abiotic elicitations and precursor feeding in cell suspensions of latex-less variety of *Papaver somniferum* with their gene expression studies and upscaling in bioreactor. Protoplasma 2014; 251(6): 1359-71.
[http://dx.doi.org/10.1007/s00709-014-0638-8] [PMID: 24677097]

[225] Ahmed SA, Baig MMV. Biotic elicitor enhanced production of psoralen in suspension cultures of *Psoralea corylifolia* L. Saudi J Biol Sci 2014; 21(5): 499-504.
[http://dx.doi.org/10.1016/j.sjbs.2013.12.008] [PMID: 25313287]

[226] Tahsili J, Sharifi M, Safaie N, Esmaeilzadeh-Bahabadi S, Behmanesh M. Induction of lignans and phenolic compounds in cell culture of *Linum album* by culture filtrate of *Fusarium graminearum*. J Plant Interact 2014; 9(1): 412-7.
[http://dx.doi.org/10.1080/17429145.2013.846419]

[227] Gadzovska Simic S, Tusevski O, Maury S, *et al*. Fungal elicitor-mediated enhancement in phenylpropanoid and naphtodianthrone contents of *Hypericum perforatum* L. cell cultures. Plant Cell Tissue Organ Cult 2015; 122(1): 213-26.
[http://dx.doi.org/10.1007/s11240-015-0762-y]

[228] Ebrahimi MA, Zarinpanjeh N. Bio-elicitation of β-carboline alkaloids in cell suspension culture of *Peganum harmala* L. J. Med Plant 2015; 14(55): 43-57.

[229] Urdová J, Rexová M, Mučaji P, Balažová A. Elicitation – a tool to improve secondary metabolites production in *Melissa Officinalis* L. Suspension cultures / Elicitácia ako nástroj na zlepšenie produkcie sekundárnych metabolitov v suspenzných kultúrach *Melissa Officinalis* L. Acta Fac Pharm Univ Comen 2015; 62(s9) (Suppl. IX): 46-50.
[http://dx.doi.org/10.1515/afpuc-2015-0012]

[230] Park W, Arasu M, Al-Dhabi N, *et al*. Yeast extract and silver nitrate induce the expression of phenylpropanoid biosynthetic genes and induce the accumulation of rosmarinic acid in *Agastache rugosa* cell culture. Molecules 2016; 21(4): 426.
[http://dx.doi.org/10.3390/molecules21040426] [PMID: 27043507]

[231] Biswas T, Kalra A, Mathur AK, Lal RK, Singh M, Mathur A. Elicitors influenced differential ginsenoside production and exudation into medium with concurrent Rg3/Rh2 panaxadiol induction in *Panax quinquefolius* cell suspensions. Appl Microbiol Biotechnol 2016; 100(11): 4909-22.
[http://dx.doi.org/10.1007/s00253-015-7264-z] [PMID: 26795963]

[232] Kumar P, Chaturvedi R, Sundar D, Bisaria VS. *Piriformospora indica* enhances the production of pentacyclic triterpenoids in *Lantana camara* L. suspension cultures. Plant Cell Tissue Organ Cult 2016; 125(1): 23-9.
[http://dx.doi.org/10.1007/s11240-015-0924-y]

[233] Guízar-González C, Monforte-González M, Vázquez-Flota F. Yeast extract induction of sanguinarine biosynthesis is partially dependent on the octadecanoic acid pathway in cell cultures of *Argemone mexicana* L., the Mexican poppy. Biotechnol Lett 2016; 38(7): 1237-42.
[http://dx.doi.org/10.1007/s10529-016-2095-2] [PMID: 27094843]

[234] Netala VR, Kotakadi VS, Gaddam SA, Ghosh SB, Tartte V. Elicitation of gymnemic 1150 acid production in cell suspension culture of *Gymnema sylvestre* R. Br through endophytic fungi. 3 Biotech 2016; 6(2): 232.
[http://dx.doi.org/10.1007/s13205-016-0555-y]

[235] Deepthi S, Satheeshkumar K. Enhanced camptothecin production induced by elicitors in the cell suspension cultures of *Ophiorrhiza mungos* Linn. Plant Cell Tissue Organ Cult 2016; 124(3): 483-93.
[http://dx.doi.org/10.1007/s11240-015-0908-y]

[236] Owis A, Abdelwahab N, Abul-Soad A. Elicitation of phenolics from the micropropagated endangered medicinal plant *Calligonum polygonoides* L. (Polygonaceae). Pharmacogn Mag 2016; 12(47) (Suppl. 4): 465.
[http://dx.doi.org/10.4103/0973-1296.191458] [PMID: 27761076]

[237] Salehi M, Moieni A, Safaie N. Elicitors derived from Hazel (*Corylus avellana* L.) cell suspension culture enhance growth and paclitaxel production of *Epicoccum nigrum.* Sci Rep 2018; 8(1): 12053.
[http://dx.doi.org/10.1038/s41598-018-29762-3] [PMID: 30104672]

[238] Salehi M, Karimzadeh G, Naghavi MR. Synergistic effect of coronatine and sorbitol on artemisinin production in cell suspension culture of *Artemisia annua* L. cv. Anamed. Plant Cell Tissue Organ Cult 2019; 137(3): 587-97.
[http://dx.doi.org/10.1007/s11240-019-01593-8]

[239] Açıkgöz MA. Establishment of cell suspension cultures of *Ocimum basilicum* L. and enhanced production of pharmaceutical active ingredients. Ind Crops Prod 2020; 148: 112278.
[http://dx.doi.org/10.1016/j.indcrop.2020.112278]

[240] Vijendra PD, Jayanna SG, Kumar V, Sannabommaji T, J R, Gajula H. Product enhancement of triterpenoid saponins in cell suspension cultures of *Leucas aspera* Spreng. Ind Crops Prod 2020; 156(2): 112857.
[http://dx.doi.org/10.1016/j.indcrop.2020.112857]

[241] Mahendran G, Iqbal Z, Kumar D, Verma SK, Rout PK, Rahman L. Enhanced gymnemic acids production in cell suspension cultures of *Gymnema sylvestre* (Retz.) R.Br. ex Sm. through elicitation. Ind Crops Prod 2021; 162: 113234.
[http://dx.doi.org/10.1016/j.indcrop.2020.113234]

[242] Rajashekar J, Kumar V, Poornima DV, Hari G, Sannabommaji T, Raghuramulu D. Dose dependent effect of silver nitrate on enhanced production of gymnemic acid in cell 1174 suspension cultures of *Gymnema sylvestre* R. Br Biomedicine 2021; 41(1): 16-22.
[http://dx.doi.org/10.1007/978-1-4939-3332-7_16]

[243] Mahood HE. Effect of mannitol and peg on the accumulation of rutin in cell suspension culture of *Ruta graveolens.* Plant Cell Biotechnol Mol Biol 2021; 22(17&18): 12-8.

[244] Kieran PM, MacLoughlin PF, Malone DM. Plant cell suspension cultures: some engineering considerations. J Biotechnol 1997; 59(1-2): 39-52.
[http://dx.doi.org/10.1016/S0168-1656(97)00163-6] [PMID: 9487717]

[245] Yue W, Ming Q, Lin B, *et al.* Medicinal plant cell suspension cultures: pharmaceutical applications and high-yielding strategies for the desired secondary metabolites. Crit Rev Biotechnol 2016; 36(2):

215-32.
[http://dx.doi.org/10.3109/07388551.2014.923986] [PMID: 24963701]

[246] Shasmita Singh NR, Rath SK, Behera S, Naik SK. *In vitro* secondary metabolite 1183 production through fungal elicitation: an approach for sustainability. In: Prasad R, Ed. In: Fungal Nanobionics: 1184 Principles and Applications. Springer 2018.

[247] Naik SK, Behera S, Rath SK, Patra JK. A comprehensive scientific overview of *Blepharispermum subsessile* DC. (Asteraceae), a conservation concern medicinal plant with promising pharmaceutical potential. Indian J Tradit Knowl 2020; 19(1): 208-17.

[248] Weathers PJ, Arsenault PR, Covello PS, McMickle A, Teoh KH, Reed DW. Artemisinin production in *Artemisia annua*: studies *in planta* and results of a novel delivery method for treating malaria and other neglected diseases. Phytochem Rev 2011; 10(2): 173-83.
[http://dx.doi.org/10.1007/s11101-010-9166-0] [PMID: 21643453]

[249] Moscatiello R, Baldan B, Navazio L. Plant cell suspension cultures. In: Yehuda S, Mostofsky DI, Eds. Plant mineral nutrients Totowa. Humana Press 2013; pp. 77-93.
[http://dx.doi.org/10.1007/978-1-62703-152-3_5]

[250] Ye M, Ning L, Zhan J, Guo H, Guo D. Biotransformation of cinobufagin by cell suspension cultures of *Catharanthus roseus* and *Platycodon grandiflorum*. J Mol Catal, B Enzym 2003; 22(1-2): 89-95.
[http://dx.doi.org/10.1016/S1381-1177(03)00011-0]

[251] Zhang X, Ye M, Dong Y, *et al.* Biotransformation of bufadienolides by cell suspension cultures of *Saussurea involucrata*. Phytochemistry 2011; 72(14-15): 1779-85.
[http://dx.doi.org/10.1016/j.phytochem.2011.05.004] [PMID: 21636103]

[252] Linh TM, Mai NC, Hoe PT, *et al.* Development of a cell suspension culture system for promoting alkaloid and vinca alkaloid biosynthesis using endophytic fungi isolated from local *Catharanthus roseus*. Plants 2021; 10(4): 672.
[http://dx.doi.org/10.3390/plants10040672] [PMID: 33807415]

[253] Radman R, Saez T, Bucke C, Keshavarz T. Elicitation of plants and microbial cell systems. Biotechnol Appl Biochem 2003; 37(1): 91-102.
[http://dx.doi.org/10.1042/BA20020118] [PMID: 12578556]

[254] Kamada H, Okamura N, Satake M, Harada H, Shimomura K. Alkaloid production by hairy root cultures in *Atropa belladonna*. Plant Cell Rep 1986; 5(4): 239-42.
[http://dx.doi.org/10.1007/BF00269811] [PMID: 24248236]

[255] Yoshikawa T, Furuya T. Saponin production by cultures of *Panax ginseng* transformed with *Agrobacterium rhizogenes*. Plant Cell Rep 1987; 6(6): 449-53.
[http://dx.doi.org/10.1007/BF00272780] [PMID: 24248930]

[256] Parr AJ, Peerless ACJ, Hamill JD, Walton NJ, Robins RJ, Rhodes MJC. Alkaloid production by transformed root cultures of *Catharanthus roseus*. Plant Cell Rep 1988; 7(5): 309-12.
[http://dx.doi.org/10.1007/BF00269925] [PMID: 24241871]

[257] Bhadra R, Vani S, Shanks JV. Production of indole alkaloids by selected hairy root lines of *Catharanthus roseus*. Biotechnol Bioeng 1993; 41(5): 581-92.
[http://dx.doi.org/10.1002/bit.260410511] [PMID: 18609590]

[258] Palazón J, Cusidó RM, Bonfill M, *et al.* Elicitation of different *Panax ginseng* transformed root phenotypes for an improved ginsenoside production. Plant Physiol Biochem 2003; 41(11-12): 1019-25.
[http://dx.doi.org/10.1016/j.plaphy.2003.09.002]

[259] Komaraiah P, Reddy GV, Reddy PS, Raghavendra AS, Ramakrishna SV, Reddanna P. Enhanced production of antimicrobial sesquiterpenes and lipoxygenase metabolites in elicitor-treated hairy root cultures of *Solanum tuberosum*. Biotechnol Lett 2003; 25(8): 593-7.
[http://dx.doi.org/10.1023/A:1023038804556] [PMID: 12882150]

[260] Yan Q, Hu Z, Tan RX, Wu J. Efficient production and recovery of diterpenoid tanshinones in *Salvia miltiorrhiza* hairy root cultures with *in situ* adsorption, elicitation and semi-continuous operation. J Biotechnol 2005; 119(4): 416-24.
[http://dx.doi.org/10.1016/j.jbiotec.2005.04.020] [PMID: 15963590]

[261] Esmaeilzadeh Bahabadi S, Sharifi M, Ahmadian Chashmi N, Murata J, Satake H. Significant enhancement of lignan accumulation in hairy root cultures of *Linum album* using biotic elicitors. Acta Physiol Plant 2014; 36(12): 3325-31.
[http://dx.doi.org/10.1007/s11738-014-1700-z]

[262] Sharifi S, Sattari TN, Zebarjadi A, Majd A, Ghasempour H. The influence of *Agrobacterium rhizogenes* on induction of hairy roots and ß-carboline alkaloids production in *Tribulus terrestris* L. Physiol Mol Biol Plants 2014; 20(1): 69-80.
[http://dx.doi.org/10.1007/s12298-013-0208-0] [PMID: 24554840]

[263] Gai QY, Jiao J, Luo M, *et al.* Establishment of hairy root cultures by *Agrobacterium rhizogenes* mediated transformation of *Isatis tinctoria* L. For the efficient production of flavonoids and evaluation of antioxidant activities. PLoS One 2015; 10(3): e0119022.
[http://dx.doi.org/10.1371/journal.pone.0119022] [PMID: 25785699]

[264] Hasanloo T, Eskandari S, Kowsari M. *Trichoderma* strains - *Silybum marianum* hairy root cultures interactions. Res J Pharmacogn 2015; 2(2): 33-46.

[265] Sivanandhan G, Arunachalam C, Selvaraj N, Sulaiman AA, Lim YP, Ganapathi A. Expression of important pathway genes involved in withanolides biosynthesis in hairy root culture of *Withania somnifera* upon treatment with *Gracilaria edulis* and *Sargassum wightii*. Plant Physiol Biochem 2015; 91: 61-4.
[http://dx.doi.org/10.1016/j.plaphy.2015.04.007] [PMID: 25885356]

[266] Belabbassi O, Khelifi-Slaoui M, Zaoui D, *et al.* Synergistic effects of polyploidization and elicitation on biomass and hyoscyamine content in hairy roots of *Datura stramonium*. Biotechnol Agron Soc Environ 2016; 20(3): 408-16.
[http://dx.doi.org/10.25518/1780-4507.13164]

[267] Moharrami F, Hosseini B, Sharafi A, Farjaminezhad M. Enhanced production of hyoscyamine and scopolamine from genetically transformed root culture of *Hyoscyamus reticulatus* L. elicited by iron oxide nanoparticles. *In Vitro* Cell Dev Biol Plant 2017; 53(2): 104-11.
[http://dx.doi.org/10.1007/s11627-017-9802-0] [PMID: 28553065]

[268] Sharan S, Sarin NB, Mukhopadhyay K. Elicitor-mediated enhanced accumulation of ursolic acid and eugenol in hairy root cultures of *Ocimum tenuiflorum* L. is age, dose, and duration dependent. S Afr J Bot 2019; 124: 199-210.
[http://dx.doi.org/10.1016/j.sajb.2019.05.009]

[269] Barba-Espín G, Chen ST, Agnolet S, *et al.* Ethephon-induced changes in antioxidants and phenolic compounds in anthocyanin-producing black carrot hairy root cultures. J Exp Bot 2020; 71(22): 7030-45.
[http://dx.doi.org/10.1093/jxb/eraa376] [PMID: 32803264]

[270] Li J, Li B, Luo L, *et al.* Increased phenolic acid and tanshinone production and transcriptional responses of biosynthetic genes in hairy root cultures of *Salvia przewalskii* Maxim. treated with methyl jasmonate and salicylic acid. Mol Biol Rep 2020; 47(11): 8565-78.
[http://dx.doi.org/10.1007/s11033-020-05899-1] [PMID: 33048323]

[271] Balasubramani S, Ranjitha Kumari BD, Moola AK, *et al.* Enhanced production of β-Caryophyllene by farnesyl diphosphate precursor-treated callus and hairy root cultures of *Artemisia vulgaris* L. Front Plant Sci 2021; 12: 634178.
[http://dx.doi.org/10.3389/fpls.2021.634178] [PMID: 33859659]

[272] Dowom AS, Abrishamchi P, Radjabian T, Salami SA. Elicitor-induced phenolic acids accumulation in *Salvia virgata* Jacq.hairy root cultures. Plant Cell Tissue Organ Cult 2021.

[http://dx.doi.org/10.1007/s11240-021-02170-8]

[273] Gutierrez-Valdes N, Häkkinen ST, Lemasson C, *et al.* Hairy root cultures - a versatile tool with multiple applications. Front Plant Sci 2020; 11: 33.
[http://dx.doi.org/10.3389/fpls.2020.00033] [PMID: 32194578]

[274] Srivastava M, Misra P. Enhancement of medicinally important bioactive compounds in hairy root Cultures of *Glycyrrhiza, Rauwolfia*, and *Solanum* through *in vitro* stress application. In: Malik S, Ed. Production of Plant Derived Natural Compounds through Hairy Root Culture. Cham: Springer 2017.
[http://dx.doi.org/10.1007/978-3-319-69769-7_6]

[275] Guillon S, Trémouillaux-Guiller J, Pati PK, Rideau M, Gantet P. Hairy root research: recent scenario and exciting prospects. Curr Opin Plant Biol 2006; 9(3): 341-6.
[http://dx.doi.org/10.1016/j.pbi.2006.03.008] [PMID: 16616871]

[276] Rekha K, Thiruvengadam M. Secondary Metabolite Production in Transgenic Hairy Root Cultures of Cucurbits. Reference Series in Phytochemistry 2017; 2017: 267-93.
[http://dx.doi.org/10.1007/978-3-319-28669-3_6]

[277] Häkkinen ST, Moyano E, Cusidó RM, Oksman-Caldentey KM. Exploring the metabolic stability of engineered hairy roots after 16 years maintenance. Front Plant Sci 2016; 7: 1486.
[http://dx.doi.org/10.3389/fpls.2016.01486] [PMID: 27746806]

[278] Hu ZB, Du M. Hairy root and its application in plant genetic engineering. J Integr Plant Biol 2006; 48(2): 121-7.
[http://dx.doi.org/10.1111/j.1744-7909.2006.00121.x]

[279] Thwe A, Valan Arasu M, Li X, *et al.* Effect of different *Agrobacterium rhizogenes* strains on hairy root induction and phenylpropanoid biosynthesis in tartary buckwheat (*Fagopyrum tataricum* Gaertn). Front Microbiol 2016; 7: 318.
[http://dx.doi.org/10.3389/fmicb.2016.00318] [PMID: 27014239]

[280] Pillai DB, Jose B, Satheeshkumar K, Krishnan PN. Optimization of inoculum density in hairy root culture of *Plumbago rosea* L. for enhanced growth and plumbagin production towards scaling-up in bioreactor. Indian J Biotechnol 2015; 14(14): 264-9.

[281] Srivastava S, Srivastava AK. Effect of elicitors and precursors on azadirachtin production in hairy root culture of *Azadirachta indica.* Appl Biochem Biotechnol 2014; 172(4): 2286-97.
[http://dx.doi.org/10.1007/s12010-013-0664-6] [PMID: 24357500]

[282] Saravanakumar A, Aslam A, Shajahan A. Development and optimization of hairy root culture systems in *Withania somnifera* (L.) Dunal for withaferin-A production. Afr J Biotechnol 2012; 11(98): 16412-20.

[283] Su W W, Lee KT. Plant cell and hairy root cultures–Process characteristics, products, 1289 and applications. Bioprocessing for value-added products from renewable resources 2007; 263-92.
[http://dx.doi.org/10.1016/B978-044452114-9/50011-6]

[284] Giri A, Narasu ML. Transgenic hairy roots. Biotechnol Adv 2000; 18(1): 1-22.
[http://dx.doi.org/10.1016/S0734-9750(99)00016-6] [PMID: 14538116]

[285] Halder M, Roychowdhury D, Jha S. A critical review on biotechnological interventions for production and yield enhancement of secondary metabolites in hairy root cultures: an effective tool of plant biotechnology. Hairy roots 2018; 21-44.
[http://dx.doi.org/10.1007/978-981-13-2562-5_2]

[286] Weathers PJ, Bunk G, McCoy MC. The effect of phytohormones on growth and artemisinin production in *Artemisia annua* hairy roots. *In Vitro* Cell Dev Biol Plant 2005; 41(1): 47-53.
[http://dx.doi.org/10.1079/IVP2004604]

[287] Mannan A, Shaheen N, Arshad W, Rizwana AQ, Zia M, Mirza B. Hairy roots induction and artemisinin analysis in *Artemisia dubia* and *Artemisia indica.* Afr J Biotechnol 2008; 7: 3288-92.

[288] Patra N, Srivastava AK, Sharma S. Study of various factors for enhancement of artemisinin in *Artemisia annua* hairy roots. Int J Chem Eng Appl 2013; 4(3): 157-60.
[http://dx.doi.org/10.7763/IJCEA.2013.V4.284]

[289] Ahlawat SP, Saxena P, Alam P, Mohd A, Abdin MZ. Influence of *Agrobacterium rhizogenes* on induction of hairy roots for enhanced production of artemisinin in *Artemisia annua* L. plants. Afr J Biotechnol 2012; 11: 8684-91.

[290] Verma PC, Singh H, Negi AS, Saxena G, Rahman L, Banerjee S. Yield enhancement strategies for the production of picroliv from hairy root culture of *Picrorhiza kurroa* Royle ex Benth. Plant Signal Behav 2015; 10(5): e1023976.
[http://dx.doi.org/10.1080/15592324.2015.1023976] [PMID: 26039483]

[291] Bhagat P, Verma SK, Yadav S, Singh AK, Aseri GK, Khare N. Optimization of nutritive factors in culture medium for the growth of hairy root and ajmalicine content in sarpgandha, *Rauwolfia serpentina.* J Environ Biol 2020; 41(5): 1018-25.
[http://dx.doi.org/10.22438/jeb/41/5/MRN-1316]

[292] Santos PAG, Figueiredo AC, Lourenço PML, *et al.* Hairy root cultures of *Anethum graveolens* (dill): establishment, growth, time-course study of their essential oil and its comparison with parent plant oils. Biotechnol Lett 2002; 24(12): 1031-6.
[http://dx.doi.org/10.1023/A:1015653701265]

[293] Verma PC, Singh D, Rahman L, Gupta MM, Banerjee S. *In vitro* -studies in *Plumbago zeylanica* : rapid micropropagation and establishment of higher plumbagin yielding hairy root cultures. J Plant Physiol 2002; 159(5): 547-52.
[http://dx.doi.org/10.1078/0176-1617-00518]

[294] Keil M, Härtle B, Guillaume A, Psiorz M. Production of amarogentin in root cultures of *Swertia chirata.* Planta Med 2000; 66(5): 452-7.
[http://dx.doi.org/10.1055/s-2000-8579] [PMID: 10909267]

[295] Huffman GA, White FF, Gordon MP, Nester EW. Hairy-root-inducing plasmid: physical map and homology to tumor-inducing plasmids. J Bacteriol 1984; 157(1): 269-76.
[http://dx.doi.org/10.1128/jb.157.1.269-276.1984] [PMID: 6690423]

[296] Huang SH, Vishwakarma RK, Lee TT, Chan HS, Tsay HS. Establishment of hairy root lines and analysis of iridoids and secoiridoids in the medicinal plant *Gentiana scabra.* Bot Stud (Taipei, Taiwan) 2014; 55(1): 17-25.
[http://dx.doi.org/10.1186/1999-3110-55-17] [PMID: 28510924]

[297] Miao Y, Hu Y, Yi S, Zhang X, Tan N. Establishment of hairy root culture of *Rubia yunnanensis* Diels: Production of Rubiaceae-type cyclopeptides and quinones. J Biotechnol 2021; 341: 21-9.
[http://dx.doi.org/10.1016/j.jbiotec.2021.09.004] [PMID: 34536456]

[298] Tiwari RK, Trivedi M, Guang ZC, Guo GQ, Zheng GC. Genetic transformation of *Gentiana macrophylla* with *Agrobacterium rhizogenes*: growth and production of secoiridoid glucoside gentiopicroside in transformed hairy root cultures. Plant Cell Rep 2007; 26(2): 199-210.
[http://dx.doi.org/10.1007/s00299-006-0236-0] [PMID: 16972092]

[299] Giri A, Ravindra ST, Dhingra V, Narasu ML. Influence of different strains of *Agrobacterium rhizogenes* on induction of hairy roots and artemisinin production in *Artemisia annua.* Curr Sci 2001; 81(4): 378-82.

[300] Swarna J, Ravindhran R. *Agrobacterium rhizogenes* - mediated hairy root induction of *Momordica charantia* L. and the detection of charantin, a potent hypoglycaemic agent in hairy roots. Res J Biotechnol 2012; 7(4): 227-31.

[301] Mohammad RA, Ismanizan I, Zamri Z. Expression analysis of the 35S CaMV promoter and its derivatives in transgenic hairy root cultures of cucumber (*Cucumis sativus*) generated by *Agrobacterium rhizogenes* infection. Afr J Biotechnol 2011; 10(42): 8236-44.

[http://dx.doi.org/10.5897/AJB11.130]

[302] Sheikholeslam SN, Weeks DP. Acetosyringone promotes high efficiency transformation of *Arabidopsis thaliana* explants by *Agrobacterium tumefaciens.* Plant Mol Biol 1987; 8(4): 291-8.
[http://dx.doi.org/10.1007/BF00021308] [PMID: 24301191]

[303] Dutt M, Grosser JW. Evaluation of parameters affecting Agrobacterium-mediated transformation of citrus. Plant Cell Tissue Organ Cult 2009; 98(3): 331-40.
[http://dx.doi.org/10.1007/s11240-009-9567-1]

[304] Kim OT, Bang KH, Shin YS, *et al.* Enhanced production of asiaticoside from hairy root cultures of *Centella asiatica* (L.) Urban elicited by methyl jasmonate. Plant Cell Rep 2007; 26(11): 1941-9.
[http://dx.doi.org/10.1007/s00299-007-0400-1] [PMID: 17632725]

[305] Spollansky TC, Pitta-Alvarez SI, Giulietti AM. Effect of jasmonic acid and aluminium on production of tropane alkaloids in hairy root cultures of *Brugmansia candida.* Electron J Biotechnol 2000; 3(1): 31-2.

[306] Shi M, Kwok KW, Wu JY. Enhancement of tanshinone production in *Salvia miltiorrhiza* Bunge (red or Chinese sage) hairy-root culture by hyperosmotic stress and yeast elicitor. Biotechnol Appl Biochem 2007; 46(Pt 4): 191-6.
[PMID: 17014425]

[307] Smetanska I, Tonkha O, Patyka T, *et al.* The influence of yeast extract and jasmonic acid on phenolic acids content of *in vitro* hairy root cultures of *Orthosiphon aristatus.* Potravinárstvo 2021; 15: 1-8.
[http://dx.doi.org/10.5219/1508]

[308] Choi YE, Kim YS, Paek KY. Types and designs of bioreactors for hairy root culture. In: Gupta SD, Ibarki Y, Eds. Plant Tissue Culture Engineering Focus on Biotechnology. Springer 2006; 6.

[309] Suttipanta N, Pattanaik S, Kulshrestha M, Patra B, Singh SK, Yuan L. The transcription factor CrWRKY1 positively regulates the terpenoid indole alkaloid biosynthesis in *Catharanthus roseus.* Plant Physiol 2011; 157(4): 2081-93.
[http://dx.doi.org/10.1104/pp.111.181834] [PMID: 21988879]

[310] Pickens LB, Tang Y, Chooi YH. Metabolic engineering for the production of natural products. Annu Rev Chem Biomol Eng 2011; 2(1): 211-36.
[http://dx.doi.org/10.1146/annurev-chembioeng-061010-114209] [PMID: 22432617]

[311] Duraisamy GS, Mishra AK, Kocabek T, Matoušek J. Identification and characterization of promoters and cis-regulatory elements of genes involved in secondary metabolites production in hop (*Humulus lupulus.* L). Comput Biol Chem 2016; 64: 346-52.
[http://dx.doi.org/10.1016/j.compbiolchem.2016.07.010] [PMID: 27580343]

[312] Umemura M, Kuriiwa K, Dao LV, Okuda T, Terai G. Promoter tools for further development of *Aspergillus oryzae* as a platform for fungal secondary metabolite production. Fungal Biol Biotechnol 2020; 7(1): 3.
[http://dx.doi.org/10.1186/s40694-020-00093-1] [PMID: 32211196]

[313] Shkryl YN, Veremeichik GN, Makhazen DS, *et al.* Increase of anthraquinone content in *Rubia cordifolia* cells transformed by native and constitutively active forms of the AtCPK1 gene. Plant Cell Rep 2016; 35(9): 1907-16.
[http://dx.doi.org/10.1007/s00299-016-2005-z] [PMID: 27251124]

[314] Moyano E, Jouhikainen K, Tammela P, *et al.* Effect of *pmt* gene overexpression on tropane alkaloid production in transformed root cultures of *Datura metel* and *Hyoscyamus muticus.* J Exp Bot 2003; 54(381): 203-11.
[http://dx.doi.org/10.1093/jxb/erg014] [PMID: 12493848]

[315] Lodhi AH, Bongaerts RJM, Verpoorte R, Coomber SA, Charlwood BV. Expression of bacterial isochorismate synthase (EC 5.4.99.6) in transgenic root cultures of *Rubia peregrina.* Plant Cell Rep 1996; 16(1-2): 54-7.

[http://dx.doi.org/10.1007/BF01275449] [PMID: 24178654]

[316] Sazegari S, Niazi A, Shahriari-Ahmadi F, Moshtaghi N, Ghasemi Y. CrMYC1 transcription factor overexpression promotes the production of low abundance terpenoid indole alkaloids in *Catharanthus roseus*. Plant Omics 2018; 11(1): 30-6.
[http://dx.doi.org/10.21475/poj.11.01.18.pne1020]

[317] Singh P, Prasad R, Tewari R, *et al.* Silencing of quinolinic acid phosphoribosyl transferase (QPT) gene for enhanced production of scopolamine in hairy root culture of *Duboisia leichhardtii*. Sci Rep 2018; 8(1): 13939.
[http://dx.doi.org/10.1038/s41598-018-32396-0] [PMID: 30224763]

[318] Baghalian K, Hajirezaei MR, Schreiber F. Plant metabolic modeling: achieving new insight into metabolism and metabolic engineering. Plant Cell 2014; 26(10): 3847-66.
[http://dx.doi.org/10.1105/tpc.114.130328] [PMID: 25344492]

[319] Hill CB, Czauderna T, Klapperstück M, Roessner U, Schreiber F. Metabolomics, standards, and metabolic modeling for synthetic biology in plants. Front Bioeng Biotechnol 2015; 3: 167.
[http://dx.doi.org/10.3389/fbioe.2015.00167] [PMID: 26557642]

[320] Yamazaki Y, Kitajima M, Arita M, *et al.* Biosynthesis of camptothecin. *In silico* and *in vivo* tracer study from [1-13C]glucose. Plant Physiol 2004; 134(1): 161-70.
[http://dx.doi.org/10.1104/pp.103.029389] [PMID: 14657405]

[321] Li CY, Leopold AL, Sander GW, Shanks JV, Zhao L, Gibson SI. CrBPF1 overexpression alters transcript levels of terpenoid indole alkaloid biosynthetic and regulatory genes. Front Plant Sci 2015; 6: 818.
[http://dx.doi.org/10.3389/fpls.2015.00818] [PMID: 26483828]

[322] Gani U, Vishwakarma RA, Misra P. Membrane transporters: the key drivers of transport of secondary metabolites in plants. Plant Cell Rep 2021; 40(1): 1-18.
[http://dx.doi.org/10.1007/s00299-020-02599-9] [PMID: 32959124]

[323] Lv H, Li J, Wu Y, Garyali S, Wang Y. Transporter and its engineering for secondary metabolites. Appl Microbiol Biotechnol 2016; 100(14): 6119-30.
[http://dx.doi.org/10.1007/s00253-016-7605-6] [PMID: 27209041]

[324] Shitan N. Secondary metabolites in plants: transport and self-tolerance mechanisms. Biosci Biotechnol Biochem 2016; 80(7): 1283-93.
[http://dx.doi.org/10.1080/09168451.2016.1151344] [PMID: 26940949]

[325] Larsen B, Xu D, Halkier BA, Nour-Eldin HH. Advances in methods for identification and characterization of plant transporter function. J Exp Bot 2017; 68(15): 4045-56.
[http://dx.doi.org/10.1093/jxb/erx140] [PMID: 28472492]

[326] Tang RJ, Luan M, Wang C, *et al.* Plant membrane transport research in the post-genomic era. Plant Commun 2020; 1(1): 100013.
[http://dx.doi.org/10.1016/j.xplc.2019.100013] [PMID: 33404541]

[327] Nogia P, Pati PK. Plant secondary metabolite transporters: diversity, functionality, and their modulation. Front Plant Sci 2021; 12: 758202.
[http://dx.doi.org/10.3389/fpls.2021.758202] [PMID: 34777438]

[328] Wang Y, Yang B, Zhang M, Jia S, Yu F. Application of transport engineering to promote catharanthine production in *Catharanthus roseus* hairy roots. Plant Cell Tissue Organ Cult 2019; 139(3): 523-30.
[http://dx.doi.org/10.1007/s11240-019-01696-2]

[329] Yu F, De Luca V. ATP-binding cassette transporter controls leaf surface secretion of anticancer drug components in *Catharanthus roseus*. Proc Natl Acad Sci USA 2013; 110(39): 15830-5.
[http://dx.doi.org/10.1073/pnas.1307504110] [PMID: 24019465]

[330] Pyne ME, Narcross L, Martin VJJ. Engineering plant secondary metabolism in microbial systems.

Plant Physiol 2019; 179(3): 844-61.
[http://dx.doi.org/10.1104/pp.18.01291] [PMID: 30643013]

[331] Srinivasan P, Smolke CD. Engineering cellular metabolite transport for biosynthesis 1416 of computationally predicted tropane alkaloid derivatives in yeast. Proc Natl Acad Sci USA 2021; 118(25): e2104460118.
[http://dx.doi.org/10.1073/pnas.2104460118]

[332] Yamada Y, Urui M, Oki H, *et al.* Transport engineering for improving the production and secretion of valuable alkaloids in *Escherichia coli.* Metab Eng Commun 2021; 13: e00184.
[http://dx.doi.org/10.1016/j.mec.2021.e00184] [PMID: 34567974]

SUBJECT INDEX

T

Techniques 2, 30, 62, 63, 66, 80, 110, 121,
      152, 178, 184, 185, 192
  biotechnological 2
  hairy root 192
  proteomic 110
Technologies, integrated omics 300
Thymus plants 64
Tobacco, smoking 230
Transcription factors (TF) 47, 96, 98, 101,
      109, 110, 150, 299
Transcriptional machinery 99
Transcriptomics 80
Transporter genes 101
Tryptamine accumulation 50, 55

V

Vindoline 44, 47, 49, 51, 53, 54
    biosynthesis 51
    pathway 47, 49, 53, 54
    synthesis 44, 49
Virus-induced gene silencing (VIGS) 301

Y

Yeast extract (YE) 1, 3, 4, 5, 9, 191, 207, 286,
      287, 290, 291, 294, 297, 298, 299

www.ingramcontent.com/pod-product-compliance
Lightning Source LLC
Chambersburg PA
CBHW050807220326
41598CB00006B/136